Understanding
Acid-Base

Understanding Acid-Base

Benjamin Abelow, M.D.
Lecturer in Medicine
Yale School of Medicine

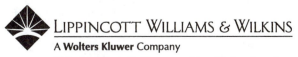
LIPPINCOTT WILLIAMS & WILKINS
A **Wolters Kluwer** Company

Philadelphia · Baltimore · New York · London
Buenos Aires · Hong Kong · Sydney · Tokyo

Editor: Paul Kelly
Managing Editor: Crystal Taylor
Copy Editor: Klemie Bryte
Design Coordinator: Mario Fernández
Product Coordinator: Marette D. Magargle-Smith
Cover Designer: Benjamin Abelow and Susan Hochgraf
Manufacturing: Marette D. Magargle-Smith

Williams & Wilkins
351 West Camden Street
Baltimore, Maryland 21201 USA

Rose Tree Corporate Center
1400 North Providence Road
Building II, Suite 5025
Media, Pennsylvania 19063-2043 USA

Notice. The author and the publisher have taken care to ensure that the information presented in this book is accurate. However, because human error can occur, and because progress in medical science is sometimes rapid, neither the author nor publisher nor any other party can guarantee the accuracy of everything contained herein. Readers are especially encouraged to consult with therapeutic manuals, guides to toxicology, and other frequently updated sources when making specific treatment decisions for particular patients.

Printed in the United States of America

Library of Congress Cataloging in Publication Data

Understanding Acid-Base / Benjamin Abelow—1st ed.
    p. cm.—Understanding Acid Base
    First Edition: Understanding Acid-Base / Abelow, Benjamin
    Includes bibliographical references and index.
    ISBN 0-0683-18272-2
    1. Subject–Understanding Acid-Base. 2. Subject–Understanding Acid-Base.
    I. Abelow, Benjamin Understanding Acid-Base. [DNLM: 1. Subject of Diseases-textbook. WG00 Cooo]
    RC000.H000 1007
    000.0'0-dc00
    DNLM/DLC
    for Library of Congress   97-00000
                                                                              CIP

To purchase additional copies of this book, call our customer service department at **(800) 638-0672** or fax orders to **(800) 447-8438**. For other book services, including chapter reprints and large quantity sales, ask for the Special Sales department.

Canadian customers should call **(800) 268-4178**, or fax **(905) 470-6780**. For all other calls originating outside of the United States, please call **(410) 528-4223** or fax us at **(410) 528-8550**.

Visit Williams & Wilkins on the Internet: **http://www.wwilkins.com** or contact our customer service department at **custserv@wwilkins.com**. Williams & Wilkins customer service representatives are available from 8:30 am to 6:00 pm, EST, Monday through Friday for telephone access.

                                                                              00
                                                            3 4 5 6 7 8 9

Table of Contents

To the Reader...

Acid-base is one of the most important and difficult areas in medicine. Students and residents study it intensely yet too often come away without the clarity and confidence they want and need. Why is this?

Acid-base involves many organs. Kidney, lung, gut, liver, and blood all play essential roles. As a result, students typically learn the basic science in piecemeal fashion, often using several different texts. Medical school faculty attempt to integrate the various concepts in their lectures, but the limited time available can leave both teacher and student frustrated.

Learning the clinical aspects of acid-base proves equally problematic. Without a firm grasp of the basics, it is almost impossible to master diagnosis and treatment. In addition, many students and residents find that standard texts do not provide the clear, detailed explanations they need when learning a new subject.

Understanding Acid-Base was written to address these problems. It is designed to let medical students and residents master the essentials of acid-base quickly, efficiently, and thoroughly. The book's unique approach is based on six innovative features:

1. *Reader-Friendly.* The text reads like a private tutorial. Complex ideas are presented step by step using clear language and simple illustrations. There is no jargon or "textbook-ese." The reader comes away from each topic with a deep, conceptual understanding of all the essentials—and a real sense of confidence and mastery.

2. *Review of Fundamentals.* The text opens with an optional review of fundamentals, which ensures that all readers start with a solid foundation. This concise but careful review provides students with a refresher for essential material learned during their premedical training. Topics include ionic solutions, pH, moles and equivalents, Brønsted-Lowry theory, and steady state. Readers can devote as much or as little time to this optional review as they need.

3. *Stand-Alone Sections.* The text has five sections: chemistry, physiology, pathophysiology, diagnosis, and treatment. Each is short (50–60 pages), self-contained, and can be read by itself. Students learning acid-base physiology can read just the physiology section. Those studying disease mechanisms can read the pathophysiology section. The diagnosis section is a complete course, ideal for both medical students and residents. Sections can also be combined to meet individual or classroom needs. For example,

sequential reading of the chemistry, physiology, and pathophysiology sections provides an integrated tutorial on preclinical acid-base.

4. *Self-Assessment Quizzes.* Each of the five sections ends with a detailed self-assessment quiz, with answer key. These quizzes are not mere spot checks but are designed to cover all core concepts. The quizzes provide an integrative learning experience that clarifies and reinforces all essential information presented in a given section. Taken together, each section and its quiz forms a carefully-structured learning experience.

5. *Optional Footnotes.* Special footnotes provide additional information. Some give mnemonics for confusing terms. Some give extra help to keep readers on track. And some give clinical details. Because all the essentials are contained in the main text, these footnotes are completely optional. To help readers decide at a glance if they want to read a particular note, each begins with a descriptive title, such as "Mnemonic," "Clinical note," or "Going further."

6. *Continuing Education.* A detailed appendix lets aspiring specialists and other motivated readers explore selected topics in greater depth. Each topic is presented clearly and thoroughly. Placing these topics in an appendix lets readers of the main text focus on essentials, without being distracted by advanced or esoteric material.

These features all have a single goal: To help the reader master the essentials of medical acid-base—and to do so quickly, efficiently, and enjoyably.

Good luck and . . . enjoy!

Review of Fundamentals

This chapter reviews key concepts and terms needed to study acid-base. It is specially designed for medical students who are just beginning their studies—but it can provide a helpful refresher for any reader. Depending on your needs, it can be skimmed, read selectively, or studied with care from start to finish. We start with elementary concepts and build rapidly.

Molecules and ions

By definition, a molecule is electrically neutral whereas an ion carries a charge. Thus, glucose ($C_6H_{12}O_6$) is a molecule whereas chloride (Cl^-) is an ion. To specify whether an ion's charge is positive or negative, the terms cation (+) and anion (−) are used. For example, the sodium ion (Na^+) is a cation whereas the bicarbonate ion (HCO_3^-) is an anion. Also, an ion can be either organic, which means it has a carbon-hydrogen backbone, or inorganic, which means it does not. For instance, acetate (CH_3COO^-) is organic whereas Na^+ is inorganic.*

"Sodium" and "potassium"

Sodium and potassium, two key substances in physiology and medicine, exist in the body almost exclusively as ions (Na^+, K^+). For this reason, it is acceptable to drop the word *ion* when discussing them. Thus, phrases like "sodium concentration" and "potassium levels" always refer to the concentrations of the ions, not the molecular forms. Calcium (Ca^{2+}), magnesium (Mg^{2+}), and a number of other important substances also exist almost exclusively in their ionized forms. *Ion* can be dropped when discussing them as well.

Hydrogen ions

The common hydrogen atom consists of one proton and one electron. If the electron is lost, a hydrogen ion, symbolized H^+, results. Because H^+ is nothing but a bare proton, the terms "hydrogen ion" and "proton" can be used interchangeably.

---

* **Mnemonic.** If you confuse *anion* and *cation,* here's a mnemonic: The "n" in anion is the first letter of the word negative. The "t" in cation is like a stretched-out "+" sign.

What is meant by "acid-base"?

"Acid-base" refers to anything having to do with the concentration of hydrogen ions in water or aqueous (i.e., water-based) solutions. In medical acid-base, the major areas include (1) the chemistry and physiology that keep the body's H^+ concentration stable during health, (2) the pathologic processes that alter H^+ concentration during disease (these are called either "acid-base disorders" or "acid-base disturbances"), and (3) the diagnosis and treatment of these disorders.

Ionic solutions

Certain uncharged chemical substances, upon being dissolved in a solvent, break apart into ions (e.g., $NaCl \rightarrow Na^+ + Cl^-$). This process is referred to as ionization or dissociation. A substance that ionizes when dissolved is referred to as an electrolyte, because the resulting solution can conduct an electrical current. An electrolyte can be either strong or weak. A strong electrolyte is one that dissociates virtually 100%, leaving only an infinitesimal quantity in its original form. A weak electrolyte dissociates incompletely, so that both the original and ionized forms exist in appreciable quantities.

Ionic solutions (i.e., solutions that contain ions) are generally named after the electrolyte from which they are prepared. They are named this way even if none of the electrolyte remains in its original, undissociated form. For example, a patient receiving an intravenous "sodium chloride" infusion is actually receiving an aqueous solution containing free ions of Na^+ and Cl^-, but essentially no NaCl. Similarly, solutions of "sodium bicarbonate" and "potassium chloride" contain virtually no $NaHCO_3$ or KCl in their undissociated form. The electrolytes in body fluids are also almost entirely dissociated. For example, there is virtually no NaCl in blood plasma, only Na^+ and Cl^-.

Moles and equivalents

A *mole* (pronounced like the animal, abbreviated mol) refers to a specific quantity. It is like saying "dozen" for 12 or "gross" for 144. In this case, the quantity is 6.023×10^{23} (i.e., 602,300,000,000,000,000,000,000). Thus, while a solution containing a dozen bicarbonate ions has 12 ions, a solution containing a mole of bicarbonate ions has 6.023×10^{23} ions.

"Equivalent" is a related term. It refers to a *mole of ionic charges*. For example, the bicarbonate ion, HCO_3^-, carries a single charge, so a mole of HCO_3^- carries a mole of charges. Therefore, a mole of bicarbonate equals "an equivalent." However, if the ion carries a charge that is greater than one, the numbers are no longer equal. For example, a mole of calcium ions (Ca^{2+}) equals two equivalents. The relationship between moles and equivalents is expressed by the formula Moles × Valence = Equivalents.

When do you use the term "moles" and when do you use "equivalents?" Molecules must be quantified in moles (e.g., "a mole of glucose") because they carry no charge. To say "an equivalent of glucose" makes no sense. Ions, however, can be quantified in either moles or equivalents (e.g., "a mole of Na^+" or "an equivalent of Na^+"). Incidentally, when using the term equivalent, it doesn't matter if the ion is negative or positive: a mole of Na^+ and a mole of Cl^- are both an equivalent.

Most molecules and ions in the body exist in relatively low concentrations. For instance, a liter of blood plasma contains about 0.004 moles of K^+. To avoid long decimal numbers, it is standard practice in medicine to use the prefix *milli-*, which refers to 1/1000 of the unit that follows (as in *millimeter*). Thus, quantities are generally expressed in millimoles (abbreviated mmol) and milliequivalents (abbreviated meq). For example, instead of saying 0.004 moles, we would say 4 mmol. Similarly, concentrations are given in millimoles per liter (mmol/l) and milliequivalents per liter (meq/l).

Since ionic concentrations can be expressed in either mmol/l or meq/l, the choice of units is somewhat arbitrary. In this book, we generally use mmol/l. We use meq/l only when doing so makes things clearer or simpler.*

[Brackets]

Brackets indicate concentrations. Typically, we bracket the chemical symbol. Thus, [Na^+] refers to sodium concentration and [H^+] refers to free proton concentration. However, it is sometimes convenient to bracket the written name. For example, [aldosterone] indicates aldosterone concentration, and [organic anion] indicates the total concentration of all organic anions in solution.

The pH scale

Aqueous solutions can have [H^+] values ranging from greater than 0.1 moles per liter to less than 0.000000000000001 moles per liter. The pH scale lets you express this wide range of values using just a few digits. The following table shows a series of [H^+] values (given in both decimal and exponential form) along with the corresponding pH values.

---

* **Going further.** For very small quantities or concentrations, prefixes other than *milli-* are sometimes used: *micro-* (μ) = one millionth, *nano-* (n) = one billionth, and *pico-* (p) = one trillionth. Thus, 1 mol = 10^3 mmol = 10^6 μmol = 10^9 nmol = 10^{12} pmol.

[H⁺] (moles/liter)	[H⁺] (moles/liter)	pH
0.1	10^{-1}	1
0.01	10^{-2}	2
0.001	10^{-3}	3
0.0001	10^{-4}	4
0.00001	10^{-5}	5
0.000001	10^{-6}	6
0.0000001	10^{-7}	7
0.00000001	10^{-8}	8
0.000000001	10^{-9}	9
0.0000000001	10^{-10}	10
0.00000000001	10^{-11}	11
0.000000000001	10^{-12}	12
0.0000000000001	10^{-13}	13
0.00000000000001	10^{-14}	14

This table illustrates five important characteristics of the pH scale. As you read about each, refer to the table so as to better grasp the idea.

First, notice that an increase in pH means [H⁺] is decreasing, and that a decrease in pH means [H⁺] is increasing. This backward or *inverse* relationship is the first important characteristic of the pH scale.

Second, notice that a one-unit change in pH represents a ten-fold change in [H⁺]. For example, look at the second row (0.01 moles/liter). If you reduce [H⁺] by a factor of ten (moving down one row in the table to 0.001 moles/liter), pH rises by one unit. If you reduce [H⁺] by another factor of ten (down two rows from the original starting point), pH is now two units above its original value. This "factor-of-ten" relationship means the pH scale is a *base-10 logarithmic scale*. It is often referred to simply as a "log scale."

Third, look at the middle column. Notice that the negative of the exponent is the same as the pH. For example, if [H⁺] is 10^{-3} moles/liter, pH is 3. If [H⁺] is 10^{-4} moles/liter, pH is 4. Thus, to convert an [H⁺] value into its corresponding pH, first express [H⁺] in exponential form, then extract the exponent and change its sign. This process can be described more formally as taking the negative of the log of [H⁺], which can be symbolized like this: $-\log$ [H⁺]. In fact, the mathematical definition of pH is:

$$pH = -\log [H^+]$$

For example, if [H⁺] is 0.00001 moles per liter, then

$$pH = -\log [H^+]$$
$$pH = -\log 0.00001$$

$$pH = -\log 10^{-5}$$
$$pH = -(-5)$$
$$pH = 5$$

Because the negative log of x is the same as the positive log of $1/x$, we can also define pH like this: $pH = \log 1/[H^+]$. The two definitions are mathematically identical, so either can be used.

Fourth, notice that in the table $[H^+]$ is given in moles per liter. This fact is important. For the mathematical definitions of pH just given to be valid, $[H^+]$ must always be expressed in moles per liter. For example, if $[H^+]$ is 1 *millimole* per liter, we must convert it to 0.001 *moles* per liter before plugging it into the pH equation.

Fifth, and finally, notice that we do not write or say (for example) "pH = 5 moles per liter" but simply "pH = 5." That is, the pH scale has no units. Even though we begin with $[H^+]$ expressed in moles per liter, the units drop away when we switch to pH. Numbers that have no units are described, formally, as "dimensionless." A simpler term would be "unitless," but this term is not used. Thus, the pH scale is dimensionless.

In summary, the pH scale is inverse, base-10 logarithmic, defined by $-\log [H^+]$ expressed in moles per liter, and dimensionless.*

So far, we have looked only at values of $[H^+]$ that are multiples of ten (e.g., 0.01 mol/l). These values are easy to convert to pH. When $[H^+]$ is not a simple multiple of ten, the principle is the same, but you need a calculator or a log table to find pH. For example, in health, $[H^+]$ of arterial blood plasma is 0.00000004 (or 4×10^{-8}) moles per liter. This value can be expressed as $10^{-7.4}$. Thus, the pH of normal arterial blood is 7.4.

It is not important to be able to mentally convert pH values into their corresponding $[H^+]$. For example, you don't need to know that pH 7.1 represents an $[H^+]$ of 8×10^{-8} mol/l. However, one simple fact is worth remembering: the log of 2 is 0.3 (i.e., $2 = 10^{0.3}$). This fact means that a pH change of 0.3 units corresponds to a doubling or halving of $[H^+]$. For example, if arterial pH falls from 7.4 to 7.1, you know that $[H^+]$ is twice its normal value. If it falls by another 0.3 units, down to 6.8, $[H^+]$ is four times normal. If pH rises to 7.7, $[H^+]$ is one-half normal. If it falls to 7.25, $[H^+]$ is somewhere between normal and twice normal (but *not* exactly half way, because logs are non-linear).

** **Hint for the reader.** If the pH scale seems strange to you, it may help to realize that two other logarithmic scales are widely used: the Richter scale for measuring earthquakes and the decibel scale for measuring sound. Although neither of these scales is inverse, both have other twists. The Richter scale is essentially base 30, which means that an earthquake of 5 is 30 times more powerful than one of 4, and 900 (i.e., 30^2) times more powerful than one of 3. The decibel scale, like pH, is base 10, but after the log of the sound intensity is calculated, the number is then multiplied by ten. Thus, an increase of 10 db, say from 60 db to 70 db, represents a ten-fold increase in intensity.*

In the chemistry section of this book, we sometimes describe proton concentrations using the pH scale, and at other times we use $[H^+]$. Thus, in one sentence you may read that "pH fell by one unit" and in the next sentence you may see this same change described as a "ten-fold increase in $[H^+]$." This is done to help you develop a feel for the relationship between changes in pH and the actual alterations in $[H^+]$ to which they refer.

Protons are often said to exist "free" in solution, and pH is therefore said to signify "free hydrogen ion concentration." This usage is a standard part of acid-base terminology. In reality, however, hydrogen ions do *not* exist free in solution; they are highly reactive and almost instantaneously form complexes with water molecules. The symbol H_3O^+ (the hydronium ion) is sometimes used, instead of H^+, to indicate this water-bound status. In fact, even this symbol is too simple, because a single proton can combine with several water molecules. To be accurate, you would need to write $\{H:(H_2O)_n\}^+$, which indicates that a "free" proton is actually bound to an indeterminate number of water molecules. However, because this formula is so unwieldy, it is almost never used. In this book, we use standard terms and symbols like hydrogen ion, H^+, free proton, or, occasionally, H_3O^+.

A final note. Some authors italicize the p in pH, like this: *p*H. The meaning is exactly the same, whether italicized or not.

Neutral, acidic, and basic

The term *neutral* can be used in two ways: electrical neutrality and acid-base neutrality. Electrical neutrality is considered later in this chapter. In this discussion, *neutral* refers to acid-base neutrality.

The terms neutral, acidic, and basic all refer to aqueous solutions. By definition, a solution is neutral if it contains an equal concentration of H^+ and OH^-. Thus, at acid-base neutrality, $[H^+] = [OH^-]$. *Acidic* and *basic* are defined relative to neutrality. Acidic means that $[H^+]$ is greater than $[OH^-]$. Basic means that $[H^+]$ is less than $[OH^-]$. *Alkaline* is commonly used as a synonym for basic. Thus, alkaline and basic can be used interchangeably. Note: OH^- is called either the hydroxyl ion or hydroxide ion.

Is pH 7 neutral?

There is a popular notion that pH 7 is "neutral pH," that a pH below 7 is acidic, and that a pH above 7 is basic. Let's see if this notion is correct. Liquid water is considered an electrolyte (albeit a very weak one) because a minute fraction of the molecules naturally dissociate into protons and hydroxyl ions:

$$H-O-H \;\rightarrow\; H^+ + OH^-$$

This reaction indicates that one water molecule dissociates into one ion each of H^+ and OH^- (i.e., H^+ and OH^- are formed in a 1:1 ratio). Since, in pure water, the dissociation of H_2O is the only possible source of H^+ and OH^-, and since these ions are formed in equal quantities, we know that pure water is always acid-base neutral (i.e., $[H^+] = [OH^-]$). It doesn't matter whether the water dissociates relatively little or relatively much; it is always neutral.

The extent to which water dissociates depends on temperature. High temperatures increase dissociation and cause $[H^+]$ and $[OH^-]$ to rise. Low temperatures decrease dissociation and cause $[H^+]$ and $[OH^-]$ to fall. It has been shown empirically that at 25 degrees Celsius (about 77 degrees Fahrenheit), $[H^+]$ and $[OH^-]$ are both exactly 10^{-7} moles per liter. This $[H^+]$ can be expressed as pH 7. Because 25°C is considered "standard" temperature (an arbitrary designation used primarily for work with gases), the notion has evolved that pH 7 is "neutral pH."

But this popular notion ignores the fact that pH 7 is neutral (i.e., $[H^+] = [OH^-]$) only when the water temperature is 25°C. At other temperatures, pH 7 is not neutral. For example, in pure water at 37°C (body temperature), $[H^+]$ and $[OH^-]$ are both $10^{-6.8}$ moles per liter. Thus, the neutral pH of water at body temperature is really 6.8. A pH of 7, at this temperature, is slightly alkaline.*

As this example shows, water has no single neutral pH. Instead, there is a different neutral value for each temperature. Furthermore, these values apply only to *pure* water. In aqueous solutions (i.e., non-pure water), ions and other solutes tend to increase the dissociation slightly. Thus, even at 25°C, the neutral pH of a solution like blood plasma is not exactly 7.

The pH of normal arterial blood plasma is about 7.4. Thus, normal blood pH is basic (or alkaline). In fact, it's alkaline whether you are thinking in terms of the popular notion of neutrality (i.e., pH 7 = neutral) or the more rigorously correct notion just discussed. However, using the popular notion, you would conclude that blood is 0.4 pH units above neutrality, whereas the correct figure is closer to 0.6 units.

Acid and base

We have seen what "acidic" and "basic" mean. But what, exactly, is an acid and what is a base? Perhaps surprisingly, some disagreement exists over

---

* **Technical information.** These equilibrium values for $[H^+]$ and $[OH^-]$ come from an empirically derived constant called the ion product of water (symbolized as K_w'), which is defined as the product of the proton and hydroxyl concentrations (i.e., $[H^+] \times [OH^-]$). K_w' is a temperature-dependent constant. At 25°C, $K_w' = 10^{-14}$. At 37°C, $K_w' = 2.4 \times 10^{-14}$.

how best to define these terms. For medical purposes, it is useful to be familiar with two different sets of definitions.

The first definition was proposed by Brønsted and Lowry. They defined an acid as a substance that can "donate" (i.e., give up) a proton, and a base as a substance that can "accept" (i.e., pick up) a proton. Hydrochloric acid (HCl) is considered an acid because it releases a proton when it dissociates. Sodium hydroxide (NaOH) is considered a base because, after dissociating into sodium and hydroxyl ions ($Na^+ + OH^-$), the hydroxyl ion can accept a proton ($OH^- + H^+ \rightarrow H_2O$). When an acid donates its proton, it *becomes* a base because it now can accept a proton (i.e., to replace the one it just gave up). When a base accepts a proton it becomes an acid because it now has a proton it can donate.

Actually, Brønsted-Lowry terminology is even more specific. When an acid loses a proton, it becomes the *conjugate* base of that acid. By definition, a conjugate base is identical in every respect to the parent acid except that it is missing a proton. Here is an example of an acid and its conjugate base:

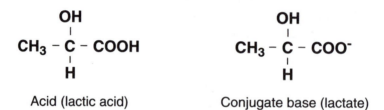

Acid (lactic acid)   Conjugate base (lactate)

When an acid and base are related through the loss or gain of a proton, they are referred to as a "conjugate acid-base pair." Examples of such pairs are lactic acid and lactate, and ammonium and ammonia (i.e., NH_4^+ and NH_3). In a conjugate pair, the acid is always more positive, by one charge unit, than its conjugate base. This charge relationship follows from the fact that the acid and base are identical except for a proton, which has a +1 charge. However, as the ammonium-ammonia pair demonstrates, there is no reason why the acid must be neutral, or why the conjugate base must be an anion. Note: for added clarity, we can apply the adjective "conjugate" to both the acid and base components of the pair. For example, when discussing the lactic acid-lactate pair, we can call lactic acid the conjugate acid and lactate the conjugate base.*

When an acid releases a proton, where does the proton go? In aqueous solutions, the proton is donated to water (recall that "free" protons are actu-

---

* **Terminology.** The verb *conjugate* means "to join together" and is related to the adjective *conjugal*, which refers to marriage, as in "the groom recited the conjugal vows." Thus, an acid is simply a conjugate base that is cohabiting with a proton.

ally bound to water). This is illustrated in the dissociation of hydrochloric acid: $HCl + H_2O \rightarrow Cl^- + H_3O^+$.

The second set of definitions for acid and base is simpler. It can be termed the "pH definition." An acid is defined as a substance that, when added to a solution, raises $[H^+]$ (i.e., lowers pH). A base is defined as a substance that, when added to a solution, lowers $[H^+]$ (i.e., raises pH). For example, HCl is an acid because it causes the pH of water to fall. And NaOH is a base because it causes the pH of water to rise. Occasionally, a substance may fulfill the criteria of one definitional scheme but not the other. For example, carbon dioxide (CO_2), which is not a Brønsted-Lowry acid because it has no protons to donate, is considered an acid under this second definitional scheme because it causes pH to fall when it is bubbled through water (we study this reaction in a later chapter).

Strong and weak acids

An acid is considered an electrolyte because it ionizes when dissolved. Therefore, the modifiers "strong" and "weak" can be applied to acids just as they are applied to other electrolytes. A strong acid is one that dissociates virtually 100% when dissolved in water, leaving essentially none of the acid in its original form. This dissociation happens because the attraction of the highly polar water molecules immediately overcomes the attraction between the proton and the rest of the acid molecule. Hydrochloric acid is an example of a strong acid.

A weak acid, in contrast, is only partially dissociated. The attraction between the proton and the rest of the acid molecule is only partly overcome by the attraction of the solvent, so only some molecules are dissociated at any given moment. Therefore, significant quantities of both the associated and dissociated acid can be found in solution. Some weak acids are weaker than others, with the weakest hardly dissociating at all and the strongest dissociating quite a bit. We can thus distinguish between very weak and moderately weak acids.

The following examples do not represent any particular acids, but should give you a better sense of what strong and weak mean. *Strong acid:* If we dissolve 1 mole of a particular strong acid, and then assay the solution, we might find that 0.99998 moles (99.998%) are dissociated; the other 0.00002 moles (0.002%) are left in the original, undissociated form. *Moderately weak acid:* If we dissolve 1 mole of a moderately weak acid, we might find that 800 millimoles (80%) are dissociated; the other 200 millimoles (20%) remain in the undissociated form. *Very weak acid:* For the same 1 mole, we might find that only 20 millimoles (2%) dissociates; the other 980 millimoles (98%) remain undissociated.

Electrical neutrality

As described above, acid-base neutrality refers to an equality of $[H^+]$ and $[OH^-]$. In contrast, electrical neutrality refers to an equality of positive and negative charges from any source. For example, a solution prepared by mixing the strong base sodium hydroxide (NaOH) with pure water is not acid-base neutral because the solution contains more hydroxyl ions than protons. However, the solution is electrically neutral because the excess of negative charges from the hydroxyl ions is exactly offset by the positive charges on sodium ions (i.e., $[H^+] + [Na^+] = [OH^-]$).

Therefore, acid-base neutrality means $[H^+] = [OH^-]$, whereas electrical neutrality means $[+]_{total} = [-]_{total}$.

It turns out that *all* solutions are electrically neutral, regardless of composition or pH. It doesn't matter whether the solution is biologic (e.g., blood plasma, urine) or non-biologic (e.g., gasoline, hydrochloric acid), or whether it is acidic or basic. This condition of electroneutrality is so inviolate that it is sometimes called the *law of electroneutrality*. Electroneutrality prevails because it takes tremendous energy to separate positive and negative charges. How much energy? Using Coulomb's law (which describes the attraction between charges), it has been calculated that to prepare just 0.01 ml of a solution that has an excess of positive over negative ionic charges of just 10^{-7} moles per liter, would require over a half million volts.

One practical implication of this law is that you cannot prepare therapeutic solutions that contain only anions or only cations. For example, if you want to give a patient intravenous bicarbonate, you must give a solution that also contains a cation such as sodium (i.e., a "sodium bicarbonate" solution).*

Body fluids and fluid compartments

In the body, all water is in the form of dilute aqueous solutions, which are referred to, generically, as *body fluids*. These fluids exist in two general locations: outside cells and inside cells. Fluid outside cells is called extracellular fluid (ECF). Fluid inside cells is called intracellular fluid (ICF). Thus, the body is sometimes said to consist of two fluid "compartments": ECF and ICF. In reality, both compartments are subdivided. For example, the cerebrospinal fluid, which surrounds the brain and spinal cord, is part of the ECF, but it is separated by membranes from the rest of the ECF. The ICF divisions are even more obvious and numerous, in that the compartment consists of billions of separate cells.

Body fluids account for about 60% of the body's total mass, equaling about

---

* **Going further.** Inside cells and cellular organelles, the law of electroneutrality is sometimes stretched a little. Because energy-driven pumps transport ions across membranes, a minute charge imbalance can be created across the membrane. This results in a small voltage difference across the membrane, usually no more than 0.1 volts. To create this small voltage difference, only an infinitesimally small concentration difference is required and, for practical purposes, electroneutrality is maintained.

42 liters in a 70 kg person (note: a liter of water has a mass of almost exactly 1 kg). ICF volume is about twice that of the ECF. That is, the compartment is twice as large. For a 70 kg person, ICF volume is about 28 liters and ECF volume is about 14 liters.

ECF

Let's focus on the ECF. The ECF has two components: intravascular and extravascular. The intravascular component is simply blood plasma (intravascular means "inside vessels"). It accounts for about 20% of ECF volume. The extravascular component ("outside blood vessels") surrounds and bathes the cells of the body. This component is often referred to as interstitial fluid because it exists in the interstices (spaces) between cells. It accounts for about 80% of ECF volume. Thus, if ECF volume is 14 liters, 3 liters are blood plasma* and 11 liters are interstitial fluid.

Blood plasma and interstitial fluid together are considered a single ECF compartment because, although they are separated by blood vessel walls, the capillaries and post-capillary venules are quite leaky. This leakage permits free exchange of all constituents of the ECF except for the membrane-bounded formed components (i.e., blood cells and platelets) and large protein molecules (e.g., albumin), which usually remain in vessels. The body fluids can be schematized like this:

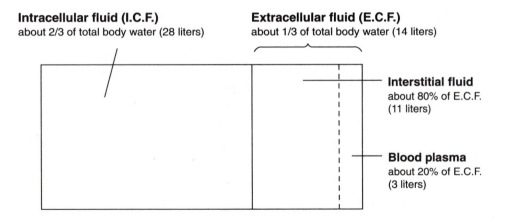

Intracellular fluid (I.C.F.)
about 2/3 of total body water (28 liters)

Extracellular fluid (E.C.F.)
about 1/3 of total body water (14 liters)

Interstitial fluid
about 80% of E.C.F.
(11 liters)

Blood plasma
about 20% of E.C.F.
(3 liters)

Human survival requires that extracellular fluid pH be maintained between 6.8 and 7.8. Health, as opposed to survival, requires a much narrower range, usually between 7.35 and 7.45. In the chemistry and physiology sections of this text, we will study, in detail, how this narrow range is maintained.

---

* **Reminder.** Total blood volume is about 5 liters. The other 2 liters consist primarily of red blood cells.

Steady state

In physiology and medicine, the concept of *steady state* plays a central role. We can illustrate this concept with a bucket of water:

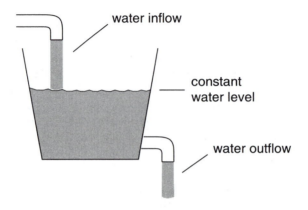

Water enters the bucket from above and exits from below. Although water in the bucket is constantly being replaced by new water, the level (i.e., the total amount of water in the bucket) does not change. We describe this situation as a "steady state" for water, which indicates a constant ("steady") level but a continuous turnover of the molecules that account for that level.

Why does the water level remain constant? The reason is that the rates of inflow and outflow are equal. It does not matter whether the total amount of water passing through the bucket (i.e., the total flux) is 1 liter per hour or 1000 liters per hour. So long as inflow equals outflow, the level remains constant. If the rates become unequal, the water level will change. Thus, if the rate of inflow exceeds the rate of outflow, the level will rise at a rate proportional to the difference.

In the body, the amounts or concentrations of many substances are regulated as steady state functions. Think of water. There is a continual inflow (via drinking and eating) and outflow (via urine, stool, breath vapor, and skin losses), but total body water remains relatively constant. The concentration of ions such as Na^+, K^+, and Cl^- in body fluids are also in steady state. These ions are ingested and excreted, with the rates of inflow and outflow being approximately equal.

Two substances crucial to acid-base regulation are also in steady state: bicarbonate ions (HCO_3^-) and dissolved carbon dioxide gas (CO_2). In later chapters, we will focus on these substances in detail.

Why is pH important in medicine?

Because opposite charges attract, protons tend to bind with negatively charged (i.e., "anionic") substances. In addition, the proton is small, which makes it highly mobile and also gives it a high "charge density" (i.e., a high ratio of charge to volume). These characteristics make the proton very reactive.

Proton binding is reversible and depends on the $[H^+]$ of the solution. When the solution's $[H^+]$ rises (i.e., when pH falls), more anionic sites in the solution are occupied by protons. These occupied sites are neutralized; that is, they lose their negative charge. When $[H^+]$ falls (i.e., when pH rises), fewer anionic sites are occupied, and these sites retain their negative charge. In this way, changes in body fluid pH affect the electrical charge on chemical substances throughout the body.

These changes in charge have important physiologic effects. Proteins are especially vulnerable because their three-dimensional structure is greatly influenced by the charges on constituent amino acids, and these structural changes affect function. Enzyme activity may be decreased, the shape of structural proteins may be altered, and the activity of trans-membrane channels and pumps may be reduced.

pH changes have other effects as well. For example, when blood pH rises, additional anionic sites on albumin and other plasma proteins are exposed. Some of these sites bind calcium ions (Ca^{2+}), lowering the concentration of physiologically active free (i.e., unbound) calcium ions. The fall in $[Ca^{2+}]$ may cause a reversible condition called tetany, which is characterized by peri-oral numbness, tingling of the fingers and toes, and spasms of the flexor muscles of the wrists and ankles ("carpopedal spasms"). pH changes can cause other problems as well, including cardiac arrhythmias.

Why focus on extracellular pH?

In clinical medicine, extracellular pH is attended to closely whereas intracellular pH is rarely discussed. Why?

First, during disease, the pH of the ECF and ICF tend to move in the same direction. For example, during diabetic ketoacidosis, acids produced in liver cells enter the interstitial fluid and then diffuse into the blood plasma. Because blood is pumped to all parts of the body, the pH of the most distant cells is rapidly affected. Sampling the ECF provides a single view of the whole body's pH status.

Second, ECF pH is easily measured whereas ICF pH is not. Measuring intracellular pH requires specialized research tools, such as microscopic probes or massive nuclear magnetic resonance instruments. In contrast, ECF pH can be assayed by simply drawing blood and analyzing the plasma's composition.

Third, emphasis on the ECF is based on therapeutic considerations. During treatment, clinicians do not try to directly manipulate each of the body's billions of cells. Instead, they help balance the ECF. Balancing the ECF provides an interstitial environment in which it is possible for cells to reestablish their own normal internal pH levels.

This completes our review of fundamentals.

Section 1
Chemistry

The study of acid-base is built on a foundation of chemistry. A clear understanding of this foundation makes acid-base physiology and pathophysiology truly comprehensible. In the *Review of Fundamentals* (Chapter 1), we explored a number of important chemical concepts. In this section, we turn to *the* central topic of acid-base chemistry: Buffers.

A buffer is a chemical substance that helps stabilize the $[H^+]$ (and hence the pH) of a solution. The word *buffer* comes from an archaic usage of the word *buff,* which means "to limit the shock of"—in this case, the shock of a pH change. A *buffered solution* is a solution that has a buffer dissolved in it. If you add strong acid to a buffered solution, pH falls much less than it would if no buffer were present; if you add strong base to the solution, pH rises much less. All body fluids are buffered solutions. The term *buffering* refers to the process by which buffers act to minimize pH changes.

This section has five chapters:

How Buffers Work: Part 1
How Buffers Work: Part 2
Non-Bicarbonate Buffers
The Bicarbonate Buffer System
Extracellular Fluid as a Multi-Buffered Solution

In the first two of these chapters, we discuss the mechanism by which buffering takes place. In the next two chapters, we describe the particular chemical substances that act as buffers in the body. In the final chapter of the section, we examine how the different buffers work together to stabilize the pH of the extracellular fluid.

How Buffers Work: Part 1

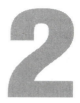

Understanding how buffers work is one of the more complex topics in acid-base. As a result, many students will find this chapter and the next quite challenging. Take your time. You need not memorize anything, but it is important to follow the progression of ideas closely. The effort you devote now will allow you to master all of acid-base, including areas of great clinical importance.*

Introduction

A buffer consists of two parts and, for this reason, is often referred to as a *buffer pair*. Even if we don't say "pair," the word is implied—just as it is implied when we speak of (a pair of) pants. What are these two parts? In human body fluids, the important buffers all consist of (1) a weak acid and (2) the conjugate base of that acid. As described earlier (p. 9), a weak acid is one that has only a modest tendency to dissociate.

For the rest of this chapter, we will work with a hypothetical weak acid, symbolized "HA." It will be our demonstration model. HA consists of a proton, H^+, and a negatively charged structure, designated "A^-" (for anion), which remains after the proton dissociates. HA is the weak acid and A^- is its conjugate base. Thus, buffered solutions contain both dissolved HA and A^-. Buffered solutions are generally prepared by mixing both HA and a salt of A^- (e.g., NaA, which dissociates into Na^+ and A^-) in water.

How do buffers work? The brief answer is as follows: When $[H^+]$ starts to rise (say, due to the addition of a strong acid, like HCl), some of the dissolved A^- combines with free protons via the reaction $A^- + H^+ \rightarrow HA$. This reaction takes some (but not all) of the added free protons out of solution, thereby minimizing the rise in $[H^+]$. Conversely, when $[H^+]$ starts to fall (say, due to the addition of a strong base, like NaOH), some of the dissolved HA dissociates and liberates, or "releases," free protons via the reaction HA $\rightarrow A^- + H^+$. This reaction replaces some (but not all) of the removed protons, thereby minimizing the fall in $[H^+]$. Both A^- and HA are needed because each plays a specific role: A^- removes protons when $[H^+]$ rises and HA donates protons when $[H^+]$ falls. Together, A^- and HA minimize changes in $[H^+]$ in either direction. We will now explore these processes in greater detail, beginning with underlying concepts and then applying these concepts to the buffering situation.

---

* **Hint for the reader.** Readers with a strong chemistry background may wish to read these two chapters more quickly.

Underlying concepts

When a weak acid (HA) is first dissolved in water, it begins to dissociate into free protons (H^+) and anions (A^-). As the concentrations of H^+ and A^- rise, the rate of random collisions between these two ions increases. These collisions allow H^+ and A^- to interact chemically, re-forming molecules of undissociated HA. Soon an equilibrium is reached, which can be represented like this:

$$HA \rightleftharpoons H^+ + A^-$$

or as two separate but simultaneously occurring reactions:

$$HA \rightarrow H^+ + A^- \text{ (called the "dissociation reaction")}$$
and
$$HA \leftarrow H^+ + A^- \text{ (called the "association reaction")}$$

At equilibrium, the rates of these two reactions are equal. Each molecule of HA that dissociates is immediately replaced by the combination ("association") of an H^+ and A^-. And each H^+ and A^- that associate into HA are immediately replaced by the dissociation of an HA. Thus, [HA], [A^-], and [H^+] all remain constant. Chemical equilibria are sometimes called *dynamic* equilibria to emphasize the fact that, even though concentrations do not change, both the association and dissociation reactions never stop.

The rates of the association and dissociation reaction are described by the *law of mass action*. This law states that rate is proportional to the product of the concentrations of the reactants. For the association reaction ($H^+ + A^- \rightarrow$ HA), the rate is proportional to [H^+] $\times$ [A^-]. For example, if [H^+] doubles but [A^-] stays the same, the reaction rate doubles. If both [H^+] and [A^-] double, the reaction rate quadruples. If both [H^+] and [A^-] are halved, the reaction rate is quartered (because $1/2 \times 1/2 = 1/4$). This "multiplicative" relationship holds because the association of two ions requires that the ions collide with each other, and the probability of a random collision between two dissolved ions is proportional to the product of their concentrations.

To better grasp this concept, consider a box containing red and yellow marbles:

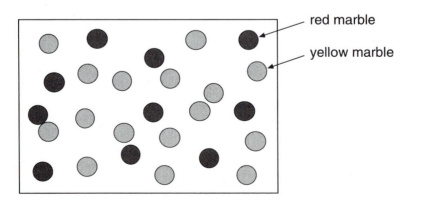

If the box is shaken, the frequency of collisions between red and yellow marbles will be proportional to the product of their numbers. For example, if the box contains ten red marbles and one yellow marble, and we add another yellow marble, the frequency of red-yellow collisions will double. The same basic idea holds for collisions between H^+ and A^- in solution.*

What about the dissociation reaction ($HA \rightarrow H^+ + A^-$)? Here the reaction rate is proportional simply to [HA]. Thus, if [HA] doubles, the reaction rate doubles. If [HA] is halved, the reaction rate is halved. This proportionality is also explained by the law of mass action, although the reason is less obvious. According to Brønsted-Lowry theory, the release of a proton from HA involves its transfer to water ($HA + H_2O \rightarrow H_3O^+ + A^-$). Because this transfer requires a collision between HA and H_2O, the rate of the dissociation reaction is proportional to $[HA] \times [H_2O]$. (When we speak of concentration, we are usually referring to solutes, but it is perfectly correct to talk about the concentration of solvents, like water, as well.) However, the concentration of water is so high, about 55.5 moles per liter, that it remains essentially constant even if small amounts of water are consumed or produced during a chemical reaction (e.g., the percentage change in $[H_2O]$ is minute even if, say, 2 millimoles of water are produced). Since $[H_2O]$ does not change, we can simplify and say that the rate of the dissociation reaction is proportional to [HA].

We can summarize the rules governing reaction rates like this:

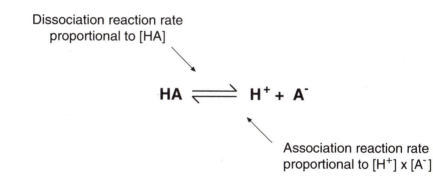

Dissociation reaction rate proportional to [HA]

$$HA \rightleftharpoons H^+ + A^-$$

Association reaction rate proportional to $[H^+] \times [A^-]$

---

* **Going further.** Actually, the reaction rate of ions is slightly lower than would be expected based on concentrations alone. Why? Neighboring ions in solution exert electrical attractions and repulsions on each other; this slightly restricts their movements, reducing the rate of collisions. Thus, the more precise term "activity" (which takes into account both concentration and the reduction in ionic mobility) is sometimes used to designate ionic reactivity. For example, it is said that the rate of the association reaction is proportional to (Activity of H^+) $\times$ (Activity of A^-). However, in dilute solutions such as body fluids, the average distance between ions is large. This keeps inter-ionic forces to a minimum, so activity is very close to estimates of reactivity based solely on concentration. It is therefore common to speak of reaction rates as being a function of concentrations, not activities.

Buffering in action

Let's now use the above ideas to explain how buffers stabilize pH. Consider a buffered solution (i.e., one containing HA and A^-) to which we add a strong acid, like hydrochloric acid, HCl. The HCl immediately and completely dissociates (HCl → H^+ + Cl^-). The rise in $[H^+]$ increases the product of $[H^+] \times [A^-]$, so the rate of the association reaction increases. H^+ and A^- are converted into HA. Thus, some of the free protons that were released from the HCl are removed. However, as the buffering reaction proceeds, $[H^+]$ and $[A^-]$ fall, and [HA] rises. As a result, the rate of the association reaction decreases while the rate of the dissociation reaction increases. When these rates become equal, a new equilibrium is reached and no more H^+ is removed. Buffering stops.

At this new equilibrium, $[H^+]$ is higher than it was before the strong acid was added, but it is much lower than it would have been if no buffer were present. Thus, buffers are said to *resist* or *mitigate* changes in pH but—this is important—not to prevent them entirely.

The following graph will clarify these processes. As you read the explanatory text, keep referring back to the graph.

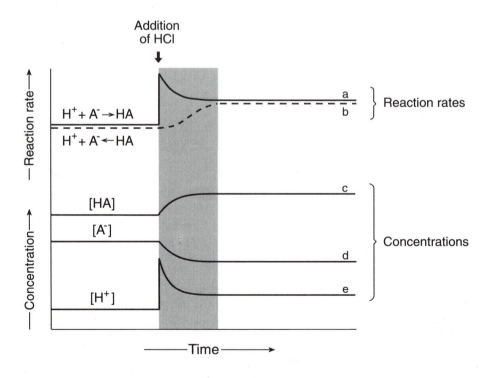

Let's get oriented. The lines labeled a (solid) and b (dotted) show the rates of the association and dissociation reactions, respectively. Lines c, d, and e show the concentrations of the reactants (HA, A^-, and H^+). The x, or horizontal, axis shows time. The y, or vertical, axis shows concentrations and reaction rates. The little bold arrow at the top marks the addition of hydrochloric acid (HCl). The gray shading indicates where the buffer system is not at equilibrium. The unshaded regions are at equilibrium. Let's now look at the buffering process.

First, before HCl is added, the system is at equilibrium. Lines a and b are superimposed (they have been separated slightly for clarity), indicating that the rates of the association and dissociation reactions are equal. Lines c, d, and e all are parallel to the x axis, indicating that $[H^+]$, $[A^-]$, and $[HA]$ are constant.

Second, when HCl is added, $[H^+]$ rises sharply, causing the rate of the association reaction to jump. The rate lines separate. Equilibrium no longer exists. As $[H^+]$ and $[A^-]$ decrease, the association reaction slows. As $[HA]$ increases, the dissociation reaction increases. The rate lines start to converge.

Third, as the rate lines converge, a new equilibrium is reached. $[H^+]$, $[A^-]$, and $[HA]$ are again constant. Although many free protons have been removed, the final $[H^+]$ is still higher than it was before HCl was added. Also, the final $[A^-]$ is lower, and the final $[HA]$ is higher, than they were before the HCl was added.*

Adding (or removing) HA and A⁻

So far, we have studied what happens in a buffered solution when we add or remove H^+. We now explore what happens if we add or remove HA or A^-. In our discussion, we will refer frequently to the (now familiar) buffer equilibrium:

$$HA \rightleftharpoons A^- + H^+$$

Adding more HA

Adding more HA to a buffered solution causes pH to fall. Why? The rise in $[HA]$ increases the rate of the dissociation reaction, liberating H^+ and A^-. The equilibrium point shifts to the right. We can also explain the fall in pH another way: although HA is a weak acid, it is still an acid, which means it liberates protons when added to water. However, unlike a strong acid such as HCl, which donates virtually all of its protons, weak acids gives up only some of their protons. Thus, the fall in pH is less than it would be if an equal quantity of strong acid were added.

---

* **Going further.** In this chapter, we base our explanation of buffering on the law of mass action. Buffering is sometimes explained in other ways. For example, *Le Chatelier's Principle*, which states that a chemical system acts to minimize a "stress" imposed on it, can be used to explain buffering by describing a change in $[H^+]$ as a stress; i.e., the buffer equilibrium shifts so as to minimize this stress. The *common ion effect* is also used to explain buffering. In reality, the underlying explanation for both Le Chatelier's Principle and the common ion effect, as they apply to buffering, is the law of mass action. This law is the reason why a stress or a common ion causes the equilibrium to shift.

Removing HA

If we remove HA from the solution, pH rises. Why? The fall in [HA] slows the dissociation reaction, so protons get consumed. The equilibrium point shifts to the left. Put differently, the removal of an acid (even a weak one) makes the solution less acidic and, therefore, more basic.

Adding more A⁻

If we add more A⁻, pH rises. The rise in [A⁻] increases the rate of the association reaction, which consumes protons. The equilibrium point shifts to the left. Put differently, adding more base makes the solution more basic.*

Removing A⁻

If we remove A⁻, pH falls. The fall in [A⁻] slows the association rate and shifts the equilibrium point to the right. Put differently, removing base makes the solution more acidic.

Simultaneous changes

Now consider what happens if we simultaneously add HA and A⁻. For example, let's double both [HA] and [A⁻]. Doubling [A⁻] causes the association rate to double. Doubling [HA] causes the dissociation rate to double. Thus, the rates increase in parallel. Although both rates are higher, they remain balanced, so no net substrate, including H^+, is produced or consumed. pH is unchanged. Similarly, pH does not change if [A⁻] and [HA] decrease in parallel.

Finally, let's add both HA and A⁻, but add slightly more HA. For example, let's increase [HA] by 99% and increase [A⁻] by 98%. What happens? The answer is that pH falls very slightly. In this example (i.e., 99% vs. 98%), the net effect on pH is the same as if we did nothing to A⁻ but increased [HA] by about 1%.

Summary

The buffers in body fluids each consist of a weak acid (symbolized HA) and its conjugate base (symbolized A⁻). HA and A⁻ are considered a buffer pair. Buffering occurs because HA liberates free protons when [H^+] falls, and A⁻ removes free protons when [H^+] rises. Buffering mitigates, but does not entirely prevent, changes in pH. The liberation and removal of protons occurs because changes in [H^+] affect the reaction rates of the $HA \rightleftharpoons H^+ + A^-$ equilibrium, and this shifts the equilibrium point. For example, a rise in [H^+]

---

* **Technical information.** The law of electroneutrality prevents us from preparing or adding just A⁻. However, we can produce the same effect by adding a salt of A⁻ (e.g., NaA or KA), which liberates A⁻ when it dissociates.

pushes the equilibrium leftward, removing free protons. These same equilibrium shifts also explain why the following occur: the addition of HA raises [H^+], the removal of HA lowers [H^+], the addition of A^- lowers [H^+], and the removal of A^- raises [H^+].

This ends the first of two foundational chapters. If the material seems abstract or boring, don't be dissuaded. The clinical relevance will soon become clear. If you are confused about anything in this chapter, please review before continuing, because the next chapter builds directly on this one.

How Buffers Work: Part 2

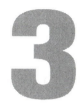

In this chapter, we explore three quantitative aspects of buffering: pK, the Henderson-Hasselbalch equation, and the concept of buffer capacity. These subjects are often explained using formal mathematical derivations, but many students find that this does not provide a "gut-level" understanding. We have therefore replaced the standard approach with a more visual, reader-friendly discussion that focuses on those aspects most relevant to medical acid-base. As noted previously, you need not memorize, but it is important to follow the progression of ideas carefully.

Background

As background for the chapter's three main topics, we need to explore the concept of "the $[A^-]/[HA]$ ratio." Once you grasp this concept, all that follows becomes much easier to understand. Imagine that we have prepared one liter of a buffered solution that contains a total of one mole of weak acid. And let's say that the weak acid is exactly half dissociated, so that 500 millimoles each of A^- and HA are dissolved in solution. We can express these two concentrations as a fraction, like this:

$$[A^-]/[HA] = 500/500 = 1/1 = 1$$

Now imagine that we gradually add a strong acid (say, hydrochloric acid, HCl), which dissociates, releasing protons. Most of these added protons are buffered, but at the new equilibrium point the $[H^+]$ is still higher than it was previously. Let's say we stop adding the HCl when the equilibrium $[H^+]$ has increased by a factor of ten (i.e., when pH has fallen by one unit). How does this pH change affect $[A^-]$ and $[HA]$?

Since adding H^+ shifts the $HA \rightleftharpoons A^- + H^+$ equilibrium to the left, we expect the new $[A^-]$ to be less than 500 mmol/l and the new $[HA]$ to be greater than 500 mmol/l. To find the actual concentrations, we do a chemical analysis of the solution. We find that $[A^-]$ is just under 91 mmol/l and $[HA]$ is just over 909 mmol/l. When we express these values in ratio form, we observe something interesting:

$$[A^-]/[HA] = 91/909 = 1/10$$

The $[A^-]/[HA]$ ratio fell by a factor of ten, from 1 to $1/10$.* Notice that the ten-fold *decrease* in the equilibrium $[A^-]/[HA]$ ratio exactly matches the ten-fold *increase* in the equilibrium $[H^+]$. The changes are precisely <u>reciprocal</u>. It makes sense that the ratio falls because the addition of H^+ from the strong acid leads to the consumption of A^-, which is the numerator, and the production of HA, which is the denominator. But why are the changes exactly reciprocal?

A detailed answer to this question is beyond the scope of this book, but this paragraph should give you the general idea. Recall that a ten-fold rise in $[H^+]$ tends to increase the rate of the association reaction by a factor of ten. Assuming no other changes, this increase in the rate of association would cause a ten-fold disparity between the association and dissociation rates. However, during buffering, free protons combine with A^-, causing $[A^-]$ to fall and $[HA]$ to rise. The fall in $[A^-]$ slows the association rate, partially offsetting the rate increase caused by the rise in $[H^+]$. The rise in $[HA]$ increases the dissociation rate, further offsetting the disparity in reaction rates (the illustration on page 22 portrays this visually). Since a fall in $[A^-]$ and a rise in $[HA]$ are both reflected as a fall in $[A^-]/[HA]$, and since these concentration changes act to offset what would otherwise be a ten-fold disparity in reaction rates, it makes sense that equilibrium is reestablished at the precise point where $[A^-]/[HA]$ falls by a factor of ten. Thus, the changes are reciprocal.

Let's look at other examples of these reciprocal changes. If we add enough HCl to a buffered solution to increase equilibrium $[H^+]$ by a factor of 100, the new $[A^-]/[HA]$ ratio will be $1/100$ its original value. If we add enough HCl to raise the equilibrium $[H^+]$ by a factor of 1000, the ratio falls by a factor of 1000. And there is nothing magical about multiple-of-ten increases in $[H^+]$. For example, if we raise the equilibrium $[H^+]$ by a factor of 7, the $[A^-]/[HA]$ ratio falls by a factor of 7. If we raise the equilibrium $[H^+]$ by a factor of 275, the $[A^-]/[HA]$ ratio falls to $1/275$ its original value.

We can describe this same phenomenon using pH values. For example, a fall of 2 pH units (a 100-fold rise in $[H^+]$) causes the $[A^-]/[HA]$ ratio to fall to $1/100$ its original value. A fall of 4 pH units causes the ratio to fall by a factor of 10,000. A fall of 0.3 pH units (a two-fold rise in $[H^+]$) halves the ratio.

If we add strong base to the buffered solution (e.g., sodium hydroxide, NaOH), instead of strong acid, the same reciprocal changes are observed. For example, if we add enough NaOH to cause the equilibrium $[H^+]$ to fall by a factor of ten, the ratio rises by ten. If we add more NaOH, say enough to reduce equilibrium $[H^+]$ to $1/123$ its starting level, the new $[A^-]/[HA]$ ratio will be 123 times its original value.

---

*Technical information.** We have rounded off all fractional numbers in this chapter to the nearest integer. Thus, in this example, the numbers given as 91 and 909 are actually closer to 90.9 and 909.1. If the actual numbers were used, the $[A^-]/[HA]$ ratio would be exactly $1/10$.

As these examples suggest, any time we change the equilibrium $[H^+]$ of a buffered solution, there is a reciprocal change in the $[A^-]/[HA]$ ratio of the buffer pair. This pattern of reciprocal changes is *not* a property of the particular buffer used. It occurs with all buffers. The pattern develops because a change in $[H^+]$ causes an inequality in the reaction rates of the buffer equilibrium, and this inequality causes $[A^-]$ and $[HA]$ to rise or fall until the reaction rates are again equal. The reciprocal change in $[A^-]/[HA]$ is an automatic (in fact, tautological) consequence of the reestablishment of equilibrium. The importance of this phenomenon will become clear as we continue.

Let's extend the example given earlier. Recall that we had a one liter solution containing a total of 1 mole HA, which was half dissociated. That is, there are 500 mmol each of HA and A^-. We can describe this weak acid as being at its "dissociation midpoint," since it is exactly half dissociated. Now let's add either strong acid (HCl) or strong base (NaOH) in quantities sufficient to produce progressive one-unit changes in the equilibrium pH. The following table shows what happens to the $[A^-]/[HA]$ ratio at each new pH level. In the table, we call our starting pH "x."

Addition of HCl		Addition of NaOH	
pH	$[A^-]/[HA]$	pH	$[A^-]/[HA]$
x	1/1	x	1/1
x − 1	1/10	x + 1	10/1
x − 2	1/100	x + 2	100/1
x − 3	1/1000	x + 3	1000/1

This table summarizes, using pH values, what we already know: that as we change the equilibrium $[H^+]$ of a buffered solution, the $[A^-]/[HA]$ ratio changes in a reciprocal fashion. If we wished, we could extend the table almost indefinitely. For example, the next row would show that a pH fall of 4 units results in a ratio of 1/10,000, and a pH rise of 4 units results in a ratio of 10,000/1 (or simply 10,000). Spend a moment studying this table so that it really makes sense to you.

To deepen our understanding, we need to introduce a visual device:

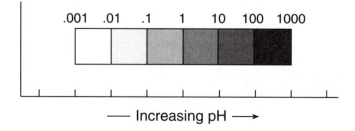

Numbers indicate [A⁻] / [HA] ratio

.001 .01 .1 1 10 100 1000

— Increasing pH ⟶

This figure is called a "dissociation bar." It visually portrays the concepts we have just been discussing. Let's see how. Start by scanning the bar from left to right. The increasing density of shading indicates that, as pH rises, an increasing fraction of the buffer exists in the A⁻ (i.e., conjugate base) form. That is, the bar shows how a fall in [H⁺] causes a reciprocal rise in [A⁻]/[HA]. Next, scan the bar from right to left. The decreasing density of shading indicates that, as pH falls, an increasing fraction of the buffer exists in the HA form. That is, the bar shows how a rise in [H⁺] causes a fall in [A⁻]/[HA]. The black vertical lines within the bar indicate where the [A⁻]/[HA] ratio has shifted by a factor of ten (corresponding to ten-fold changes in [H⁺]). This dissociation bar illustrates a pH range of six units, three on either side of the dissociation midpoint. As with the table, above, we could have extended the pH range of the bar in either direction. Pause to be sure you clearly understand the concepts portrayed by the dissociation bar.

We are now ready to apply these ideas to the three main topics of this chapter, starting with pK.

pK

Not all weak acids are equally weak: some are very weak (and dissociate just a little), some are moderately weak (and dissociate somewhat more), and some are relatively strong (and dissociate quite a bit, although not nearly as much as strong acids like HCl). In terms of the HA ⇌ H⁺ + A⁻ equilibrium, we can say that a stronger weak acid has an equilibrium point that is displaced further to the right than that of a weaker acid. All else being equal, a stronger weak acid will be more dissociated, and will therefore have a higher [A⁻]/[HA] ratio, than a weaker weak acid.

A high [H⁺] in a buffered solution tends to drive the HA ⇌ A⁻ + H⁺ equilibrium to the left, and a low [H⁺] tends to shift the equilibrium point to the right. Therefore, if we dissolve a relatively strong weak acid in solution, and we want this acid to exist at its dissociation midpoint (where [HA] = [A⁻] and [A⁻]/[HA] = 1), we would expect that a relatively high [H⁺] would be required. A weaker acid, on the other hand, would need only a low [H⁺] to maintain the system at the dissociation midpoint.* The result is that the dissociation bars of stronger weak acids are displaced to the left on the pH scale, whereas the bars of weaker acids are displaced to the right, like this:

Hint for the reader. Here's another way to make the same point. A relatively strong acid tends to be more than half dissociated, so a high [H⁺] is needed to push the equilibrium point back to the middle. In contrast, a relatively weak acid tends to be less than half dissociated, so a low [H⁺] is needed to "encourage" it to dissociate more fully.

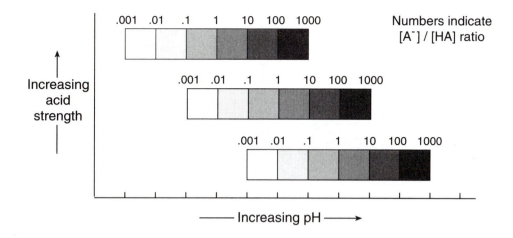

Notice that the bars are identical in terms of size and shading. This reflects the fact that all buffers respond to changes in pH in a similar way: the $[A^-]/[HA]$ ratio shifts in reciprocal fashion to changes in $[H^+]$. The only difference is that the pH value around which the ratio varies (i.e., the dissociation midpoint) is lower for stronger acids than for weaker acids. Thus, a buffer prepared from a relatively strong weak acid might be at its dissociation midpoint when the solution's pH is (for example) 4, whereas a weaker acid might be at its dissociation midpoint when the solution's pH is 7. Once again, pause to be sure that the above illustration really makes sense to you.

This kind of illustration lets you assess the relative strengths of different acids. To do so, simply compare the locations of the dissociation bars. The further a bar is displaced to the left, the stronger the acid; the further the bar is displaced to the right, the weaker the acid. This relationship between an acid's strength and the location of its dissociation bar on the pH axis suggests a concise way to describe acidic strength: we can simply name the pH value that corresponds to the middle of the bar (i.e., the dissociation midpoint). To find this pH value, drop a vertical line from the bar's midpoint to the pH axis. The pH value intersected by the drop-line numerically indicates the bar's location and hence its acidic strength. The lower the midpoint pH value, the stronger the acid; the higher the midpoint pH value, the weaker the acid. This midpoint pH value is called "pK."

This is a key concept and warrants emphasis. The pK of an acid represents the pH at which the acid is half dissociated. Put differently, pK represents the pH at which $[HA] = [A^-]$ and $[A^-]/[HA] = 1$. Similarly, when a solution's pH coincides with the acid's pK (e.g., a weak acid with a pK of 7 in a solution whose pH is 7), we know that the acid is half dissociated. Therefore, when pH = pK, $[HA] = [A^-]$ and $[A^-]/[HA] = 1$. In visual terms, pK simply tells you where the midpoint of the bar graph is located along the pH axis. Different acids have different pKs, depending on their inherent tendency to dissociate. The lower the pK, the stronger the acid; the higher the pK, the weaker the acid.

The following illustration shows how pKs can be graphically derived for a few physiologically relevant acids. Notice the dotted drop-lines and how their points of intersection with the pH axis correspond to the pK values:

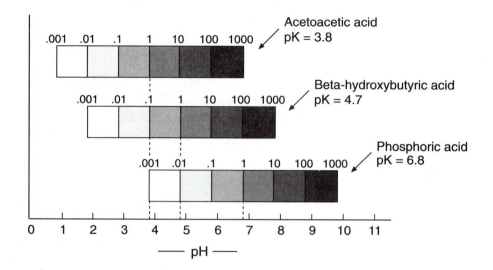

Using this illustration, convince yourself visually that when pH = pK, the acid really is half dissociated. Next, convince yourself visually that when pH > pK, the acid is more than half dissociated (e.g., an acid of pK 4 in a solution of pH 7). Also notice that when pH is more than about 2 units above pK, the acid is almost completely dissociated. Conversely, observe that when pH < pK, the acid is less than half dissociated.*

The Henderson-Hasselbalch Equation

As we have seen, the [A⁻]/[HA] ratio of a weak acid varies with pH. This fact suggests a way to determine the pH of a buffered solution. The steps are (1) measure the solution's [A⁻] and [HA] by chemical analysis and calculate the [A⁻]/[HA] ratio, (2) find the point on the appropriate dissociation bar that matches this [A⁻]/[HA] ratio, and (3) drop a line to the horizontal axis and read off the pH. To better understand this approach, use the preceding bar graph illustration (just above) to help you solve this Q & A:

Q: For a solution of acetoacetic acid, chemical analysis shows that the concentration of acetoacetate (the A⁻ form) is 100 mmol/l and that the con-

---

*Going further.** Since the degree of acidic dissociation is a function not of pK alone, but of the proximity of pK to pH, designations of acidic strength are not absolute. For example, in blood plasma, beta-hydroxybutyric acid is more than 99% dissociated (a "strong acid") whereas in acidic urine it is about half dissociated (a "weak acid"). Thus, designating an acid as strong or weak always implies a pH context, and it is not possible to make general statements like "Acids with pKs below x are strong acids" unless a pH context is assumed. This relativity with respect to pH explains why organic acids like lactic, acetoacetic, and beta-hydroxybutyric are sometimes described as strong, whereas in other contexts they are described as weak.

centration of undissociated acetoacetic acid (the HA form) is 1 mmol/l. What is the pH?

A: The [A⁻]/[HA] ratio = 100/1. Locate this ratio on the dissociation bar for acetoacetic acid. From this point, drop a line to the horizontal axis. The pH of the solution is 5.8.

All acids with the same pK have the same acidic strength and the same dissociation midpoint. As a result, acids with the same pK share the same dissociation bar. Therefore, as long as you know the pK of the buffer*, you know which dissociation bar to use. You don't have to know the acid's name. For example, if you know that a buffer has a pK of 4.7, you would use the bar whose midpoint is directly above 4.7 on the pH axis. In the preceding illustration, this bar is labeled "Beta-hydroxybutyric acid," but this same bar represents all acids whose pK is 4.7. Try this problem:

Q. If an acid has a pK of 4.7, and the [A⁻]/[HA] ratio is 1/10, what is the pH?

A. Use the bar whose dissociation midpoint is at pH 4.7. Find the point on the bar where the [A⁻]/[HA] ratio is 1/10. Drop a vertical line from that point. It intersects a pH of 3.7.

Until now we have relied heavily on the bar graph. But the bar graph is simply a visual portrayal of a logarithmic scale, with each shaded square representing a ten-fold change in [A⁻]/[HA]. When we use the bar graph to find pH, we are actually finding the log of the [A⁻]/[HA] ratio and adding it to the pK. If we could find the log of the [A⁻]/[HA] ratio by other means, we could dispense with the bar graph entirely.

To make this point, let's redo the previous two Q & A examples without looking at the bar graph. In the first example (the one about acetoacetic acid), the [A⁻]/[HA] ratio is 100/1 or, more simply, 100. Since we know that the log of 100 is 2 (because $100 = 10^2$), we don't need the bar graph. We simply add 2 to the pK of the acid, which is 3.8. This gives us a pH of 5.8, the same as we got using the bar graph. Spend a moment comparing the two ways that we solved this problem. Convince yourself that they are really the same.

In the next Q & A (the one with the pK of 4.7), the [A⁻]/[HA] ratio is 1/10, or 0.1. The log of 0.1 is −1 (since $0.1 = 10^{-1}$). So we add (−1) to 4.7, which gives us a pH of 3.7. Pause again to compare the two approaches.

We are now ready to express this non-graphic approach in a simple formula, called the Henderson-Hasselbalch equation:

$$pH = pK + \log [A^-]/[HA]$$

***Terminology.** It is common to speak about "the pK of a buffer," as we have done here. This is a short-hand way of referring to the pK of the conjugate acid of the buffer pair. Thus, a buffer with "a pK of 7" is a buffer whose HA form has a pK of 7.

There is nothing magical or new about the Henderson-Hasselbalch (or "H.H.") equation. It is just a condensed way of saying: "To find pH, determine the [A⁻]/[HA] ratio, calculate its log, and add that value to the pK." You can think of the H.H. equation as a mathematical summary of the bar-graph approach. Or you can think of the bar-graph approach as a visual expression of the H.H. equation. The key point to recognize is that the equation is simply a reflection of the fact that the [A⁻]/[HA] ratio changes as the reciprocal of the solution's [H⁺], and that this happens because changes in [H⁺] shift the equilibrium point of the HA ⇌ H⁺ + A⁻ equilibrium.

Students sometimes find it confusing that the H.H. equation has us add the *log* of the [A⁻]/[HA] ratio to pK, as opposed to simply adding the value of the ratio itself. We add the log because we are finding pH, which is logarithmic. If we added the ratio itself to pK, we would be mixing log and non-log values and would come up with absurd results. For example, if an acid had a pK of 7, and an [A⁻]/[HA] ratio of 100/1, adding the ratio would give us a pH of 107, instead of the correct value of 9.

For practice, use the Henderson-Hasselbalch equation to solve the following problems. You may wish to cover the answers.

Q: A solution of lactic acid (pK = 3.8) has an [A⁻]/[HA] (i.e., [lactate]/[lactic acid]) ratio of 1/10. What is the pH?

A: pH = pK + log [A⁻]/[HA]
    pH = 3.8 + log 0.1
    pH = 3.8 + (−1)
    pH = 3.8 − 1
    pH = 2.8

Q: In a solution containing beta-hydroxybutyric acid (pK = 4.7), chemical analysis shows that [beta-hydroxybutyrate] = 1000 mmol/l and that [beta-hydroxybutyric acid] = 1 mmol/l. What is the pH?

A: Beta-hydroxybutyrate is the dissociated form (A⁻) and beta-hydroxybutyric acid is the undissociated form (HA). Thus the [A⁻]/[HA] ratio is 1000. Therefore:

    pH = pK + log [A⁻]/[HA] = 4.7 + log 1000 = 4.7 + 3 = 7.7

In the above examples, the [A⁻]/[HA] ratios are all multiples of ten. However, in physiologic solutions, the [A⁻]/[HA] ratios can be intimidating fractions like 25.4/1.27. To reduce these fractions and find their logs requires a calculator, but the approach is identical. For example:

Q: If a weak acid has a pK of 6.1, and its concentrations in solution are [A⁻] = 25.4 mmol/l and [HA] = 1.31 mmol/l, what is the pH?

A: A calculator tells us that 25.4/1.31 = 19.4. It also tells us that the log of 19.4 is 1.29 (i.e., $19.4 = 10^{1.29}$). Therefore: pH = 6.1 + 1.29 = 7.4.

As you work through the following problems, feel free to use a calculator, remembering that we are using base-10 logs. Or, if you prefer, just follow the steps mentally.

Q: If the concentration of lactate in a solution is 160 mmol/l, and that of undissociated lactic acid is 4 mmol/l, what is the pH?

Hint: The $[A^-]/[HA]$ ratio is 160/4 , which can be reduced to 40, the log of which is 1.6.

A: pH = pK + log $[A^-]/[HA]$
pH = 3.8 + 1.6
pH = 5.4

Q: A solution contains 327 mmol/l beta-hydroxybutyrate and 327 mmol/l undissociated beta-hydroxybutyric acid. What is the pH?

A: pH = pK + log $[A^-]/[HA]$
pH = 4.7 + log 327/327
pH = 4.7 + log 1
pH = 4.7 + 0
pH = 4.7

Q: A sample of blood plasma has a lactate concentration of 1 mmol/l and a lactic acid concentration of 0.00025 mmol/l. What is the pH?

Hint: The $[A^-]/[HA]$ ratio is 1/0.00025 = 4000.
        Log 4000 = 3.6.

A: pH = pK + log $[A^-]/[HA]$
pH = 3.8 + 3.6
pH = 7.4

This concludes our introduction to the H.H. equation. We now move on to the third (and last) main topic of this chapter.

Buffer capacity

"Buffer capacity" describes how resistant a solution is to pH changes. A solution with high buffer capacity is well buffered and requires a substantial quantity of strong acid or base to alter pH by one unit; a solution with low buffer capacity is poorly buffered and requires just a small amount of strong acid or base to produce the same pH changes.

Two factors determine buffer capacity. The first is obvious: the more buffer (i.e., the higher the concentration) the greater the buffer capacity. The reason is that more buffer means greater capacity to donate or remove protons.

The second factor is not obvious: for a buffer to be effective, the pH of the solution must be fairly close to the pK of the buffer (i.e., close to the pH = pK point). Since at this point $[A^-]$ = $[HA]$ and the $[A^-]/[HA]$ ratio is 1, we can also say that, for a buffer to be effective, $[A^-]$ and $[HA]$ must not differ too much from each other, or we can say that the $[A^-]/[HA]$ ratio must not deviate too far from 1. For example, a weak acid with a pK of 5.0 (and its conjugate base) will make an effective buffer when the solution has a pH of 5.3. However, it will not be effective in a solution of pH 9.

To better understand this second factor, we will make use of an illustration. Although it may look intimidating, the illustration is simply an enlarged dissociation bar with some additional lines of information suspended above it:

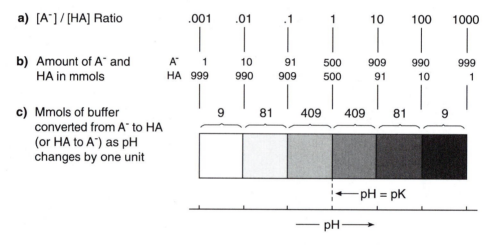

a) $[A^-]/[HA]$ Ratio   .001   .01   .1   1   10   100   1000

b) Amount of A^- and HA in mmols

| | A^- | 1 | 10 | 91 | 500 | 909 | 990 | 999 |
| | HA | 999 | 990 | 909 | 500 | 91 | 10 | 1 |

c) Mmols of buffer converted from A^- to HA (or HA to A^-) as pH changes by one unit   9   81   409   409   81   9

pH = pK

— pH —→

Note: Total buffer = 1000 mmols. Volume = 1 liter.

Let's study this figure point by point. First, notice that the dissociation bar is just like the bars presented earlier (same shape, shading, etc.). The statement beneath the bar, "Total buffer = 1,000 millimoles. Volume = 1 liter," indicates that the solution has 1000 mmol of buffer dissolved in one liter of solution. The word "Total" indicates that the 1000 mmol comprises both the A^- and HA forms. This total will not change even if A^- is converted to HA, or vice versa.

Second, note that the top line of information (labeled "a") gives the $[A^-]/[HA]$ ratio. As expected, the ratio rises as pH rises and falls as pH falls. When the pH of the solution has the same value as the pK of the buffer, the $[A^-]/[HA]$ ratio is 1.

Third, look at the middle row of information (labeled "b"). It shows the actual amounts (in millimoles) of A^- and HA in the solution. Notice that the amounts of A^- and HA change in parallel with the $[A^-]/[HA]$ ratio. Notice also that the sum of A^- and HA always equals 1000 millimoles.

Fourth, the next line of information (labeled "c") shows the quantity of buffer that is converted from A^- to HA (or from HA to A^-) as pH changes by one unit. These values are derived from the quantities in row "b." For example, if pH starts at the pH = pK point and then falls by one unit, we see that the quantities of A^- and HA change from 500 + 500 to 91 + 909. This change indicates that 409 mmol of A^- were converted to HA (because 500 − 91 = 409). Notice that the closer we are to the dissociation midpoint, the more buffer is converted, and that the farther we are from the dissociation midpoint, the less buffer is converted. In other words, the farther we are from an $[A^-]/[HA]$ ratio of 1, the less buffer must be converted to produce a ten-fold change in the ratio. Be sure you understand this concept; it is key.

This concept leads directly to our main point. The amount of buffer converted from HA to A^- is equal to the amount of protons liberated, and the amount of buffer converted from A^- to HA is equal to the amount of protons consumed. For example, if we start at the point where pK = pH, we must add 409 millimoles of HCl to lower pH by one unit. To lower pH an additional unit, only 81 mmol HCl are required. The next one-unit pH change requires just 9 mmol HCl. The next (not illustrated), less than one. The same pattern holds if we add NaOH, thus raising pH: as pH moves farther from the pH = pK point, less and less NaOH is required to produce a one-unit pH change. This pattern means that buffer capacity is greatest when pH = pK, and that it drops off as pH deviates from this point.*

We can make this point graphically:

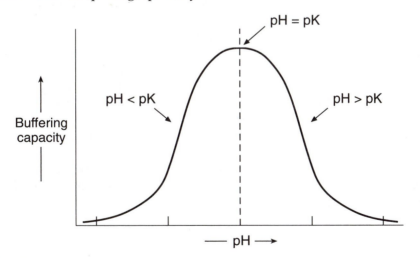

Technical information. In calculating the amount of HCl or NaOH needed to change pH by one unit, we have neglected the protons that account for the free $[H^+]$ of the solution. Except in the extremely low (and thus non-physiologic) pH range, this quantity of free protons is minuscule.

The vertical height of each point on the curve indicates buffer capacity at the corresponding pH level. The shape of the curve is the same for all buffers. This graph shows that buffer capacity is greatest when the pH of the solution equals the pK of the buffer. It also shows that buffer capacity falls off rapidly as we move away from this point in either direction. The decline is gradual and smooth, with no absolute "cut off" where a buffer becomes totally ineffective. However, for simplicity, it is often said that buffers are effective only when pH is within 1.5 units of pK.

How does this "1.5 rule" help us? It tells us that for a buffer to be effective in maintaining the pH of blood, it must have a pK within 1.5 units of 7.4. Thus, only buffers with pK values between 5.9 and 8.9 are good buffers in normal blood. Similarly, if we want to buffer the pH of urine (which has a minimum pH of about 4.5), the buffer should have a pK no lower than about 3.0.

Summary

In a buffered solution, changes in $[H^+]$ shift the equilibrium point of the HA $\rightleftharpoons H^+ + A^-$ buffer equilibrium. This shift alters $[A^-]$ and $[HA]$, and hence the ratio $[A^-]/[HA]$. When the equilibrium value of $[H^+]$ changes, the $[A^-]/[HA]$ ratio changes reciprocally. For example, if the equilibrium $[H^+]$ doubles, $[A^-]/[HA]$ is halved. pK is a measure of an acid's tendency to dissociate. Strong acids have low pKs and weak acids have high pKs. pK is defined such that when the pK of a dissolved acid has the same numerical value as the pH of the solution (e.g., a solution of pH 6 containing a dissolved acid of pK 6), the acid is exactly half dissociated. That is, when pH = pK, $[A^-] = [HA]$ and, therefore, $[A^-]/[HA] = 1$. When pH > pK, the acid is more than half dissociated, and when pH < pK, the acid is less than half dissociated. If you know the $[A^-]/[HA]$ ratio of a buffered solution, and the pK of the buffer, you can calculate the solution's pH using the Henderson-Hasselbalch equation: pH = pK + log $[A^-]/[HA]$. For example, if $[A^-]$ = 10 mmol/l, $[HA]$ = 1 mmol/l, and pK = 3, pH = 4. Buffer capacity, which refers to the effectiveness with which a buffered solution resists pH changes, is influenced by two factors: buffer concentration and the proximity of pH to pK. The higher the buffer concentration, and the closer pH to pK, the greater the buffer capacity. When pH is more than 1.5 units from pK (e.g., a solution of pH 7.4 containing a buffer of pK 5.8), buffers are largely ineffective.

Congratulations! You have just completed two of the most abstract and dense chapters in this book. If you are like most readers, you will find that, from this point on, acid-base becomes increasingly interesting and medically relevant.

Non-Bicarbonate Buffers

Up to this point, we have focused primarily on the model buffer "HA." We are now ready to discuss the actual buffers of the extracellular fluid (ECF). Although any substance with a dissociable proton can act as a buffer, we have seen that the only buffers with a quantitatively important effect are those that (1) are present in substantial concentrations and (2) have a pK close (within about 1.5 units) to 7.4, the pH of blood plasma. Four buffers in the ECF meet these criteria.

Of these four buffers, three follow the HA pattern quite closely: hemoglobin, plasma proteins, and phosphates. These three are the subject of this chapter. The fourth ECF buffer, known as the bicarbonate buffer, has several unusual properties and therefore is discussed separately, in the next chapter. Because of their differences with the bicarbonate buffer, the three buffers discussed in this chapter are sometimes referred to as non-bicarbonate buffers.

Hemoglobin

Hemoglobin is the most important of the ECF's non-bicarbonate buffers. It accounts for about 80% of non-bicarbonate buffering power. Found inside red blood cells, hemoglobin is, strictly speaking, an *intracellular* buffer. However, because of the permeability characteristics of the red blood cell's membrane, hemoglobin has a relatively important and rapid impact on the ECF. Therefore, it is often considered an extracellular buffer.

Hemoglobin, like all proteins, consists of amino acids linked by peptide bonds. Its buffering capacity comes almost entirely from the side group of the amino acid histidine. Histidine is both plentiful (it comprises 36 of hemoglobin's 574 amino acids) and has a dissociable proton with a pK that makes it a good buffer in the physiologic range. The histidine side group (the imidazole ring) looks like this:

Dissociable proton

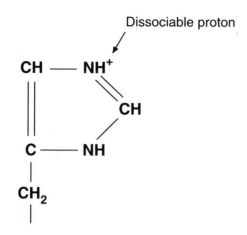

Thus, the HA $\rightleftharpoons$ A$^-$ + H$^+$ equilibrium takes the form of:

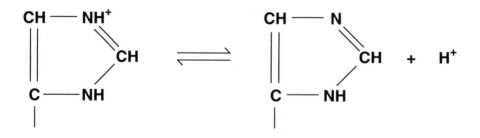

Hemoglobin buffers pH in essentially the same way as HA. When strong acid is added, the equilibrium shifts to the left, binding H$^+$. When strong base is added, the equilibrium shifts right, releasing H$^+$. Like all buffers, hemoglobin mitigates, but does not prevent, changes in pH. The pK of histidine varies somewhat, depending on its position in the protein chain, but the average pK is about 6.5.*

Plasma Proteins

The second most important non-bicarbonate buffer consists of all the various proteins in blood plasma. Of these, albumin has the highest concentration and the greatest buffer capacity. Many other proteins are present in

---

* **Going further.** A few of the histidine groups in hemoglobin have pKs that are affected by oxygen binding. In these "oxylabile" groups, pK falls as blood is oxygenated at the lung and rises as blood is deoxygenated at the tissues. These pK changes are known as the Bohr effect. The rise in pK that occurs at the tissues brings hemoglobin's average pK slightly closer to plasma pH, thus increasing buffer capacity. This increase allows hemoglobin to accept additional protons released into blood by the tissues.

lower concentrations (e.g., immunoglobulins, hormone binding proteins), and some have physiologically active buffer groups. The total buffering capacity of all plasma proteins is about 20% that of hemoglobin.

As with hemoglobin, the most important buffering sites of the plasma proteins are the side groups of histidine. Thus, conceptually, it would not be wrong to consider hemoglobin and plasma proteins as a single class of "histidine buffers." As in hemoglobin, these histidines have pKs around 6.5. The other amino acids that have buffer sites on their side groups play very minor roles.*

Plasma proteins may comprise hundreds of linked amino acids, including a dozen or more histidines (albumin has 16). Thus, a single molecule may have many buffer sites. Although located on the same molecule, each site acts independently, with no regard for the others. The fact that the sites are linked in a chain makes no fundamental difference.

Phosphate

Phosphoric acid is a triprotic acid, meaning it has three dissociable protons (triprotic means "three protons"). The formula for the undissociated acid is H_3PO_4. It looks like this:

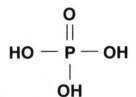

As the protons dissociate, the formula becomes $H_2PO_4^{1-}$ (the diprotic form) then HPO_4^{2-} (monoprotic form) then PO_4^{3-} (completely dissociated). Because each dissociation adds a negative charge, which attracts the remaining protons with increased avidity, the order of acidic strength is $H_3PO_4 >$ $H_2PO_4^{1-} > HPO_4^{2-}$. The pK of the second dissociation,

$$H_2PO_4^{1-} \rightleftharpoons H^+ + HPO_4^{2-}$$

is about 6.8, making it a good ECF buffer. This equilibrium represents the third main non-bicarbonate buffer. In terms of the HA model, $H_2PO_4^{1-}$ represents HA (the conjugate acid) and HPO_4^{2-} represents A^- (the conjugate

---

*Technical information. . . . a fact indicated by the side-group pK values: aspartic acid = 3.9, glutamic acid = 4.3, tyrosine = 10.1, lysine = 10.6, cysteine = 10.8, arginine = 12.5.

base). The pKs of the other forms of phosphoric acid are either too high or low for them to be good ECF buffers.*

Phosphate is the least important of the major non-bicarbonate buffers in the ECF. Although the pK of 6.8 is relatively close to extracellular pH, the concentrations of $H_2PO_4^{1-}$ and HPO_4^{2-} are low. In fact, the combined ECF concentration of all forms of phosphoric acid is just over 1 mmol/l. The buffering power of phosphate in the ECF is only a few percent of that of hemoglobin.

A final note

Buffers are also present *inside* cells. These intracellular fluid (ICF) buffers help keep the internal pH of cells stable when stressed by cellular processes (e.g., protons liberated by cellular metabolism) or by pH changes transmitted from the ECF across cell membranes. Two key ICF buffers are protein molecules and phosphate groups, both of which are similar to their ECF counterparts, although their concentrations in the ICF are higher. The cellular proteins, like plasma proteins, get most of their buffering capacity from histidine. As for the phosphate groups, one difference between ICF and ECF phosphates is that most ICF phosphates are incorporated into the structure of organic molecules. Two examples are glucose-6-phosphate and adenosine triphosphate (ATP), molecules that have important non-buffer functions as well. These phosphorylated molecules are called "organic phosphates," in contrast to the simple "inorganic phosphates" discussed and illustrated above.

Summary

The pH of extracellular fluid (ECF) is stabilized by four main buffer pairs, which are of two general types: non-bicarbonate and bicarbonate. The major non-bicarbonate buffers are (in descending order of importance) hemoglobin, plasma proteins, and phosphate. Hemoglobin and plasma proteins are effective because they contain histidine, whose average pK (about 6.5) is near physiologic pH. Phosphate is effective because the second dissociation of phosphoric acid ($H_2PO_4^{1-} \rightleftharpoons H^+ + HPO_4^{2-}$) has a pK of 6.8. Buffering also takes place inside cells, where proteins and organic phosphates exist in high concentration and play a key role.

---

* **Technical information.** pK for the H_3PO_4 dissociation is 2.0. pK for the HPO_4^{2-} dissociation is 12.4.

The Bicarbonate Buffer System

Unlike the three extracellular fluid (ECF) buffers discussed in the previous chapter, the bicarbonate buffer does not neatly fit the "HA" model. The buffer pair consists of the bicarbonate ion (HCO_3^-), which is the conjugate base, and carbon dioxide (CO_2), which acts as the conjugate acid. Bicarbonate is an anion and a proton acceptor, so it fits the standard pattern for "A^-." But it is not at all obvious how CO_2, which has no protons to donate and commonly exists as a gas, can act as HA.

Our goal in this chapter is to develop a solid understanding of this unusual buffer. As we will see, the bicarbonate system is the most important buffer in the body and, for this reason, we will be especially thorough in our presentation. Our first step is to understand how carbon dioxide gas dissolves in water.

How carbon dioxide dissolves in water

Atmospheric pressure at sea level is 760 mm Hg (pronounced "millimeters of mercury"), which means that the pressure exerted by air (on the ground, on this book, on our skin, etc.) is sufficient to support a 760 mm column of mercury. This pressure results from a vast number of rapidly and randomly moving gas molecules, which strike the surface of objects.

Dalton's Law states that, in a mixture of gases, the pressure exerted by any one gas is proportional to the fraction of the total number of molecules accounted for by that gas. This pressure is called the *partial pressure* because it is the part of the total pressure due to that one gas. For example, because the atmosphere is 79% nitrogen (i.e., 79% of all molecules in the atmosphere are N_2), the partial pressure of nitrogen at sea level is $0.79 \times 760 = 600$ mm Hg. Partial pressure is symbolized "P." Thus, we can say that atmospheric PN_2 = 600 mm Hg or, more simply, "600" (with no units).*

Let's focus on carbon dioxide. Visualize an air-tight chamber filled with CO_2 gas. If a glass of pure water is placed into the chamber, molecules of

---

*__Hint for the reader.__ Although molecules may have different masses (e.g., $CO_2 > O_2$), the pressures exerted by equal numbers of molecules are always equal. Why? At a given temperature, small molecules move more rapidly than large ones, and collision force is determined by both mass and velocity.

CO_2 will randomly strike the water's surface. Some molecules bounce off, but some molecules penetrate the surface and are dissolved in the water. As more CO_2 molecules penetrate the surface, the concentration of dissolved CO_2 (which can be written as $[CO_2]_{dissolved}$ or, simply, $[CO_2]$) rises. As the solution's $[CO_2]$ rises, some of the CO_2 molecules diffuse back to the surface, exit the water, and reenter the gas in the chamber. Eventually an equilibrium is reached, with the rates of molecules entering and leaving the water becoming equal. When this equilibrium is reached, the solution's $[CO_2]$ becomes constant. (Notice that we speak of the *concentration* of dissolved CO_2, just as we would for other solutes in solution. The fact that CO_2 was a gas before solvation is irrelevant.)

When this equilibrium is reached, what is the concentration of dissolved CO_2? Henry's Law helps provide the answer. This law says that, once equilibrium is reached, the concentration of a dissolved gas is proportional to the partial pressure of the gas in contact with the liquid. Thus, if PCO_2 in the chamber is 100 mm Hg, and we raise it to 200 mm Hg, the solution's $[CO_2]$ will double. If we reduce PCO_2 to 50 mm Hg, the solution's $[CO_2]$ will fall to half its initial level.

Understanding this proportionality helps, but we still do not know the actual concentration of dissolved CO_2. For example, at a chamber PCO_2 of 100 mm Hg, is the solution's $[CO_2]$ 1000 mmol/l, or 0.001 mmol/l, or somewhere in between? To find out, we need to know the *solubility constant*. This constant tells us how much gas dissolves for each mm Hg of partial pressure in contact with the solution. Since we are interested in (aqueous) ECF at body temperature, we need to know the solubility of CO_2 in water at 37 °C. That solubility is:

$$0.03 \text{ mmol/l/mm Hg}$$

This solubility value tells us that for each 1 mm Hg partial pressure of CO_2 in contact with water, the equilibrium concentration of dissolved CO_2 will be 0.03 millimoles per liter. Thus, if PCO_2 is 100 mm Hg, the solution's $[CO_2]$ will be 3 mmol/l. If PCO_2 is 50 mm Hg, $[CO_2]$ will be 1.5 mmol/l.*

Until now, we have used the term partial pressure to describe the pressure exerted by a gas on a surface. But the term partial pressure can also be used to talk about the *concentration* of a gas dissolved in solution. To use the term in this way, we simply state the partial pressure that would have been required to produce the concentration in question. Thus, if we place a glass of water into a gas-filled chamber with a PCO_2 of 50 mm Hg, and allow it to equilibrate, we can say that the PCO_2 of the water is 50 mm Hg. This is just

---

*Hint for the reader.** Solubility constants vary with temperature and are specific for each combination of gas and solvent. For instance, at 37 °C, the solubility of O_2 in water is only 1/24 of what it is for CO_2. The low solubility of oxygen in water is why hemoglobin is necessary for O_2 transport.

a shorthand way of saying that $[CO_2]$ is 1.5 mmol/l (because $50 \times 0.03 = 1.5$). In arterial blood, normal PCO_2 is 40 mm Hg. Therefore, arterial $[CO_2]$ is 1.2 mmol/l (because $0.03 \times 40 = 1.2$). When we say that a patient with lung disease has a PCO_2 of 80, we are indicating that the concentration of dissolved CO_2 in his blood plasma is twice normal, or 2.4 mmol/l.

It is important to realize that a liquid can have several different gases dissolved in it (just as it can have several non-gaseous solutes dissolved in it). Furthermore, each dissolved gas may have a different partial pressure. For example, arterial blood plasma typically has a PCO_2 of 40 and a PO_2 of 100. With this background, we can now move on to the next stage of our presentation.

How dissolved carbon dioxide reacts with water to produce bicarbonate and protons

When carbon dioxide (CO_2) dissolves in water, it remains carbon dioxide. Its environment is different but its molecular structure is unchanged. However, once dissolved, CO_2 can react chemically with the water, like this:

$$CO_2 + H_2O \rightarrow H_2CO_3$$

The product of this reaction, H_2CO_3, is called carbonic acid. It has a tendency to give up protons, like this:

$$H_2CO_3 \rightarrow H^+ + HCO_3^-$$

Recall that HCO_3^- is called the bicarbonate ion (or simply "bicarbonate"). When we combine the above two reactions, we get:

$$CO_2 + H_2O \rightarrow H_2CO_3 \rightarrow H^+ + HCO_3^-$$

Thus, when CO_2 dissolves in water, it reacts chemically with water molecules, forming bicarbonate and protons, with carbonic acid acting as an intermediary. It is important to recognize, however, that only a small fraction of the dissolved CO_2 reacts in this way. The rest remains just as it was, as dissolved CO_2.

The two-step reaction just shown is quite slow. It can actually take several minutes to occur (the formation of carbonic acid is the slow step). However, the rate can be greatly increased by a particular enzyme, called carbonic anhydrase. With carbonic anhydrase, the predominant reaction route is altered. The pathway looks like this:

$$H_2O \rightarrow H^+ + OH^-$$
$$CO_2 \longrightarrow HCO_3^-$$

In this reaction, carbonic acid is never produced. Instead, water is split, producing a proton and a hydroxyl ion, and this hydroxyl ion combines directly with CO_2, producing HCO_3^-. Whether or not carbonic anhydrase is present, the reactants are water and carbon dioxide, and the final products are bicarbonate and protons. (Recall that, by definition, a catalyst alters the reaction pathway but not the net reaction). Thus, the net reaction in both the catalyzed and uncatalyzed reaction is:

$$CO_2 + H_2O \rightarrow H^+ + HCO_3^-$$

Looking at this net reaction, we see that carbon dioxide acts as an acid, with bicarbonate acting as its conjugate base. Since only a fraction of the dissolved carbon dioxide reacts this way, we can think of CO_2 as a *weak* acid.

How dissolved carbon dioxide and bicarbonate act as a buffer

We have just seen that CO_2 acts as a weak acid and that HCO_3^- acts as its conjugate base. CO_2 and HCO_3^- thus fulfill the definition of a buffer pair: a weak acid and its conjugate base. Although CO_2 and HCO_3^- both play essential roles, it is usual to call the buffer, simply, the bicarbonate buffer. It is the fourth major ECF buffer:

$$CO_2 + H_2O \; \rightleftharpoons \; H^+ + HCO_3^-$$

Although this buffer system does not closely fit the standard buffer pattern (i.e., $HA \rightleftharpoons H^+ + A^-$), it reacts to pH changes in a similar fashion. A rise in $[H^+]$ due to the addition of a strong acid, such as HCl, will drive the equilibrium to the left, consuming protons and liberating CO_2 and H_2O. A fall in $[H^+]$ will pull the equilibrium to the right, consuming CO_2 and H_2O, and releasing protons and bicarbonate.

Notice also from this buffer equilibrium that changes in $[CO_2]$ or $[HCO_3^-]$ will affect $[H^+]$ and, thus, pH. For example, a rise in $[CO_2]$ will drive the equilibrium to the right, raising $[H^+]$, and a fall in $[CO_2]$ will pull the equilibrium to the left, lowering $[H^+]$. Similarly, a rise in $[HCO_3^-]$ drives the equilibrium to the left, raising pH, and a fall in $[HCO_3^-]$ pulls the equilibrium to the right, lowering pH.

In health, the body maintains extracellular $[HCO_3^-]$ at about 24 mmol/l and $[CO_2]$ at 1.2 mmol/l, equal to a PCO_2 of 40 mm Hg. The pK of this equilibrium is 6.1.* As we have seen, the Henderson-Hasselbalch equation lets you find the pH of a buffered solution (p. 32). You simply plug concentration values for the conjugate acid and base forms of the buffer into the equation, and solve. We can apply this approach to the bicarbonate buffer system. For

----

*Going further.** Put differently, the acid CO_2 has an effective pK of 6.1.

example, taking normal plasma values for $[HCO_3^-]$ and $[CO_2]$, and the pK of 6.1, we can find pH:

$$pH = pK + \log [A^-]/[HA]$$
$$pH = 6.1 + \log [HCO_3^-]/[CO_2]$$
$$pH = 6.1 + \log (24/1.2)$$
$$pH = 6.1 + \log 20$$
$$pH = 6.1 + 1.3$$
$$pH = 7.4$$

In the hospital and other clinical settings, $[CO_2]$ is always reported in terms of PCO_2. The mmol/l value is never mentioned. The Henderson-Hasselbalch equation requires that CO_2 and HCO_3^- be in the same units. Therefore, to use the equation clinically, you must first convert PCO_2 into mmols per liter. Since the CO_2 solubility constant is 0.03 mmol/l/mm Hg, you can simply multiply PCO_2 by 0.03. To save a step, the solubility constant is usually incorporated into the equation, like this:

$$pH = 6.1 + \log [HCO_3^-]/0.03PCO_2$$

This modification lets you directly input PCO_2 values. For example, if $[HCO_3^-]$ is 25 mmol/l and PCO_2 is 44 mm Hg, you solve the equation like this:

$$pH = 6.1 + \log [25/(0.03 \times 44)]$$
$$pH = 6.1 + \log (25/1.32)$$
$$pH = 6.1 + \log 18.9$$
$$pH = 6.1 + 1.28$$
$$pH = 7.38$$

The importance of the bicarbonate buffer

The bicarbonate buffer is, under many circumstances, the most powerful and important of all ECF buffers. This fact may seem strange because, at a plasma pH of 7.4, the buffer's pK of 6.1 is near the 1.5 unit "cut off" for buffer effectiveness. Three factors explain the apparent contradiction.

First, the total concentration of the buffer pair (i.e., $[CO_2] + [HCO_3^-]$) is quite high, about 26 mmol/l (i.e., 24 + 1.2).

Second, the body holds the $[CO_2]$ of arterial blood constant at 1.2 mmol/l, or 40 mm Hg. It maintains this constant level by increasing alveolar ventilation when CO_2 production rises, and decreasing ventilation when CO_2 production falls. To understand the importance of this constancy of $[CO_2]$, do (with your imagination) the following experiment: Take two identical one-liter jars and fill them to the brim with extracellular fluid (i.e., $[HCO_3^-]$ = 24 mmol/l, $[CO_2]$ = 1.2 mmol/l). Seal one jar with an air-tight lid. Leave the other jar open and place it inside a chamber filled with CO_2 gas whose partial pressure is 40 mm Hg. Next, to each jar add 5 mmol of hydrochloric acid, HCl. What happens? In each jar, the HCl dissociates, releasing 5 mmol of H^+. These protons combine with 5 mmol of HCO_3^-, producing 5 mmol of CO_2 and causing $[HCO_3^-]$ to fall by 5 mmol/l, to 19 mmol/l. In the sealed jar, the CO_2 cannot escape but remains dissolved in the ECF, raising $[CO_2]$ to 6.2 mmol/l (equal to a PCO_2 of 186 mm Hg). Plugging these values into the Henderson-Hasselbalch equation, we see that pH falls sharply:

$$pH = pK + \log [HCO_3^-]/[CO_2] = 6.1 + \log (19/6.2) = 6.6$$

In the open jar, the situation is very different. The 5 mmol of newly generated CO_2 diffuses out of the fluid and into the chamber. $[CO_2]$ remains at 1.2 mmol/l. The new pH is

$$pH = pK + \log [HCO_3^-]/[CO_2] = 6.1 + \log (19/1.2) = 7.30$$

Whereas pH 6.6 is lethal, pH 7.30 is just 0.1 units below normal. The open jar has greatly increased buffering efficiency. The body, like the second jar, is an "open system" because excess CO_2 is excreted by the lung (CO_2 diffuses out of pulmonary capillary blood and into the alveolar airspaces just as it diffuses out of the open jar and into the chamber). Because it is an open system, the bicarbonate buffer has greater power than would be suspected based on its concentration and pK alone.

Third, as if the above two factors were not enough, the kidneys actually replace HCO_3^- that is lost during the buffering process. This replacement of HCO_3^- normalizes pH even more. (To prove this to yourself, input a higher value for $[HCO_3^-]$ into the Henderson-Hasselbalch equation, above.) In the physiology section, we will study in detail how the lung and kidney regulate PCO_2 and $[HCO_3^-]$. For now, it is enough just to be aware that this regulation exists.*

Summary

In the bicarbonate buffer system, bicarbonate (HCO_3^-) is the conjugate base (A^-) and dissolved carbon dioxide gas (CO_2) acts as the conjugate acid (HA). The buffer equilibrium, which is sometimes catalyzed by the enzyme carbonic anhydrase, is $CO_2 + H_2O \rightleftharpoons H^+ + HCO_3^-$. Normal arterial $[HCO_3^-]$ is about 24 mmol/l. Normal arterial dissolved $[CO_2]$ is about 1.2 mmol/l, which can also be expressed as a PCO_2 of 40 mm Hg (the solubility of CO_2 in water is 0.03 mmol/l/mm Hg; $40 \times 0.03 = 1.2$). In the clinical setting, acid-base status is assessed with reference to the bicarbonate buffer

---

*Going further. Although our main focus is on the ECF, intracellular fluids also contain bicarbonate and dissolved CO_2, just as they contain organic phosphate buffers. Thus, the bicarbonate buffer helps mitigate pH changes inside cells as well as outside.

system, using the Henderson Hasselbalch equation in the form: $pH = 6.1 + \log [HCO_3^-]/0.03PCO_2$. Under most circumstances, the bicarbonate system is the most powerful buffer in the ECF, a fact explained by its high concentration and by the physiologic regulation of PCO_2 and $[HCO_3^-]$ (by, respectively, the lung and kidney).

Extracellular Fluid as a Multi-Buffered Solution

In this final chapter of the chemistry section, we look at solutions, like the extracellular fluid, that contain more than one buffer ("multi-buffered" solutions).

Introduction

To understand multi-buffered solutions, you need to remember just one thing: all buffers in a solution are in equilibrium with the same hydrogen ion concentration. In the extracellular fluid (ECF), for example, all buffers are in equilibrium with an $[H^+]$ of about 40 nanomoles per liter (i.e., 40×10^{-9} mol/l), described by a pH of 7.4. This idea is so important that it receives a special name: the isohydric principle (from the Greek "isos," meaning same or equal, and "hydric," which refers to hydrogen). Since all buffers are in equilibrium with the same $[H^+]$, they are all indirectly in equilibrium with one another. Thus, any time something influences one buffer pair, all the buffer pairs are affected. This idea will become clearer as you continue to read.

Adding strong acid or strong base

If we add a strong acid, like HCl, to a multi-buffered solution, the protons that are liberated raise $[H^+]$. This rise in $[H^+]$ increases the rate of collisions between protons and the conjugate bases (i.e., the A^- forms) of each of the buffers in solution. As a result, all the buffers undergo a net conversion from conjugate base to conjugate acid (i.e., some of the A^- is converted to HA). This net conversion to conjugate acid is reflected in a fall in the $[A^-]/[HA]$ ratios of all the buffer pairs. If we add a strong base, the opposite happens: all of the buffers undergo a net conversion from conjugate acid to conjugate base, and all the $[A^-]/[HA]$ ratios rise.

When we raise or lower the $[H^+]$ of a multi-buffered solution, each buffer responds independently, as if the others were not even present. As a result, the total buffering power of a solution equals the combined power of all the individual buffers in it. For example, consider a solution containing two different buffers. Assume that one buffer has a pK and concentration such that, were it the only buffer present, 25 mmol of strong acid would be required to lower the equilibrium pH by one unit. And assume that the other buffer has a pK and concentration such that, were it the only buffer present, 50 mmol of strong acid would be required to lower the equilibrium pH by one unit. In this solution, 75 (i.e., 25 + 50) mmol of strong acid are required to lower pH by one unit.

Changing the concentration of either HA or A⁻

We saw elsewhere (p. 23) that if we take a buffered solution and add more of the HA form of the buffer, pH falls. And if we add more of the A⁻ form, pH rises. In a multi-buffered solution, the same effect is observed: adding the HA or A⁻ forms of any of the buffers changes the pH of the entire solution. In addition, this change in pH affects all the other buffer pairs. Let's look at an example.

Consider a sample of extracellular fluid. If we add bicarbonate to the sample, $[HCO_3^-]$ rises, and this rise in $[HCO_3^-]$ increases the $[HCO_3^-]/[CO_2]$ ratio. The added bicarbonate also consumes protons, so $[H^+]$ falls. Because $[H^+]$ falls, the HA forms of the other buffers in solution release protons and, in doing so, undergo net conversion to the A⁻ forms. As a result, the $[A^-]/[HA]$ ratios of the other buffer pairs also increase. In fact, these ratios increase in parallel with the ratio of the bicarbonate system. Thus if we add enough HCO_3^- to double the equilibrium $[HCO_3^-]$, and hence to double the $[HCO_3^-]/[CO_2]$ ratio, then we know that the equilibrium ratio of, for example, the phosphate buffer (i.e., $[HPO_4^{2-}]/[H_2PO_4^{1-}]$) will also double.

In this example, it is important to recognize that more bicarbonate had to be added than you would expect based simply on the final change in $[HCO_3^-]$. For example, to raise the $[HCO_3^-]$ of one liter of ECF from 12 to 24 mmol/l requires a good deal more than 12 mmol of HCO_3^-. Why? Because some of the added HCO_3^- gets consumed by combining with protons that are liberated from the other buffers during their transformation from HA to A⁻. For example, as $H_2PO_4^{1-}$ is converted into HPO_4^{2-}, protons are liberated, and some of these protons combine with, and consume, some of the added bicarbonate.

Now consider what happens if, instead of adding HCO_3^-, we raise $[CO_2]_{dissolved}$. (We could raise $[CO_2]_{dissolved}$ by increasing the partial pressure of CO_2 gas in contact with the solution.) Raising $[CO_2]$ lowers the $[HCO_3^-]/[CO_2]$ ratio and raises $[H^+]$, which, in turn, drives the conversion of the other buffers from the A⁻ to the HA forms. The initial fall in the $[A^-]/[HA]$ ratio of the bicarbonate system is therefore paralleled by a fall in the ratio of all the other buffers.

All the ideas discussed so far in this chapter can be expressed symbolically, like this:

$$pH = pK_1 + \log [A^-_1]/[HA_1] = pK_2 + \log [A^-_2]/[HA_2] = pK_3 + \log [A^-_3]/[HA_3] \ldots$$

This equation looks intimidating, but it is simply a bunch of Henderson-Hasselbalch equations set equal to the same pH (which is exactly what happens in a multi-buffered solution). The subscripts 1, 2, and 3 designate different buffer pairs. This formula shows that (since each of the pKs remains constant) the logs of the [A⁻]/[HA] ratios, and hence the ratios themselves, must change in parallel. Thus, if the new equilibrium value for one of the ratios is doubled, all will be doubled; if one of the ratios is halved, all will be halved.

If you're confused, this analogy should help. Think of a multi-buffered solution as a collection of gears that mesh together, like in a fine watch. When one gear turns, all the gears turn. And if you want to turn one gear by a given amount, you must use enough force to turn all the gears. You can visualize the gears like this:

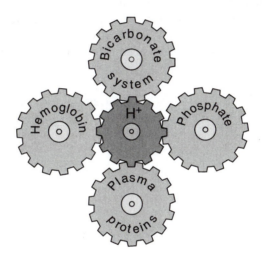

In this illustration, each of the outer gears represents one buffer in the blood plasma, a multi-buffered solution. The middle gear represents the [H⁺] of the solution, which is in equilibrium with all the buffers and thus links them together (the isohydric principle). The movement of each outer gear is like a shift in the buffer's equilibrium point and hence its [A⁻]/[HA] ratio. Just as the outer gears always must move together, so must the [A⁻]/[HA] ratios of the different buffers change in parallel.

Calculating pH in a multi-buffered solution

As we saw elsewhere (p. 32), to find the pH of a buffered solution, you simply plug values for [A⁻], [HA], and pK into the Henderson-Hasselbalch equation. The same is true for a multi-buffered solution. In fact, you can use the values from any one of the buffer pairs, because all the buffers are in equilibrium with the same [H⁺]. For example, to find the pH of blood plasma, you could, in theory, use data on phosphate, plasma protein, he-moglobin, or the bicarbonate buffer as inputs for the equation. However, it is standard practice (p. 47) to use data on the bicarbonate buffer, like this:

$$pH = 6.1 + \log [HCO_3^-]/0.03PCO_2$$

Summary

The ECF is "multi-buffered," meaning it has several buffers dissolved in it. All the buffers are in equilibrium with the same $[H^+]$ and are thus, indi-rectly, in equilibrium with each other. When a strong acid or base is added to a multi-buffered solution, the combined capacities of the buffers come into play, and the $[A^-]/[HA]$ ratios of all the buffer pairs change in parallel. The buffers are like gears in a machine, all turning together. You can find pH by applying the Henderson Hasselbalch equation to data (pK, $[A^-]$, $[HA]$) from any of the buffer pairs in the ECF. However, in the clinical setting, all calculations are done using the bicarbonate buffer system (6.1, $[HCO_3^-]$, PCO_2).

This completes the chemistry section. If you have understood the main con-cepts, you possess all the background needed to master acid-base physiol-ogy.*

---

*Getting a preview.** For students reading this section as part of a biochemistry course: If you want to see how the chemical principles presented in this section apply to acid-base physiology, but don't yet wish to explore physiology in depth, you can read just Chapter 7. It provides a brief overview of acid-base physiology.

Self-Assessment Quiz

This quiz tests your knowledge of core concepts and facts. More importantly, the process of taking and correcting the quiz will strengthen your understanding of the essentials. To get the most from this process, answer all questions in writing. Use a separate answer sheet if you wish. Take your time. When you finish, check your answers against the key. It doesn't matter whether you ace this quiz or fail it. The important thing is to grapple with the questions and then, for those that you miss, to study the correct answers carefully.

1. Use the following symbols to write a model buffer equilibrium: HA, A^-, H^+ (note: write the equilibrium so that HA is on the left). Which symbol designates the weak acid? Which designates the conjugate base? The symbol A^- is an abbreviation for the word _____.

2. Refer to the equilibrium you've just written. If you lower pH, does the equilibrium point shift right or left? Does [HA] rise or fall? Does [A^-] rise or fall?

3. Using the symbols [HA], [A^-], and [H^+]: What is the rate of the association reaction proportional to? What is the dissociation reaction proportional to?

4. When HCl is added to a buffered solution, is the final [H^+] lower than, higher than, or the same as the original value?

5. Follow-up question. How does this final [H^+] compare to what [H^+] would have been if no buffer had been present?

6. If you raise the [A^-] of a buffered solution, what happens to [H^+]?

7. If you raise the [HA] of a buffered solution, what happens to pH?

8. In a buffered solution, if the solution's pH has the same numerical value as the buffer's pK (e.g., pH = 5.4, pK = 5.4), will [A^-] be higher than, lower than, or equal to [HA]?

9. An acid is dissolved in solution. The pK of the acid is much lower than the pH of the solution. Is the acid highly dissociated or highly associated?

10. Consider a buffered solution in which the weak acid is exactly half dissociated. In this solution, what is the [A^-]/[HA] ratio? If we add HCl, thereby lowering the solution's pH, does [A^-]/[HA] rise or fall?

11. Consider a buffered solution in which the [A^-]/[HA] ratio is 1. We add

HCl and let the system equilibrate. We then measure pH and find it has fallen by 2 units from its starting point. What is the [A⁻]/[HA] ratio now? Using a percentage figure, approximately how dissociated is this acid?

12. If a solution has a pH of 7.4, and it contains a dissolved acid whose pK is 4.4, what is the [A⁻]/[HA] ratio of that acid? Approximately what percent dissociated is the acid? If [HA] = 0.1 mmol/l, what is [A⁻]?

    If you need a hint: the log of 1000 is 3.

13. The Henderson-Hasselbalch ("H.H.") equation contains the following elements: log, [HA], =, pK, pH, /, +, [A⁻]. Write the equation.

14. Consider a solution in which [A⁻] = 1000 mmol/l, [HA] = 10 mmol/l, and pK = 6.1. Use the H.H. equation to find pH.

    If you need a hint: The answer to the previous question is pH = pK + log [A⁻]/[HA].

15. In the previous problem, what is the [A⁻]/[HA] ratio? What is the log of that ratio? What is the sum of that log value plus the pK value? How does this value compare with the pH value you found using the H.H. equation?

16. Consider a solution in which [lactate] = 100 mmol/l and [lactic acid] = 1 mmol/l. Lactic acid has a pK of 3.8. Use the H.H. equation to find pH.

17. You are concerned that a patient may have lactic acidosis, a condition in which lactic acid is overproduced. You send a blood sample to the hospital laboratory and ask it to perform a "lactate" assay. Why wouldn't you ask for a "lactic acid" assay? If you made the mistake of asking for a lactic acid assay, do you think the lab would actually determine [lactic acid]?

18. In normal blood plasma, about what percentage of "total lactic acid" is in the form of lactate? Choose your answer from among the following: 88, 90, 98, 99, 99.98.

19. What are the two main categories of extracellular buffers?

20. List the three major non-bicarbonate buffers.

21. Two of the non-bicarbonate buffers are localized to the blood. Which are they? What feature of the vasculature allows these buffers to help stabilize the pH of the entire extracellular compartment?

22. Phosphoric acid exists in four forms, depending on its level of dissocia-

tion: H_3PO_4, $H_2PO_4^{1-}$, HPO_4^{2-}, PO_4^{3-}. Which two of these species exist in an equilibrium whose pK is 6.8? In the extracellular fluid, which two species exist in the highest concentrations?

23. You send a blood sample to the hospital laboratory and ask the lab to determine the plasma concentration of "phosphate." Can you guess which of the four forms of inorganic phosphate the lab will measure?

24. In both hemoglobin and plasma protein buffers, the major buffer sites consist of the side group of this amino acid: _____.

25. In the bicarbonate buffer system, which species acts as the conjugate acid? Which acts as the conjugate base?

26. When CO_2 dissolves in water, does most of the CO_2 react chemically with the water, or does most simply remain as CO_2?

27. Follow-up question. Of the CO_2 that dissolves in water but does not react, does its chemical structure change? In the hospital setting, if you want to quantify the concentration of this dissolved CO_2, you will probably use the term _____.

28. Follow-up question. Of the CO_2 that does react chemically with water, what is the reaction pathway when no enzymatic catalyst is present?

29. The correct answer to the previous question includes five chemical species. Which of these five is not present when carbonic anhydrase acts as a catalyst? (Write both the formula and the name.)

30. What summary reaction can be used to describe both the catalyzed and uncatalyzed reaction of $CO_2 + H_2O$?

31. CO_2 acts as a weak acid. It is considered an acid because, when it dissolves in water, pH falls. Why is it considered weak?

32. The summary equilibrium formula for the bicarbonate buffer system includes four chemical species. Write this equilibrium. What is its pK?

33. If you know the PCO_2 of blood plasma, and you want to find the value for dissolved $[CO_2]$ in mmol/l, what conversion factor can you use?

34. What is the technical name for this sort of conversion factor? The numerical value of this factor depends on all of the following except: the type of gas, the type of solvent, the temperature, the partial pressure of the gas.

35. In an unopened bottle of soda water, is the gas pressure (ie., partial pressure) above the liquid higher, lower, or the same as that in the liquid?

36. Follow-up question. In this same bottle, assume that the gas pressure above the liquid is twice atmospheric pressure, and that all the gas is carbon dioxide. What is the PCO_2 of the liquid? What is dissolved $[CO_2]$ in mmol/l, assuming the soda water is at body temperature

    If you need a hint: the solubility constant of CO_2 in water at 37 °C is 0.03.

37. What is the PCO_2 of normal arterial blood? What is this value expressed in mmol/l?

38. If plasma PCO_2 is 90 mm Hg, what is $[CO_2]$ in mmol/l? If you halve PCO_2, what is $[CO_2]$?

39. In the previous question, we used the term "$[CO_2]$." If we had instead used the term "$[CO_2]_{dissolved}$," would this have changed the meaning of the question?

40. What is the normal value of arterial $[HCO_3^-]$ in mmol/l? What is this value in milliequivalents per liter (meq/l)?

41. Write the Henderson-Hasselbalch equation as it applies to the bicarbonate buffer system. Use "$[HCO_3^-]$" and "$[CO_2]$" (*not* "PCO_2") to designate, respectively, the conjugate base and weak acid. Use 6.1 as the pK.

42. In answering question 41, you should not have included "0.03" as part of the H.H. equation. Why not?

43. Use the H.H. equation you just wrote to find pH in the following patient: $[CO_2] = 1.2$ mmol/l, $[HCO_3^-] = 12$ mmol/l.

44. Write the H.H. equation for the bicarbonate buffer system in a form that lets you directly plug PCO_2 values into the equation. Use the following elements: pH, $[HCO_3^-]$, =, 0.03, 6.1, log, +, /, PCO_2.

45. In writing this equation, you probably left the units unstated. What are the units for each of the following: $[HCO_3^-]$, PCO_2, 0.03, 6.1.

46. Using the H.H. equation you just wrote, solve the following: If a patient has a PCO_2 of 100 and an $[HCO_3^-]$ of 30, what is pH?

47. Follow-up question. If you halve the previous values for both PCO_2 and $[HCO_3^-]$, what is pH?

48. Buffer capacity (or "buffer power") refers to a solution's capacity to resist pH changes when stressed with a strong acid or strong base. This capacity depends on the proximity of the buffer's pK to the solution's pH. What "rule" is useful when thinking about this proximity relationship? On what other factor does buffer capacity depend?

49. Buffer capacity is highest when solution pH equals buffer pK, i.e., when pH = pK. At this point, $[A^-]$ and $[HA]$ will be _____. Also, the $[A^-]/[HA]$ ratio will be _____.

50. For a buffer to be effective in normal arterial blood plasma, within what numerical range must its pK value lie? For a buffer to be effective in urine of pH 4.5, within what numerical range must its pK value lie?

51. What is meant by a "multi-buffered solution"? The buffering power of a multi-buffered solution is equal to the _____ power of buffers in the solution.

52. You can calculate plasma pH by plugging measured values for PCO_2 and $[HCO_3^-]$ into the Henderson-Hasselbalch equation. When doing so, do you need to alter the equation in any way to adjust for the fact that the bicarbonate buffer system is in equilibrium with other buffers?

53. If you have a sample of extracellular fluid, and you hold PCO_2 constant but add enough bicarbonate to double the equilibrium $[HCO_3^-]$, what happens to the $[A^-]/[HA]$ ratio for the bicarbonate system? What happens to the ratio of $[HPO_4^{2-}]/[H_2PO_4^{1-}]$?

54. Follow-up question. In the previous example, does pH rise or fall?

Answer Key

1. $HA \rightleftharpoons A^- + H^+$. HA is the weak acid, A^- the conjugate base. Anion.

2. Left. Rise. Fall.

3. $[A^-] \times [H^+]$. [HA].

4. Higher.

5. Lower.

6. It falls.

7. It falls

8. Equal.

9. Dissociated.

10. 1 or 1/1. Fall.

11. 1/100. About 1%.

12. 1000. 99.9%. 100 mmol/l.

13. $pH = pK + \log [A^-]/[HA]$.

14. 8.1.

15. 100. 2. 8.1. The same.

16. 5.8.

17. At plasma pH, lactic acid is almost completely dissociated. No; they would do the same assay.

18. 99.98.

19. Bicarbonate and non-bicarbonate.

20. Hemoglobin, plasma proteins, phosphate.

21. Hemoglobin, plasma proteins. Permeability of the capillary and post-capillary venule to ions such as bicarbonate and protons.

22. $H_2PO_4^{1-}$, HPO_4^{2-}. Same two.

23.   Sum of all four.

24.   Histidine.

25. CO_2. HCO_3^-.

26.   Most remains as CO_2.

27.   No. PCO_2.

28. $CO_2 + H_2O \rightarrow H_2CO_3 \rightarrow HCO_3^- + H^+$.

29. H_2CO_3, carbonic acid.

30. $CO_2 + H_2O \rightarrow HCO_3^- + H^+$.

31.   Only a fraction of dissolved CO_2 reacts with water.

32. $CO_2 + H_2O \rightleftharpoons HCO_3^- + H^+$. 6.1.

33   0.03 mmol/l/mm Hg

34.   Solubility constant. Partial pressure (the final $[CO_2]$ value depends on the pressure; the constant does not).

35.   Same.

36.   1520 mm Hg. 45.6 mmol/l.

37.   40 mm Hg. 1.2 mmol/l.

38.   2.7 mmol/l. 1.35 mmol/l.

39.   No. When discussing an aqueous solution, "$[CO_2]$" implies "dissolved."

40.   Approximately 24. The same.

41. $pH = 6.1 + \log [HCO_3^-]/[CO_2]$.

42.   The solubility constant is used to convert PCO_2 values into mmol/l; the equation already incorporates the mmol/l form.

43.   7.1.

44. $pH = 6.1 + \log [HCO_3^-]/0.03PCO_2$.

45.   mmol/l, mm Hg, mmol/l/mm Hg. pK, like pH, is dimensionless; it has no units.

46.   7.1.

47.   7.1.

48.   The 1.5 rule. Total buffer concentration (i.e., sum of HA and A^- forms).

49.   Equal. 1 or 1/1.

50.   5.9–8.9. 3.0–6.0.

51.   A solution with more than one buffer in it. Combined.

52.   No; the ratio of each buffer pair will, at equilibrium, independently reflect pH.

53.   It will double. It will double.

54.   Rise.

Section 2
Physiology

This section explains how the body regulates pH during health. Understanding this regulatory process is fascinating for its own sake. It also provides the essential foundation for understanding what goes wrong during disease. Like each of the main sections of this text, the Physiology section is designed to stand alone. It can be read by itself—as if it were a short, reader-friendly monograph on acid-base physiology.

The section begins with a brief chapter titled *Introduction to Acid-Base Physiology*. This chapter gives an overview of the body's entire pH regulatory apparatus. It lets you see how the whole system works, without having to worry about details. Next come five core chapters, which flesh out the framework provided by the introduction. These chapters are:

Regulation of Arterial PCO_2
Bicarbonate Reabsorption
Endogenous Acid Production
Acid Excretion (a.k.a. Bicarbonate Regeneration)
Renal Bicarbonate Handling: An Integrated View

The final chapter is a short *Concluding Overview*, which integrates key concepts presented in the section. A detailed self-assessment quiz, with answer key, follows this final chapter.

It is not our aim in this section to present every last detail of acid-base physiology. Instead, we focus on the essentials and build a deep, conceptual understanding. This conceptual understanding will let you think clearly about both the basic science and clinical aspects of acid-base.*

---

* **Hint for the reader.** This section presumes a basic knowledge of acid-base chemistry. Readers who lack this knowledge are encouraged to review the Chemistry section by reading the section opener (p. 17) and the summaries at the end of each chapter. Chapter 5, which explains the all-important bicarbonate buffer system, should be read in its entirety.

Introduction to Acid-Base Physiology

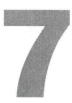

In health, the body keeps arterial blood PCO_2 constant at about 40 mm Hg and $[HCO_3^-]$ constant at about 24 mmol/l. If we plug these values into the Henderson-Hasselbalch equation, we see that normal arterial pH is 7.4:

$$pH = pK + \log [HCO_3^-]/0.03PCO_2$$
$$pH = 6.1 + \log 24/(0.03 \times 40)$$
$$pH = 6.1 + \log 24/1.2$$
$$pH = 6.1 + \log 20$$
$$pH = 6.1 + 1.3$$
$$pH = 7.4$$

As this equation suggests, pH is determined by PCO_2 and $[HCO_3^-]$. So long as PCO_2 and $[HCO_3^-]$ are normal, pH will be normal as well. We can analogize this situation to a balance:

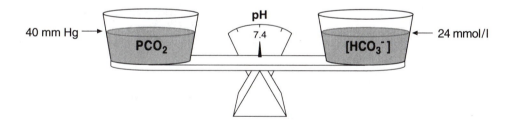

If the body were a simple container, like a glass beaker, regulating pH would be easy. You would simply adjust the concentrations of dissolved carbon dioxide and bicarbonate, and seal off the opening. PCO_2 and $[HCO_3^-]$ would stay constant and pH would never change.

But the body is not a simple container. Body fluids are exposed to stresses that affect both $[HCO_3^-]$ and PCO_2. These stresses are a byproduct of the organism's normal functioning and are always present. For example, sulfuric acid is generated when dietary protein is metabolized by the liver. The protons liberated from this acid consume bicarbonate and cause pH to fall. Thus, the regulation of pH is a dynamic balancing act between processes that alter $[HCO_3^-]$ and PCO_2 and processes that return them to their normal values. This interplay of opposing processes is the essence of acid-base physiology.

The kidney and the lung are the two major organs of acid-base regulation. The lung regulates PCO_2 and the kidney regulates $[HCO_3^-]$. It is by modulating pulmonary and renal activity that the body keeps arterial pH in the normal range. So important are the kidney and lung to the regulation of pH that the Henderson-Hasselbalch equation is sometimes represented (half-jokingly) like this:

$$pH = pK + kidney/lung$$

As described in the section opener (p. 65), this section has five core chapters. Each explores an important aspect of acid-base physiology. To provide a framework within which detailed learning can take place, let's briefly preview these chapters.

Regulation of Arterial PCO₂. In health, the concentration of dissolved carbon dioxide (PCO_2) in blood plasma is held constant. The body maintains this constant level by carefully matching the rates of CO_2 production and CO_2 excretion. Because CO_2 production varies with physical activity, the body must constantly change the rate of excretion. It does this by altering ventilatory rate.

Bicarbonate Reabsorption. As part of normal renal function, bicarbonate ions are filtered from blood at the glomerulus and enter the lumen of the renal tubule. These ions are returned to the blood via "reabsorption" across the tubule wall. If reabsorption did not occur, filtered bicarbonate would spill into the urine, and plasma $[HCO_3^-]$ would rapidly fall.

Endogenous Acid Production. As part of its normal function, the body generates small amounts of strong acids, such as sulfuric acid. This process is known as "endogenous acid production." Most of this acid is created as a byproduct of food metabolism. In addition, some net acid is generated by the gut during the secretion of digestive fluid. All these acids enter the extracellular fluid, where they consume bicarbonate via the reaction $H^+ + HCO_3^- \rightarrow CO_2 + H_2O$. Thus, normal body function results in a gradual loss of bicarbonate. This bicarbonate must be replaced.

Acid Excretion. Renal "acid excretion" (also known as "bicarbonate regeneration") refers to the process by which the kidneys produce new bicarbonate to replace bicarbonate consumed while buffering endogenously produced acids. Acid excretion occurs via two mechanisms: titratable acid excretion and ammonium excretion. We will study both these mechanisms.

Renal Bicarbonate Handling: An Integrated View. The kidney "handles" bicarbonate in several ways: filtration, reabsorption, and regeneration. If plasma $[HCO_3^-]$ is to remain constant, these processes must be carefully coordinated. This chapter shows how this coordination takes place.

If we had to condense this entire section into one sentence, we could say the following: acid-base physiology describes (1) how the lung regulates arterial PCO_2 in the face of variable carbon dioxide production and (2) how the kidney regulates arterial $[HCO_3^-]$ by reabsorbing filtered bicarbonate and replacing bicarbonate that is lost in buffering endogenously produced strong acids. As we have seen, the main goal of these processes is to hold PCO_2 constant at 40 mm Hg and $[HCO_3^-]$ constant at 24 mmol/l, thus keeping pH at 7.4.

If at any point in this section you lose the "big picture" and need to get reoriented, reread this brief overview.

Regulation of Arterial PCO$_2$

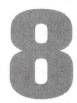

Introduction

Inside cells, molecules of foodstuffs (carbohydrate, fat, and protein) are broken down into acetyl-CoA and fed into the tricarboxylic acid, or Kreb's, cycle. This cycle, which is the body's main source of ATP, produces carbon dioxide (CO$_2$) as a byproduct. Because the body's storage capacity for ATP is very low, ATP must be generated as the need arises. As a result, except for short anaerobic bursts, the rate of CO$_2$ production closely parallels moment-by-moment energy requirements.

What happens to this carbon dioxide? First, it diffuses out of cells, where it is produced, into the interstitial fluid, and from there into capillaries. Arterial blood, and hence blood entering tissue capillaries, contains dissolved carbon dioxide at a partial pressure (designated "PCO$_2$") of about 40 mm Hg. The diffusion of CO$_2$ into capillaries raises capillary blood PCO$_2$ to about 45 mm Hg. PCO$_2$ remains at this level in the veins, the right side of the heart, and the pulmonary arteries, which deliver the blood to the lungs.*

Alveolar air has a PCO$_2$ of about 40 mm Hg, so a 5 mm Hg diffusion gradient drives the exit of CO$_2$ from pulmonary capillary blood into the lung's air spaces. Because carbon dioxide is highly permeant across biologic membranes, it passes easily through the capillary wall, into the pulmonary interstitium, and then across the alveolar wall into the air spaces. As blood moves through the pulmonary capillary bed, CO$_2$ exits and the blood's PCO$_2$ falls. By the end of the capillary, equilibration between blood and alveolar air is complete, so pulmonary vein PCO$_2$ is about 40 mm Hg. PCO$_2$ remains at this level in the left side of the heart and the systemic arteries, which deliver blood to the tissue capillaries. Take a moment to study the following illustration, which summarizes these ideas and provides an overview of CO$_2$ dynamics in the body:

---

* **Hint for the reader.** Like CO$_2$ in an unopened soda bottle, but at a much lower pressure, CO$_2$ in blood is fully dissolved; there are no bubbles. To specifically indicate the PCO$_2$ of arterial plasma, some texts use the term PaCO$_2$. If you wish to review how CO$_2$ dissolves in water and what PCO$_2$ means, see the opening pages of Chapter 5.

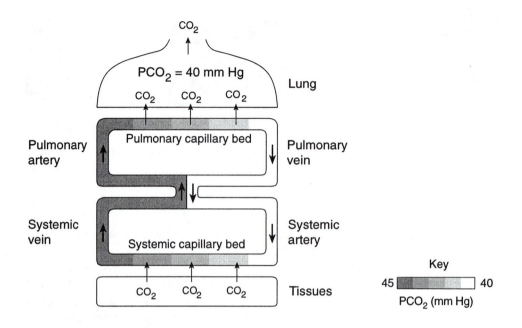

With this background, we can proceed to the main subject of the chapter: how the body regulates arterial PCO_2.

Ventilatory rate and PCO_2

To hold the PCO_2 of blood constant, the body must keep the rates of CO_2 production and CO_2 excretion closely matched. That is, it must maintain a steady state for CO_2. Because CO_2 production varies with changes in activity, the steady state can be maintained only if the body continually readjusts the rate of excretion. It readjusts the rate of excretion by changing the rate of alveolar ventilation. To understand how ventilation affects CO_2 excretion, hold your breath (or just imagine that you do) as you read the next paragraph.

At this moment, carbon dioxide from your pulmonary capillaries is diffusing into the alveolar air spaces. This CO_2 does not normally raise alveolar PCO_2 because new atmospheric air (which contains virtually no CO_2) is continually inhaled and mixed with the CO_2-rich alveolar gas. However, with the breath held, atmospheric air does not enter the lung, alveolar PCO_2 rises and, as a result, the blood-to-alveoli gradient for carbon dioxide diffusion is reduced. The reduced gradient slows the efflux of CO_2 from the blood and, as a result, the blood has an abnormally high PCO_2 when it leaves the lung and enters the systemic arteries.

Assuming you have resumed breathing, you will probably be doing so more rapidly and deeply than usual, which gives you a high ventilatory rate. Now what is happening? Atmospheric air is entering the lung at a high rate, diluting the carbon dioxide-rich alveolar gas. This dilution reduces alveolar

PCO$_2$, which increases the blood-to-alveoli CO$_2$ gradient, thus speeding the efflux of CO$_2$ from the blood. Therefore, the PCO$_2$ of blood leaving the lung falls to normal. If the high rate of ventilation continued, PCO$_2$ would soon fall below normal.

This "experiment" shows that arterial PCO$_2$ responds inversely to ventilatory rate: a low rate of alveolar ventilation yields high PCO$_2$ and a high rate of ventilation yields low PCO$_2$. Let's now deepen this understanding by finding out exactly what rate of ventilation yields a PCO$_2$ of 40 mm Hg.

Maintaining PCO$_2$ at 40 mm Hg

Because pulmonary capillary PCO$_2$ equilibrates with alveolar air, if we wish to understand how arterial PCO$_2$ is maintained at 40 mm Hg, we need to see how alveolar air PCO$_2$ is held at 40 mm Hg.

The pharynx, trachea, and pulmonary airways are open passages that connect the outside air, via the nose and mouth, with the alveolar air spaces. For this reason, air pressure in the alveoli is about the same as atmospheric pressure, 760 mm Hg. If alveolar PCO$_2$ is 40 mm Hg, and the total alveolar air pressure is 760 mm Hg, the fraction of alveolar air comprised of carbon dioxide is 40/760, or about 1/19. Therefore, alveolar air consists of one part CO$_2$ and 18 parts of other gases (mainly nitrogen and oxygen). As long as this 1/19 ratio is maintained, alveolar PCO$_2$ will be 40 mm Hg and, as a result, arterial PCO$_2$ will also be 40 mm Hg.

Let's see how this 1/19 mixture is produced. In general, the rate at which carbon dioxide enters alveolar air is equal to the rate of its production at the tissues (i.e., a steady state). In adults, this rate is usually about 10–12 millimoles per minute. At body temperature and atmospheric pressure, 10–12 mmol of gas occupies a volume of around 250 milliliters (as calculated by PV = nRT). Thus, each minute, about 250 ml of CO$_2$ enters the alveoli. If, during the same minute, we introduce about 18 times that volume of a CO$_2$-free gas into the lung (about 4.5 liters, because 18 × 0.25 = 4.5), we will achieve the desired 1/19 ratio. This process is what occurs during normal breathing, which, at rest, involves an alveolar ventilation rate in the general range of 4.5 liters per minute.*

Increased physical activity raises CO$_2$ production, and decreased activity lowers CO$_2$ production. To hold alveolar (and hence arterial) PCO$_2$ constant, ventilatory rate must be adjusted so that the 1/19 ratio is maintained. For ex-

---

* **Technical information.** The numbers in this discussion have been slightly simplified. For example, we neglect the relatively minor effects of water vapor in alveolar air (about 47 mm Hg) and of ongoing diffusion of oxygen from the alveolar air spaces into blood. Actual alveolar ventilation is closer to 5 liters per minute. This *alveolar* ventilation is achieved when *total* (or "minute") ventilation is about 7.5 liters per minute.

ample, if CO_2 production rises four fold, the steady-state efflux of CO_2 from blood increases to 1 liter per minute. To maintain the 1/19 ratio, alveolar ventilation must therefore rise to 18 liters. If CO_2 production falls by 20%, alveolar ventilation must also fall by 20%. In all cases, arterial PCO_2 is held constant by matching the changes in CO_2 production with proportional changes in alveolar ventilation.

Physiologic control

How does the body match ventilatory rate to carbon dioxide production? Matching is achieved by feedback from PCO_2-sensitive chemoreceptors, the most important of which are located in the medulla of the brainstem. The carotid bodies, located near the bifurcation of the common carotid arteries, provide additional feedback. The chemoreceptors innervate respiratory centers in the brainstem, which control the rate and depth of breathing. Thus, any change in arterial blood PCO_2 is rapidly sensed and corrected.

In addition to these feedback systems, there may also be mechanisms that *anticipate* changes in CO_2 production. These mechanisms, which may include movement sensors in joints and muscles, alter ventilation even before PCO_2 changes. For example, it is known that during strenuous exercise, where both CO_2 production and ventilatory rate are greatly elevated, arterial PCO_2 stays constant or may even fall slightly. If only feedback mechanisms were present, one would expect at least a small increase in arterial PCO_2 to precede any increase in ventilatory rate.

Summary

Through a combination of feedback and anticipatory mechanisms, the body automatically adjusts breathing rate and depth so that alveolar ventilation is closely matched to carbon dioxide production. The goal of this matching is to ventilate the alveoli with CO_2-free air at about 18 times the rate at which CO_2 enters the alveoli from pulmonary capillary blood. This ratio results in an alveolar and arterial PCO_2 of about 40 mm Hg. At rest, about 250 ml of CO_2 enter the alveoli each minute, and alveolar ventilation is around 5 liters per minute. If CO_2 production increases, alveolar ventilation increases proportionately.

Bicarbonate Reabsorption

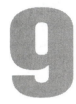

Review of the nephron

We begin this chapter with a brief review of the nephron, which is the fuctional unit of the kidney. Each kidney contains about 1,000,000 nephrons. A nephron consists of a tubule (a skinny little tube) and an associated capillary tuft. Here is one nephron, greatly enlarged:

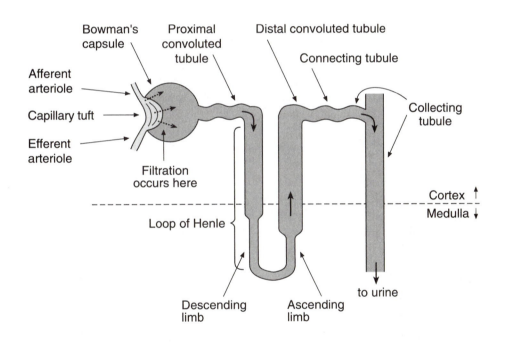

Blood from the afferent arteriole enters the glomerular capillary tuft. There, some of the plasma is filtered into Bowman's capsule, which is the wide part of the tubule that abuts the tuft. During filtration, water and small solutes (e.g., sodium, glucose, urea) pass freely into Bowman's capsule, whereas large proteins (e.g., albumin), as well as cells and platelets, remain in the capillaries. Because it gets there by filtration, fluid in Bowman's capsule is known as filtrate or (because the glomerular filter is so fine) ultrafiltrate. Elsewhere in the tubule, the fluid is referred to simply as tubular fluid. Notice that the proximal and distal portions of the nephron are oriented along the outer part, or cortex, of the kidney, whereas the loop of Henle dips towards the central part, or medulla.*

The entry of filtrate into Bowman's capsule creates a one-way fluid flow toward the collecting tubule. As fluid moves "down" the tubule, its composition is altered by reabsorption (transport of substances out of the fluid) and secretion (transport of substances into the fluid). Examples of substances that are either reabsorbed or secreted are sodium, potassium, water, urea, glucose, chloride, and various amino acids. The tubule is wider at some points than others, and it is twisted (or "convoluted") at some points and straight at others. However, it is a hollow tube throughout. Thus, a cross section at any point along the tubule's length is roughly circular, like this:

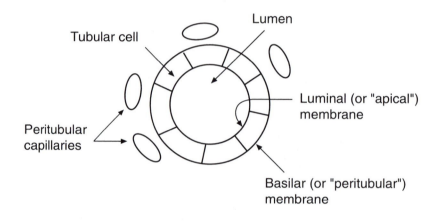

Notice that the tubule wall consists of a single layer of cells, which are known as renal tubular cells or, simply, tubular cells. It is these cells that carry out reabsorption and secretion. Capillaries (also seen here in cross section) run along the outside of the tubule. Many substances that are reabsorbed from the tubular fluid enter these capillaries and are carried away in venous blood.

The central space of the tubule is called the lumen; hence, tubular fluid is sometimes called luminal fluid. The inner wall of the tubule, which faces the lumen, is called the luminal surface. The surface that faces outward, toward the adjacent capillaries, is called the peritubular ("around the tubules") surface. Notice that the renal cells have a slightly triangular shape, with the luminal side narrower than the peritubular side. Because of this shape, the

---

* **Terminology.** If you confuse cortex and medulla, understanding etymologies can help. *Cortex* comes from the Latin word root meaning "bark" (*cork*, which comes from tree bark, has the same root). Therefore, cortex means "bark-side" (or "cork-side"), which is, of course, the outside. *Medulla*, on the other hand, has the same root as *marrow*, as in the center of a bone.

cell's peritubular surface is also known as the basilar surface (from the word *base*), whereas the luminal surface is also known as the apical surface (from the word *apex*). The base and sides of the cells are sometimes considered together as a single "basolateral" surface.

We now move from microscopic to macroscopic. Many nephrons feed into each collecting tubule; many collecting tubules drain into a calyx; and all the calyces drain into a single dilated area in the kidney's central medulla known as the pelvis. A ureter connects the pelvis with the bladder. Each day, a total (both kidneys) of about 180 liters of filtrate enter the tubules. Most is reabsorbed, so only about a liter of actual urine is produced and excreted.

This completes our review. We now focus on the main subject of this chapter, bicarbonate reabsorption.

Introduction to bicarbonate reabsorption

Since glomerular filtration rate is about 180 liters per day, and normal plasma $[HCO_3^-]$ is about 24 millimoles per liter, approximately 4,320 millimoles (i.e., 180×24) of bicarbonate leave the blood and enter the renal tubules each day. To keep plasma $[HCO_3^-]$ from falling, this filtered bicarbonate must be returned to the blood, i.e., it must be reabsorbed. As we will see shortly, reabsorption occurs by a surprising mechanism, one that does *not* involve the direct transfer of bicarbonate from lumen to blood.

Bicarbonate reabsorption takes place at two major sites along the nephron. About 85% of the filtered bicarbonate is reabsorbed in the proximal tubule ("proximal reabsorption"). Much of the remaining 15% is reabsorbed in the collecting tubule, in the distal nephron ("distal reabsorption"). The reabsorptive processes at these two sites are similar but not identical. To emphasize the similarities without obscuring the differences, we will study reabsorption in two stages. First, we'll look at processes common to both proximal and distal reabsorption. Then, we'll look at the two sites individually, emphasizing the differences.

A generic bicarbonate-reabsorbing cell

The following illustration shows key cellular processes that are present in both proximal and distal reabsorption. First, scan the illustration. Then, as you read the numbered paragraphs that follow, keep glancing back to the illustration to visually locate what is being described.

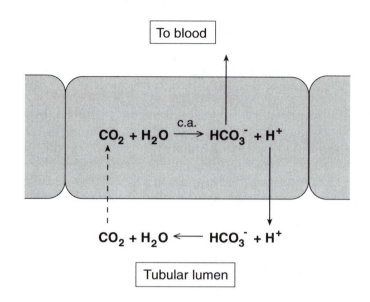

1. Inside the cell, new protons and bicarbonate ions are produced by the reaction $CO_2 + H_2O \rightarrow HCO_3^- + H^+$. This reaction is catalyzed by carbonic anhydrase ("c.a.").

2. The newly-produced protons are secreted across the luminal membrane. This secretion acidifies the tubular fluid (i.e., raises $[H^+]$). The newly-produced bicarbonate crosses the basolateral membrane and enters the blood. These bicarbonate ions replace, one-for-one, those filtered at the glomerulus.

3. In the lumen, filtered bicarbonate combines with secreted protons and is converted to carbon dioxide and water. This reaction is the reverse of the intracellular reaction of CO_2 and H_2O.

4. Carbon dioxide generated in the lumen diffuses back into the tubular cells. Inside the cell, some of this CO_2 is "recycled" into bicarbonate via the reaction with H_2O.

5. Note that bicarbonate is not actually transported out of the lumen. Thus, "bicarbonate reabsorption" is not reabsorption in the usual sense of the word. However, for each filtered bicarbonate that "disappears" from the tubular fluid (via conversion to CO_2 and H_2O), a new bicarbonate is returned to the blood. The net effect is as if direct lumen-to-blood bicarbonate transfer had occurred.

6. The secretion of protons into the lumen (described in 2., above) keeps intracellular $[H^+]$ from building up. This is important because a high intracellular $[H^+]$ would slow the $CO_2 + H_2O \rightarrow HCO_3^- + H^+$ reaction, thereby slowing bicarbonate production.

To integrate these ideas, look back to the illustration and mentally run through the entire process without looking at the text.

Proximal reabsorption

With this background, we can now see how reabsorption occurs in actual cells. We begin with reabsorption by the proximal tubule, because it is quantitatively most important. As you scan the following illustration, notice that all the previously described processes are present, albeit in modified form.

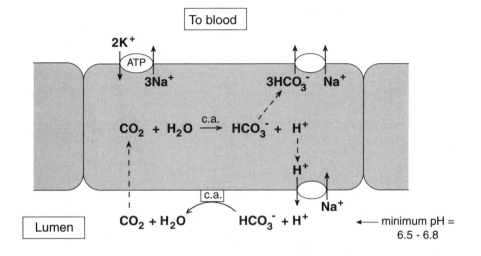

1. Protons are secreted in one-for-one exchange with sodium ions via Na^+-H^+ exchangers in the luminal membrane. Because Na^+ is freely filtered at the glomerulus, luminal $[Na^+]$ is about 140 mmol/l, the same as in blood plasma. Inside cells, $[Na^+]$ is about one-tenth that value, because the basolateral $Na^+-K^+-ATPase$ actively removes Na^+. Thus, there is a steep, inward-directed sodium gradient. This gradient provides the driving force for Na^+-H^+ exchange.*

2. Bicarbonate that enters the blood crosses the basolateral membrane via a cotransporter that carries three bicarbonate ions and one sodium ion. Because each "cycle" of this cotransporter carries a net charge of -2 out of the cell (i.e., $-3 + 1 = -2$), the normal negative charge of the cell's interior helps drive the transporter via charge repulsion.

3. The luminal Na^+-H^+ exchanger can pump protons against only a modest concentration gradient. When the pH of the luminal fluid drops much below 6.8, net proton secretion stops. Thus, the minimum pH of proximal tubule fluid is between 6.5 and 6.8.

---

* **Terminology.** Proximal proton secretion is an example of "secondary active transport." Active, because ATP provides the ultimate driving force. Secondary, because ATP energy does not directly effect proton secretion but, instead, establishes the driving gradient.

4. Carbonic anhydrase is present both inside tubular cells and on the luminal membrane (where it catalyzes the $HCO_3^- + H^+ \rightarrow CO_2 + H_2O$ reaction in the luminal fluid).

Distal reabsorption

Distal reabsorption is similar to proximal reabsorption. In both locations, the secreted proton and the "reabsorbed" bicarbonate are produced inside the tubular cell. In both locations, the proton acidifies the luminal fluid. And in both locations, bicarbonate enters the blood and replaces, one-for-one, bicarbonate lost during filtration. The following illustration shows the details:

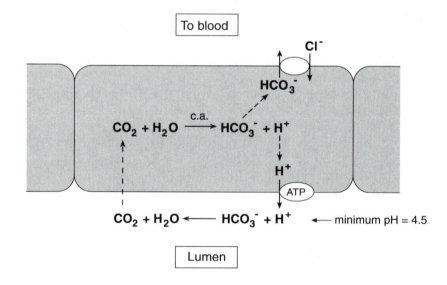

1. Protons are secreted across the luminal membrane by an ATP-consuming structure known as the H^+–ATPase or, simply, the proton pump. There is no exchange for sodium.

2. Bicarbonate enters the blood via an HCO_3^-–Cl^- exchanger.

3. The proton pump can generate a steep pH gradient. It can reduce luminal fluid pH to 4.5 (this is why urine pH can be as low as 4.5).

4. Carbonic anhydrase (c.a.) is present inside cells. However, there is little or no c.a. on the luminal membrane, as there is in the proximal tubule. Thus, the $HCO_3^- + H^+ \rightarrow H_2O + CO_2$ reaction in the luminal fluid is a slow one.

In one glance

The following schematic of the nephron shows key aspects of proximal and distal reabsorption. Take a moment to review it; this will help you place the details described above in their anatomic context. For the sake of clarity, cells are drawn much larger than scale:

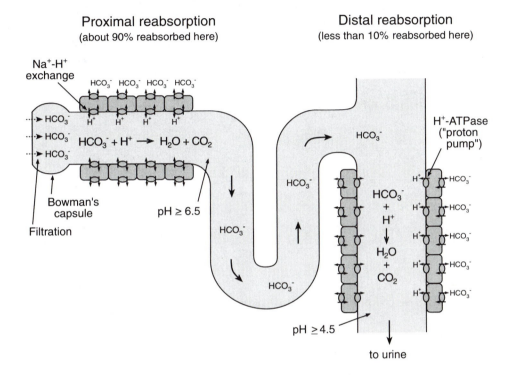

Quantitative aspects and regulation

How much bicarbonate is reabsorbed at the different tubular sites? Under normal conditions, about 3.0 mmol of bicarbonate are filtered from the blood each minute. Proximal reabsorption returns about 2.6 mmol to the blood each minute. Distal reabsorption returns much of the rest.

How is reabsorption regulated? In health, the kidney adjusts reabsorption to a level appropriate to the body's needs. When plasma $[HCO_3^-]$ is normal, the kidneys reabsorb nearly all (over 99%) of the filtered bicarbonate, thus helping maintain bicarbonate stores. If plasma $[HCO_3^-]$ is abnormally low, reabsorption comes even closer to 100%. This homeostatic increase in the re-absorptive fraction helps keep $[HCO_3^-]$ from falling further. Conversely, if plasma $[HCO_3^-]$ starts to rise, the reabsorptive fraction falls. Some bicar-bonate that would otherwise have been reabsorbed remains in the lumen and is ultimately "spilled" into the urine. As a result, plasma $[HCO_3^-]$ falls toward normal. We say more about regulation later in this section.

Summary

The reabsorption of filtered bicarbonate takes place indirectly. New bicarbonate and protons are generated inside renal tubular cells via the reaction $CO_2 + H_2O \rightarrow HCO_3^- + H^+$. The new bicarbonate crosses the basolateral membrane and enters the blood; this is the "reabsorbed" bicarbonate. The new H^+ is secreted into the lumen, where it combines with filtered bicarbonate via the reaction $H^+ + HCO_3^- \rightarrow CO_2 + H_2O$. In the proximal tubule, where most reabsorption takes place, proton secretion occurs in exchange for Na^+ via the Na^+-H^+ exchanger. In the distal tubule, protons are secreted via an $H^+-ATPase$ ("proton pump"). Because filtered bicarbonate "disappears" from the lumen when it combines with secreted protons, and new bicarbonate enters blood and replaces filtered bicarbonate in a 1:1 ratio, the net effect is as if filtered bicarbonate had passed directly from lumen to blood.

Endogenous Acid Production

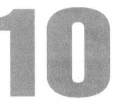

Acidification of body fluids

There are two main processes that acidify body fluids. The first is the production of carbon dioxide (CO_2) by the tissues. Because this CO_2 dissolves into aqueous body fluids, where it reacts with water and liberates protons (via the reaction $CO_2 + H_2O \rightarrow HCO_3^- + H^+$), CO_2 is considered an acid. Because only a fraction of the dissolved CO_2 reacts in this way (the rest remains, chemically unaltered, as dissolved CO_2), CO_2 is considered a *weak* acid. (This first acidifying process is described in depth in Chapter 5.)

The second acidifying process involves the production of *strong* acids, including sulfuric acid. It is referred to as endogenous acid production (EAP). A number of mechanisms are responsible for this strong acid production and, by definition, EAP comprises all these mechanisms. In fact, we can say that EAP comprises all acidifying processes in the body *except* CO_2 production. In this chapter, we explore endogenous acid production in detail.*

We begin with a question: Why distinguish between EAP and carbon dioxide production? One important reason is that the acids comprising EAP all cause the plasma bicarbonate level to fall. For example, endogenously produced sulfuric acid (H_2SO_4) liberates two protons and consumes two bicarbonates, via the reaction $H^+ + HCO_3^- \rightarrow CO_2 + H_2O$. In contrast, the production of CO_2 does not lower plasma $[HCO_3^-]$.

The acids produced during EAP include both organic acids, like lactic and beta-hydroxybutyric acid, and inorganic acids, like sulfuric and hydrochloric. Although the organic acids are not as strong as the inorganic acids, their pKs are still substantially lower than the pH of body fluids, so they dissociate almost completely. Thus, mole for mole, the organic acids release about the same quantity of protons as inorganic acids, so from the body's "perspective" they are just about as strong.

There are various ways to conceptualize EAP. One useful approach, which we follow in this book, is to think of EAP as having two distinct compo-

---

* **Terminology.** *Endo-* comes from *endon,* Greek for "within." *Genous* refers to birth or creation, as in gene, generate, and the book of Genesis. EAP, therefore, refers to "acid created within" the body.

nents: a metabolic one and a gastrointestinal one. The metabolic component consists of acids generated as waste products of metabolic pathways. It is sometimes called metabolic acid production (MAP). The gastrointestinal component consists of the net secretion of protons into the blood by the gastrointestinal tract. This process, which is part of normal gut function, can be termed gastrointestinal acid production (GAP). We can summarize these ideas by saying:

$$EAP = MAP + GAP$$

Let's now study these two components of EAP in detail, beginning with MAP.

Metabolic acid production (MAP)

Introduction to MAP

All metabolic reactions in the body do one of three things: (1) liberate protons as a waste product, (2) consume protons as a reactant, or (3) neither liberate nor consume protons. The reactions that liberate protons increase free $[H^+]$ and acidify the body fluids. The reactions that consume protons decrease free $[H^+]$ and alkalinize the body fluids. The reactions that neither consume nor liberate protons have no effect on $[H^+]$.

When strong acids are produced by metabolism, most of the protons are buffered by bicarbonate (i.e., $H^+ + HCO_3^- \rightarrow CO_2 + H_2O$). For this reason, proton-liberating reactions are often called bicarbonate-consuming reactions. Conversely, when metabolism consumes protons, the reverse buffering reaction ($CO_2 + H_2O \rightarrow HCO_3^- + H^+$), replaces lost H^+. Because a new bicarbonate is produced during this buffering reaction, proton-consuming reactions are often called bicarbonate-producing reactions. Reactions that neither liberate nor consume protons do not produce or consume bicarbonate.

Over the next few pages, we will learn to determine whether a given reaction produces protons, consumes protons, or does neither. We will do this by becoming familiar with five major types of metabolic reactions that occur in the body. However, before looking at these five types, it is useful to recognize a simple fact about chemical reactions: that protons can act to equalize the electrical charge of reactants and products. For example, consider the unbalanced reaction:

$$Glucose \rightarrow 2\ Lactate^-$$

We know that total electrical charge cannot be altered, yet this reaction appears to create two negative charges. So something must be missing: protons. The balanced reaction is:

$$Glucose \rightarrow 2\ Lactate^- + 2\ H^+$$

As this example suggests, the number of protons can be predicted by the difference in charge: we know that two protons are needed because two negative charges must be neutralized. Protons can therefore be thought of as "charge balancers." Keep this notion in mind as you continue to read.

Five reaction types

To learn the five reaction types, start by scanning the following summary table:

Summary of Five Main Reaction Types

Substrate	Product	Acid-Base Effect
Organic cations	Neutral molecules	Protons liberated
Sulfur-containing amino acids	Sulfuric acid	Protons liberated
Neutral molecules	Organic acids	Protons liberated
Organic anions	Neutral molecules	Protons consumed
Neutral molecules	Neutral molecules	No effect

As this table indicates, three different reaction types liberate protons (and thus consume bicarbonate), whereas only one reaction type consumes protons (and thus produces bicarbonate). Let's now look at these five reactions in detail.

1. Organic cations to neutral products

When organic cations (i.e., positively charged organic ions) are metabolized to neutral products, protons are liberated. The hepatic conversion of ammonium to urea by the urea cycle is an important example:

$$NH_4^+ \rightarrow CO(NH_2)_2$$

To balance the charge, we add a proton to the product side:

$$NH_4^+ \rightarrow CO(NH_2)_2 + H^+$$

This charge-balanced equation indicates that each ammonium liberates one proton. The fully balanced equation is:

$$2NH_4^+ + CO_2 \rightarrow CO(NH_2)_2 + H_2O + 2H^+$$

In this equation, we inserted carbon dioxide and water to balance the mass. Because CO_2 and H_2O are neutral, they do not affect charge balance. Each ammonium still liberates one proton.

Another example is the metabolism of the amino acid arginine. This reaction yields either glucose (during gluconeogenesis) or carbon dioxide and water (during cellular respiration). Urea is also produced. The balanced reaction is:

$$Arginine^{1+} \rightarrow Urea + H^+ + Glucose \text{ (or } CO_2 + H_2O)$$

Because the reactant has a positive charge, whereas urea, glucose, carbon dioxide, and water are all neutral, we know that a proton was needed on the product side.

2. Sulfur-containing amino-acids

The amino acids cysteine and methionine both have a sulfur atom in their side groups. When these amino acids are catabolized for energy, the sulfur is oxidized to sulfuric acid (H_2SO_4), which dissociates into sulfate (SO_4^{2-}) and two protons. Thus, the complete oxidation of each of these amino acids liberates two protons. The balanced reaction for methionine is:

$$2C_5H_{11}NO_2S + 15O_2 \rightarrow CO(NH_2)_2 + 7H_2O + 9CO_2 + 2SO_4^{2-} + 4H^+$$

The details of this reaction are unimportant. The essential point is that each sulfur atom causes two protons to be generated, like this:

$$S \rightarrow H_2SO_4 \rightarrow SO_4^{2-} + 2H^+$$

Because organic cations and sulfur-containing amino acids liberate protons when fully metabolized, they are sometimes referred to as "acid precursors" or "potential acid." For example, foods containing large quantities of organic cations may be described as "rich in potential acid."*

3. Neutral reactants to organic acid

Neutral carbohydrates and fats are usually metabolized to neutral products (e.g., $CO_2 + H_2O$). However, when oxidation is incomplete, organic acids are produced. Almost all endogenously produced organic acids have relatively low pKs and therefore dissociate almost completely in body fluids. An example is the conversion of glucose to lactic acid, which dissociates to lactate and protons:

$$C_6H_{12}O_6 \rightarrow 2CH_3CHOHCOOH \rightarrow 2CH_3CHOHCOO^- + 2H^+$$

4. Organic anions to neutral products

When organic anions (i.e., negatively charged organic ions) are metabolized to neutral products, protons are consumed. For example, when lactate or ace-

---

* **Going further.** Actually, when sulfur-containing amino acids are metablolized, H_2SO_4 never really exists in associated form. Instead, protons are liberated in step-wise fashion during the conversion of S into SO_4^{2-}. However, the net reaction is the same.

toacetate is metabolized to carbon dioxide and water, a proton is consumed (or "a bicarbonate is generated"). Acetoacetate is metabolized like this:

$$CH_3COCH_2COO^- + H^+ + 4O_2 \rightarrow 4CO_2 + 3H_2O$$

When multivalent anions are metabolized, electroneutrality requires that an equivalent number of protons be consumed. For example, when alpha-ketoglutarate (AKG^{2-}) is metabolized to glucose, two protons are consumed:

$$AKG^{2-} + 2H^+ \rightarrow Glucose$$

Because organic anions typically consume protons (and thus produce bicarbonate) when metabolized, they are sometimes referred to as "bicarbonate precursors" or "potential bicarbonate" or, simply, "potential base." If we wish, we can therefore rewrite these reactions in a way that shows a gain of bicarbonate instead of a loss of protons. For example, the previous reaction can be rewritten like this:

$$AKG^{2-} \rightarrow 2HCO_3^- + Glucose$$

For short, it is sometimes said that organic anions are "metabolized to bicarbonate" or "converted into bicarbonate."

5. Neutral reactants to neutral products

When neutral reactants are metabolized to neutral products, protons are neither liberated nor consumed. Therefore, the reaction has no effect on pH or [HCO_3^-]. For example:

$$Glucose \rightarrow CO_2 + H_2O$$

Other examples of neutral-to-neutral reactions include the catabolism of triglyceride to carbon dioxide and water, and the conversion of alanine, a neutral amino acid, to glucose:

$$Alanine \rightarrow Glucose + Urea$$

Effect of diet

We now use our knowledge of these five reactions to assess the impact of carbohydrate, fat, and protein metabolism on acid-base balance.

Carbohydrates

When neutral carbohydrates are completely oxidized to CO_2 and H_2O (reaction type 5, above), there is no effect on acid-base balance or [HCO_3^-]. However, when carbohydrate is oxidized incompletely, organic acids are produced, and these liberate protons (reaction type 3).

To determine the net effect of a metabolic pathway, you must follow it from the first step to the last. For example, if glucose is metabolized anaerobically to lactic acid, protons are liberated (reaction 3) and plasma $[HCO_3^-]$ falls. If the lactate anion is subsequently metabolized to neutral products, such as carbon dioxide and water, an offsetting quantity of protons is consumed (reaction 4), and this consumption returns $[HCO_3^-]$ to its starting level. The net effect is the same as if glucose had been directly metabolized to CO_2 and H_2O (reaction 5). However, if the lactate is not metabolized, but is instead excreted in the urine, acidification will not be reversed and $[HCO_3^-]$ will remain low.*

Fats

The same principles apply to fats. In general, the metabolism of neutral fats has no effect on acid-base balance. For example, the oxidation of triglycerides to CO_2 and H_2O neither liberates nor consumes protons. However, when oxidation is incomplete, triglycerides can produce acetoacetic acid and beta-hydroxybutyric acid, which dissociate. If the acetoacetate and beta-hydroxybutyrate anions are subsequently oxidized to CO_2 and H_2O, an equal number of protons will be consumed, and acidification will be reversed.

Proteins

The first step of protein metabolism is the breakdown of the protein molecule into amino acids. This step has no impact on acid-base balance. Next, the amino acids are metabolized. This step may affect acid-base balance, depending on which amino acid is involved. Recall that amino acids have the following structure:

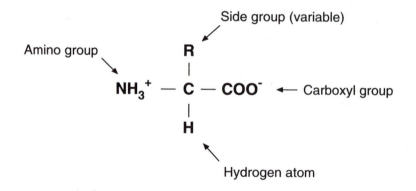

It is useful to consider amino acid metabolism as having two stages: metabolism of the side group and metabolism of the rest of the structure.

---

* **Going further.** For example, during heavy exercise, in a sequence called the Cori cycle, muscles glycolytically convert glucose to lactic acid, which dissociates. The lactate is carried via blood to the liver, where it is reconverted to glucose. Protons are liberated at the muscles and consumed at the liver, so there is no net effect on acid-base balance. However, if lactate is excreted in the urine, the cycle is interrupted and the acidification that occurs at the muscles cannot be reversed.

The side group.   To determine the acid-base effect of side group metabolism, simply decide which of the five reaction types apply. Cationic side groups (e.g., lysine and arginine) liberate protons (reaction 1), as do sulfur-containing side groups (cysteine and methionine; reaction 2). Anionic side groups (glutamate and aspartate) consume protons (reaction 4). Neutral side groups that do not contain sulfur (e.g., alanine, valine, leucine) have no effect (reaction 5).

The rest of the molecule.   At physiologic pH, the amino group is positively charged and the carboxylic acid group is negatively charged. Thus deamination yields cationic ammonium (NH_4^+) and an anionic carbohydrate skeleton (i.e., an organic anion). The ammonium is converted to urea, a reaction that liberates protons (reaction 1), and the carbohydrate anion is converted either to glucose or to CO_2 and H_2O, a reaction that consumes protons (reaction 4). Because proton liberation and consumption are matched, there is no net effect on acid-base balance.

Therefore, the acid-base effect of protein metabolism depends on the types and quantities of side groups in the protein. In most proteins, more cationic and sulfur-containing amino acids (proton liberating) are present than anionic amino acids (proton consuming). Therefore, protein metabolism tends, on balance, to liberate protons, consume bicarbonate, and acidify the body fluids.

Net effect of diet

Most dietary carbohydrates and fats are metabolized to neutral products and therefore have no effect on acid-base balance. However, a small fraction of these molecules are metabolized to organic acids (e.g., lactic, acetoacetic, beta-hydroxybutyric). Thus, normal carbohydrate and fat metabolism slightly acidifies the body fluids. Dietary proteins generally liberate H^+ when metabolized, and this process is the major source of metabolic acid. Dietary organic anions, found mostly in fruits and vegetables, are generally metabolized to neutral products, especially CO_2 and H_2O. This process produces HCO_3^- and tends to oppose the acidifying effects of the other foodstuffs.

In non-industrialized societies, the usual diet is low in meat and eggs (protein) but high in fruits and vegetables (organic anions). This diet yields low rates of metabolic acid production. In industrialized societies (e.g., North America and Europe), the usual diet is high in protein and relatively low in organic anions. This diet yields high rates of metabolic acid production.*

A common misconception

It is often said that "acidic" beverages like grapefruit juice will acidify the urine. In fact, the citric, lactic, and other acids in such juices exist primarily in

---

* **Clinical note.** Hospitalized patients who are not eating and not receiving parenteral nutrition tend to have high rates of MAP. They catabolize their own muscle protein for energy and, in essence, live on a very high protein diet.

their anionic form, especially as their Na^+ and K^+ salts (e.g., potassium citrate). Following absorption, these anions are metabolized to bicarbonate and therefore tend to alkalinize—not acidify—blood and urine. Alkalinization occurs even though the juice's pH is typically low, because the free protons are more than offset by the generated bicarbonate. For example, a liter of juice with a pH of 4 has only 0.1 mmol (i.e., 10^{-4} moles) of free protons. As long as the quantity of organic anions exceeds this small number, net alkalinization will occur.

The same applies to vitamin C (ascorbic acid), which is sometimes prescribed to acidify urine. Vitamin C is often manufactured as the dissociated anion, ascorbate, a fact indicated on the label. Ascorbate is metabolized to bicarbonate, thus alkalinizing the urine. Even the protonated form, ascorbic acid, does not lower urine pH as much as might be expected. Although the acid's dissociation acidifies, the subsequent metabolism of ascorbate to bicarbonate alkalinizes. Only to the extent that ascorbate is excreted unmetabolized will net acidification occur.

Gastrointestinal acid production (GAP)

Introduction to GAP

When "gastrointestinal" and "acid" appear in the same sentence, the topic is usually acid secretion into the stomach's lumen. However, for our purposes, gastrointestinal acid production does not refer to this process. It refers to acid secreted by the gut *into the blood*. GAP is thus like MAP: both involve the addition of strong acid to the blood and result in a fall in plasma $[HCO_3^-]$.

In many segments of the alimentary canal, either protons or bicarbonate are secreted into the gut lumen. For example, in the stomach, protons are secreted; in the colon, bicarbonate. Although secretory mechanisms vary, all bicarbonate and all protons are produced inside gut mucosa cells by the same net reaction:

$$CO_2 + H_2O \rightarrow HCO_3^- + H^+$$

Thus, any time bicarbonate is needed for secretion into the gut lumen, a proton is also generated. And any time a proton is needed for secretion, a bicarbonate is also produced. What happens to the "waste" proton or bicarbonate? It cannot enter the gut lumen, because it would react with, and thus neutralize, the secreted bicarbonate or proton (via the reaction $H^+ + HCO_3^- \rightarrow CO_2 + H_2O$), thereby preventing the intended effect on luminal pH. Also, it must not remain in the cell because this would perturb intracellular pH and eventually kill the cell. It has only one choice: leave the cell in the direction opposite to the gut lumen—that is, into the interstitial fluid and blood.

Therefore, if an organ secretes protons into the gut lumen, it must secrete bicarbonate into the blood. And if it secretes bicarbonate into the lumen, it must secrete protons into the blood. Because the $CO_2 + H_2O \rightarrow HCO_3^- + H^+$ reaction generates bicarbonate and protons in a one-to-one ratio, the effects on the blood and alimentary lumen are equal and opposite. We can present these ideas schematically:

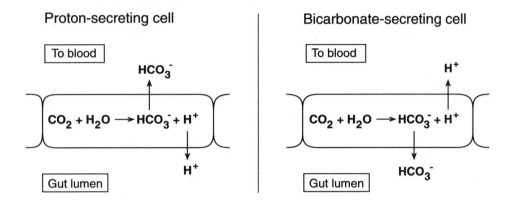

Gut segments

With this background, we can now look at the different gut segments in detail.

Stomach

Under fasting (basal) conditions, parietal cells secrete protons into the gastric lumen at about 10 millimoles per hour (mmol/h). Following meals (postprandial), the rate can reach 50 mmol/h. This secretion of protons lowers the pH of the alimentary contents (chyme) to about 1.0. Thus, the stomach liberates bicarbonate into the blood, both at rest and, especially, during meals.*

Duodenum and associated organs

Bicarbonate is secreted into duodenal chyme from three sources: pancreas, gall bladder, and duodenal mucosa. Pancreatic fluid has an $[HCO_3^-]$ of between 25 mmol/l (basal) and 150 mmol/l (postprandial). In 24 hours, total pancreatic bicarbonate secretion is about 200 mmol. Bile from the gall bladder has an $[HCO_3^-]$ of about 40 mmol/l. The duodenal mucosa also generates and secretes HCO_3^-. As expected, these organs secrete equimolar quantities of H^+ into the blood.

Jejunum, ileum, colon

The jejunum secretes small quantities of H^+ into the gut lumen, thereby alkalinizing the blood. The ileum secretes HCO_3^-, thereby acidifying the

---

* **Technical information.** This release of bicarbonate into blood results in a very slight postprandial rise in plasma $[HCO_3^-]$, which is often reflected, after a delay, in the renal spillage of bicarbonate. The rise in urinary $[HCO_3^-]$ that results is sometimes called the "alkaline tide."

blood. The colon secretes more than 200 mmol HCO_3^- per day into the lumen and thus has a major acidifying effect on blood.

Overview of gut secretion

The stomach adds protons to the gut lumen, thus acidifying its contents, and adds bicarbonate to the blood, thus alkalinizing it. Almost all the segments below the pylorus have the opposite effect: they add bicarbonate to the gut lumen and protons to the blood. We can portray this general schema pictorially:

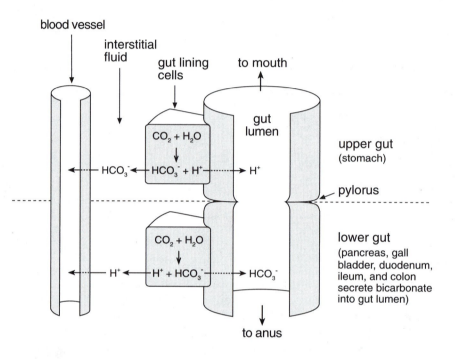

In both the gut lumen and the blood, equal quantities of secreted H^+ and HCO_3^- neutralize each other via the reaction $H^+ + HCO_3^- \rightarrow CO_2 + H_2O$. If the quantities of bicarbonate and protons entering the blood were exactly equal, the gut would have no impact on extracellular acid-base balance: plasma $[HCO_3^-]$ would not change. However, on balance, the gut secretes slightly more bicarbonate than protons into the gut lumen, so more protons than bicarbonate enter the blood. Thus, even after added protons and bicarbonate neutralize each other, some additional protons remain in the blood (hence, gastrointestinal *acid* production). These excess protons, like those released during metabolic acid production, are buffered by plasma bicarbonate, causing $[HCO_3^-]$ to fall slightly.

Quantitative aspects

Although firm data are lacking, net bicarbonate secretion (i.e., in excess of proton secretion) into the gut lumen may be in the range of 20 to 40 mmol/day. Thus, the gut may liberate roughly 20–40 mmol of net H^+ per day into the blood. Given this secretory rate, and the fact that daily stool volume is typically 0.25 liters or less, one might expect a stool bicarbonate concentration of around 80–160 mmol/l.

In fact, fecal $[HCO_3^-]$ is typically just 15–30 mmol/l. How can we explain this? In the colon, some undigested food is metabolized by bacteria to organic acids, especially acetic, propionic, and butyric acid. These acids dissociate and liberate protons, which consume stool bicarbonate via the reaction $HCO_3^- + H^+ \rightarrow CO_2 + H_2O$. The anions of these dissociated organic acids (e.g., acetate, propionate, butyrate) remain, and their combined stool concentration is often greater than 100 mmol/l. Thus, most secreted luminal bicarbonate is consumed and replaced with organic anions, resulting in low stool $[HCO_3^-]$ and high stool [organic anion].

How much endogenous acid is produced daily? Total EAP (i.e., MAP + GAP) for a healthy person eating a typical Western diet is about 70–100 milliequivalents per day (i.e., 70–100 mmol H^+ per day). Most probably comes from MAP. A small fraction, perhaps about one third of the total, comes from GAP.*

Summary

Protons are produced, and bicarbonate is consumed, when organic cations or amino acid sulfur is completely metabolized, or when fats or carbohydrates are incompletely metabolized to organic acids. Conversely, H^+ is consumed and HCO_3^- is produced when organic anions are completely metabolized. Metabolic sequences like Glucose $\rightarrow$ Lactic acid $\rightarrow CO_2 + H_2O$ have no net acid-base effect because production and consumption of H^+ exactly cancel. Gut segments produce new protons and bicarbonate via the reaction $CO_2 + H_2O \rightarrow HCO_3^- + H^+$. Because the gut segments secrete one product of this reaction into the gut lumen and the other product into the ECF, acidification of the gut lumen leads to alkalinization of the blood, and alkalinization of the gut lumen leads to acidification of the blood. Metabolism and the gut each add more H^+ than HCO_3^- to the ECF. Thus, both metabolism and gut independently acidify body fluids. Metabolism and gut together add about 70–100 mmol H^+ per day to the body fluids.

---

* **Terminology.** Since some of the acids that contribute to EAP release more than one proton (e.g., sulfuric acid), it is usual to quantify EAP in meq, not mmol.

Acid Excretion (a.k.a. Bicarbonate Regeneration)

11

Introduction

In the previous chapter, we saw that when endogenously produced acids enter the extracellular fluid (ECF), protons consume bicarbonate via the reaction $H^+ + HCO_3^- \rightarrow CO_2 + H_2O$. To keep plasma $[HCO_3^-]$ from falling, new bicarbonate must be produced to replace that which is lost. This replacement is carried out by the kidney through a process known as either acid excretion or bicarbonate regeneration.*

"Regenerated" bicarbonate is conceptually distinct from "reabsorbed" bicarbonate: regeneration replaces HCO_3^- consumed during buffering of endogenous acids, whereas reabsorption replaces HCO_3^- lost during glomerular filtration. If reabsorption is 100% effective, $[HCO_3^-]$ in the renal vein and artery will be exactly equal. In contrast, bicarbonate regeneration will (when it occurs in conjunction with efficient reabsorption) actually raise $[HCO_3^-]$ in the renal vein to a level slightly higher than that in the renal artery.

Two different mechanisms are involved in creating these new bicarbonate ions: titratable acid excretion and ammonium excretion. The meaning of these names will soon become clear. The two mechanisms have much in common. In both, the new ("regenerated") bicarbonate is produced inside renal tubular cells by the carbonic anhydrase-catalyzed reaction $CO_2 + H_2O \rightarrow HCO_3^- + H^+$. In both, the new bicarbonate exits the cell across the basolateral membrane and enters the blood. And in both, a free proton is created (during the bicarbonate-producing reaction) and must be disposed of.

These same processes are also present during bicarbonate reabsorption. The

---

* **Terminology.** As we will see, the name "acid excretion" applies because the kidney excretes various conjugate acids as part of the bicarbonate-producing process.

key difference between bicarbonate reabsorption and regeneration is how the "waste" free protons are disposed of. As we have seen, during reabsorption protons are secreted into the lumen, where they are buffered by filtered bicarbonate. The disposal of protons during bicarbonate regeneration will be a major focus of this chapter.

With this background, we can begin our study in detail. We look at titratable acid excretion first, followed by ammonium excretion.

Titratable acid excretion

In titratable acid excretion, protons are secreted into the luminal fluid, both proximally and distally, just as occurs during bicarbonate reabsorption. In fact, the same cells, and the same ion transporters, are involved. The only difference between the two processes is that during titratable acid excretion, secreted protons are buffered in the lumen not by bicarbonate, but by non-bicarbonate buffers, especially phosphate in its monoprotic form (HPO_4^{2-}).* Like bicarbonate, these non-bicarbonate buffers enter the lumen by glomerular filtration. In the proximal tubule, the process looks like this:

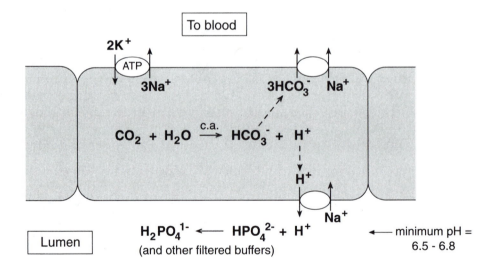

In the distal collecting tubule, where the lower pH allows additional buffering, the process is again identical to bicarbonate reabsorption except for the luminal buffer:

---

* **Hint for the reader.** The phosphate buffering reaction in the lumen is the same as in the ECF. For additional details on this reaction, see p. 41.

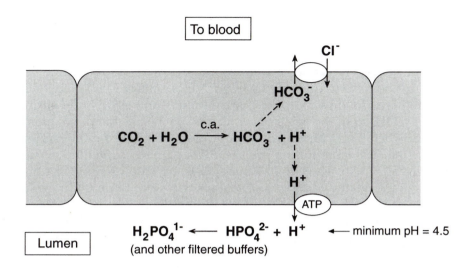

Take a moment to study these two illustrations. Compare them with each other and with those showing bicarbonate reabsorption (p. 79 and 80).

Why is titratable acid excretion important? To answer this question, let's consider what would happen if the tubular fluid contained no phosphate or other non-bicarbonate buffers. The nephron can lower the pH of luminal fluid, and hence of urine, to a minimum of 4.5, which equals an [H^+] of about 0.03 mmol/l. If one liter of urine is excreted each day, then the maximum daily excretion of free protons, and hence the maximum amount of bicarbonate regenerated (remember that H^+ and HCO_3^- are produced in equal quantities), is only about 0.03 mmol.

Compare this 0.03 mmol with the amount of bicarbonate regenerated during normal titratable acid excretion. Daily phosphate excretion is about 45 mmol. At a plasma pH of 7.4, phosphate is about 80% in the monoprotic (HPO_4^{2-}) form and 20% in the diprotic ($H_2PO_4^{1-}$) form. Thus about 36 mmol (i.e., 45×0.80) enter the tubule in a form that can buffer secreted protons. By the time tubular fluid pH falls to 5.3 (1.5 units below phosphate's pK of 6.8) almost all the phosphate has been converted to the diprotic form. Therefore, on average, about 36 mmol of protons are secreted and 36 mmol of bicarbonate are regenerated.*

In addition to phosphate, the ECF contains low concentrations of several other buffers that undergo glomerular filtration. These include urate (pK = 5.8), creatinine (pK = 5), and beta-hydroxybutyrate (pK = 4.8). As the pH of

---

* **Food for thought.** How much of the 36 mmol is regenerated proximally? Distally? Assume that minimum proximal pH is 6.8, equal to the pK of phosphate. When pH = pK, [A^-] = [HA]. Thus [HPO_4^{2-}] = [$H_2PO_4^{1-}$]. This means there are 22.5 mmol (i.e., $45 \times 1/2$) in the diprotic form at the end of the proximal tubule. Thus, 13.5 (i.e., $36 - 22.5$) mmol are regenerated proximally. The remaining 22.5 are regenerated distally.

the luminal fluid falls toward the pK values of these conjugate bases, additional proton buffering, and hence bicarbonate regeneration, occurs.

All of these non-bicarbonate buffers ultimately appear in the urine. This fact makes it possible to quantify how much bicarbonate was regenerated. The method is as follows: We take a urine sample and slowly add strong base (e.g., NaOH) until the urine pH reaches 7.4, which is the pH of glomerular filtrate when it first forms from blood plasma. This "titration" precisely reverses the original buffering reaction that occurred as the filtrate was acidified in the lumen. Thus, the amount of strong base used in the titration is equal to the quantity of secreted protons that were buffered in the luminal fluid. For example, if 45 mmol NaOH is required to raise urine pH to 7.4, we know that 45 mmol of protons were buffered and, therefore, that 45 mmol of bicarbonate was regenerated during the time that the urine was produced. The name "titratable acid" comes from this measurement process.

Notice that we cannot quantify bicarbonate regeneration simply by measuring phosphate excretion. Why? First, some phosphate is already protonated when it enters the lumen (i.e., it is already in the $H_2PO_4^{1-}$ form). Second, other non-bicarbonate buffers must be taken into account. Third, if urine pH is relatively high, a sizable fraction of the total excreted buffer will be unprotonated, indicating that it played no role in bicarbonate regeneration. Titrating the urine with strong base (i.e., measuring "titratable acid excretion") automatically takes these factors into account.

Ammonium excretion

In bicarbonate reabsorption and titratable acid excretion, protons generated by the intracellular reaction $CO_2 + H_2O \rightarrow HCO_3^- + H^+$ are secreted into the lumen. In ammonium excretion, the protons are disposed of in an entirely different way: they are fed into a metabolic pathway and consumed. As part of this process, ammonium (NH_4^+) is generated and must be excreted.*

We saw elsewhere (p. 86) that protons are consumed when organic anions are metabolized to neutral products. In ammonium excretion, it is this type of reaction that removes protons. The organic anions are derived from amino acids, especially glutamine. Glutamine is released into the blood from several sources (liver, muscle, gut, and dietary proteins), and is taken up by proximal renal tubular cells. In these cells, glutamine's two nitrogen groups are enzymatically removed as ammonium ions: one NH_4^+ comes from the amino group ("deamination"), the other NH_4^+ comes from the amide side group ("deamidation"). The remaining structure is alpha-ketoglutarate, abbreviated AKG^{2-}. As the superscript indicates, AKG^{2-} is a diva-

---

* **Mnemonic.** If you confuse ammonium (NH_4^+) and ammonia (NH_3), look at the last three letters of "ammonium" and let your vision blur. With a little imagination you will see the word "ion." Ammonium is an ion; ammonia is not.

lent anion. AKG must carry a double negative charge because glutamine is neutral, and two positive charges are removed. The breakdown of glutamine occurs in two steps, with glutamate produced as an intermediary. The process looks like this:

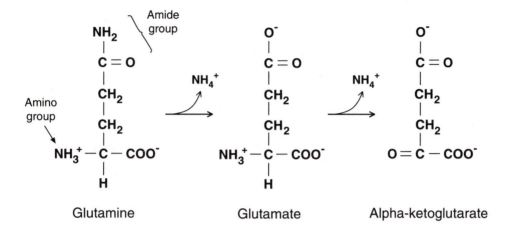

Glutamine   Glutamate   Alpha-ketoglutarate

Once produced, AKG^{2-} is metabolized in the tubular cells either to glucose or to carbon dioxide and water. Both pathways consume two protons. The ammonium is disposed of by being transported into the luminal fluid, primarily by substituting for protons on the Na^+-H^+ exchanger. The process looks like this:

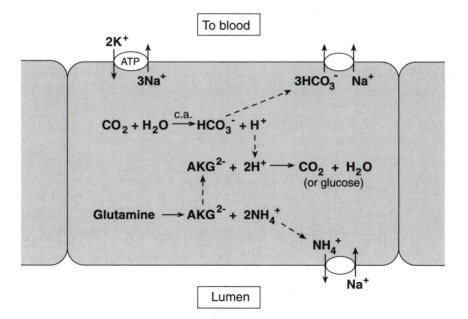

The excretion of NH_4^+ plays no direct role in removing protons: NH_4^+ is merely a side product in the formation of AKG^{2-}. Nonetheless, NH_4^+ must be excreted. Were it retained in the cell, it would eventually diffuse into the renal blood vessels, exit the kidney via the renal vein, and be carried to the liver. There, it would be converted to urea, a reaction that liberates protons (p. 85). These protons would be buffered in the body fluids by bicarbonate, canceling the gain of bicarbonate made by the kidney in metabolizing AKG^{2-}. No net bicarbonate production would occur; the whole process would be futile.

How much bicarbonate is regenerated for each ammonium that appears in the urine? Each molecule of glutamine yields two ammonium ions and two new bicarbonates, which means each urinary ammonium is a marker for one regenerated bicarbonate. For example, if 30 mmol of NH_4^+ appears in a urine sample, you can infer that 30 mmol of HCO_3^- was added to the blood during the time that the urine was produced.

Quantitative aspects and regulation

How much titratable acid and ammonium are excreted each day? Titratable acid excretion is limited by the quantity of luminal non-bicarbonate buffers, especially phosphate. This quantity is determined primarily by dietary phosphate intake, which is relatively constant. Thus, although titratable acid excretion varies (inversely) with urine pH, which tends to fall when there is a need to raise plasma $[HCO_3^-]$, it is usually fixed within a modest range of about 10–40 milliequivalents per day.*

Ammonium excretion is usually around 30–40 mmol per day. However, unlike titratable acid excretion, ammonium excretion can increase markedly. How? When the need for bicarbonate regeneration is high, all aspects of ammoniogenesis (i.e., ammonium-production) increase, including the release of more substrate glutamine into the blood. Ammonium excretion, and hence ammoniogenic bicarbonate regeneration, can increase more than ten fold, although the increase takes several days to fully develop because complex enzymatic changes are required. Therefore, when high rates of bicarbonate regeneration are necessary, ammonium excretion is usually much more important than titratable acid excretion. We say more about the regulation of titratable acid and ammonium excretion in the next chapter.

Summary

The body loses bicarbonate during buffering of endogenously produced acid. (A small amount is also lost during spillage of bicarbonate into urine

---

* **Terminology.** Because titratable acid excretion quantifies not the mmol amount of urinary phosphate and other buffers, but the quantity of buffered protons (p. 98), it is usually reported in milliequivalents (meq), not millimoles. **Clinical note.** The one condition in which titratable acid excretion increases markedly is diabetic ketoacidosis (DKA), a disorder we study later in the text. During DKA, large quantities of organic anions can spill into the urine. When urinary pH is low, some of these anions can act as buffers, and titratable acid excretion can increase more than five times.

due to incomplete reabsorption.) This lost bicarbonate is replaced by a process called either bicarbonate regeneration or acid excretion. Two mechanisms are involved: titratable acid (T.A.) excretion and ammonium (NH_4^+) excretion. In both T.A. and NH_4^+ excretion, new bicarbonate and protons are produced in renal cells by the intracellular reaction $CO_2 + H_2O \rightarrow H^+ + HCO_3^-$. The new bicarbonate crosses the basolateral membrane and enters the blood; this is the "regenerated" bicarbonate. Protons are disposed of as follows. In T.A. excretion, protons are secreted into the nephron lumen and buffered by filtered monoprotic phosphate (HPO_4^{2-}) and other non-bicarbonate buffers. In NH_4^+ excretion, glutamine is split into two NH_4^+ ions, which are excreted in the urine, and alpha-ketoglutarate (AKG^{2-}), which is metabolized to glucose or $H_2O + CO_2$ via a reaction that consumes two protons. When the need for bicarbonate regeneration is high, ammonium excretion can increase greatly, whereas titratable acid excretion can increase only modestly.

Renal Bicarbonate Handling: An Integrated View

12

In this chapter, we bring together essential ideas presented in the previous three chapters (Chapters 9–11). Our goal is to develop an integrated understanding of renal bicarbonate handling, and to see how the component processes are regulated during health.

The kidney: quantitative aspects

The kidney carries out four processes that affect plasma bicarbonate level: bicarbonate filtration, bicarbonate reabsorption, ammonium excretion, and titratable acid excretion. Let's determine the net effect of these processes.

The excretion of ammonium (NH_4^+) and of titratable acid (T.A.) lead to the production of new bicarbonate. Since urinary NH_4^+ and T.A. are both one-for-one markers of regenerated bicarbonate, we can say:

Renal bicarbonate regeneration = Urinary NH_4^+ + Urinary T.A.

Thus, if a urine sample contains 10 mmol NH_4^+ and 5 meq T.A., bicarbonate regeneration was 15 mmol during the time the urine was produced.

We have also seen that not quite all filtered bicarbonate is reabsorbed. The daily load of filtered bicarbonate is typically just over 4000 mmol. If 99.5% of this bicarbonate is reabsorbed, then 0.5%, or about 20 mmol of bicarbonate, will appear in the urine each day. This urinary bicarbonate spillage tends to gradually lower plasma $[HCO_3^-]$. Therefore, if we wish to quantify the *net* effect of the kidney on bicarbonate balance, we must subtract this lost urinary bicarbonate from our value for bicarbonate regeneration, like this:

$$\text{Net renal bicarbonate regeneration} = \text{Urinary } NH_4^+ + \text{T.A.} - HCO_3^-$$

Because T.A. and NH_4^+ are acids (recall that NH_4^+ is the conjugate acid of NH_3) and bicarbonate is a base, it is convenient to use the term *net acid* to describe the quantity of $NH_4^+ + \text{T.A.} - HCO_3^-$. Since this urinary quantity equals net bicarbonate regeneration, it is standard practice to talk about *net acid excretion* (NAE) when we want to indicate net renal bicarbonate regeneration:

$$\text{NAE} = \text{Urinary } NH_4^+ + \text{T.A.} - HCO_3^-$$

Let's look at an example. If, over 24 hours, 4320 mmol of HCO_3^- are filtered and 99.7% is reabsorbed, then about 15 mmol of unreabsorbed HCO_3^- will appear in the urine. If, during this same 24 hours, 60 mmol NH_4^+ and 30 meq titratable acid are excreted, then NAE, and hence net bicarbonate production, during this 24-hour period can be quantified like this:

$$\begin{aligned}\text{NAE} &= \text{Urinary } NH_4^+ + \text{Urinary T.A.} - \text{Urinary } HCO_3^- \\ &= 60 + 30 - 15 \\ &= 75 \text{ meq}\end{aligned}$$

This quantity represents the total renal contribution to the body's bicarbonate balance during that 24 hour period. All else being equal, a fall in urinary NH_4^+ or T.A., or a rise in urinary HCO_3^-, means that less bicarbonate is being added to the blood.*

The kidney: mechanistic aspects

Let's continue our integration by looking at mechanisms involved in renal bicarbonate handling. The renal tubule reabsorbs bicarbonate and excretes ammonium and titratable acid. It was stated earlier that the same cells carry out these different processes. To understand this point more clearly, consider this illustration of a proximal renal tubular cell:

---

* **Terminology.** Since NAE includes T.A., and T.A. is quantified in meq, it is usual to quantify NAE in meq, not mmol. **Technical information.** Since NH_4^+-NH_3 is a conjugate acid-base pair, you might expect NH_4^+ to be quantified as part of the T.A. measurement. It isn't, because the pK of ammonium at body temperature is around 9.0, which means that almost all the ammonium remains as NH_4^+ even after the urine is titrated up to 7.4. Thus, NH_4^+ is an acid, but not a *titratable* acid.

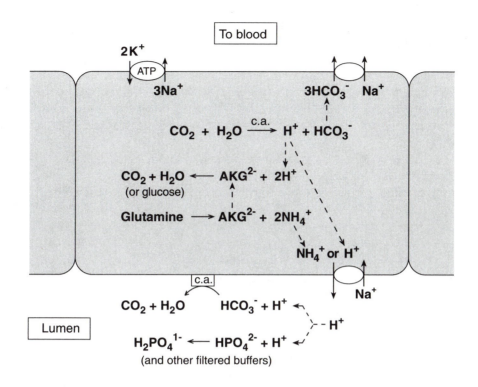

First, notice that the same Na^+-H^+ exchanger secretes protons associated with both bicarbonate reabsorption and titratable acid formation. Thus, while *we* make conceptual distinctions between bicarbonate reabsorption and titratable acid formation, the tubular cell does not: it simply secretes protons, adding bicarbonate to the blood in the process. The final disposition of these protons in the lumen is not under tubular control, but is a passive process that depends on the luminal concentrations of bicarbonate and non-bicarbonate buffers, and on the pKs of those buffers. It goes without saying that a small fraction of secreted protons remains free in the lumen, and it is this quantity that lowers pH.

Second, notice that this same Na^+-H^+ exchanger is also thought to secrete most of the NH_4^+ produced during ammonium excretion. As noted (p. 99), NH_4^+ may substitute for protons on the exchanger.

Third, notice that all bicarbonate and all protons are generated in the cell by the carbonic anhydrase-catalyzed reaction of carbon dioxide and water.

Finally, notice that all bicarbonate that enters the blood, whether it is ultimately quantified as "reabsorbed" or "regenerated," crosses the basolateral membrane on the same transporters. Thus, the proximal tubular cell acts as a multifunctional bicarbonate-producing mechanism, carrying out all three modes of bicarbonate generation: reabsorption, titratable acid excretion, and ammonium excretion.

What about the distal tubular cell? It also is an integrated, multi-functional bicarbonate handler. Protons are secreted by the H^+–ATPase. In the lumen, these protons are buffered by either bicarbonate or non-bicarbonate buffers. Protons that remain unbuffered in the lumen act to lower urine pH.*

The following schematic shows key aspects of proximal and distal bicarbonate handling. Pause for a moment to study it. It should help you integrate ideas presented in this section, and place them in their anatomic context.

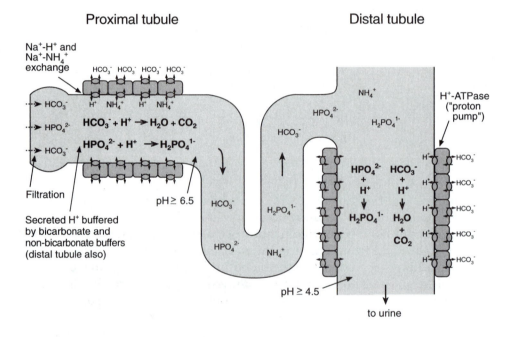

Matching bicarbonate regeneration to bicarbonate losses

Earlier in this section, we saw that endogenous acid production (EAP) quantifies the amount of strong acid added to the body fluids by physiologic processes. The protons released from these acids are buffered by bicarbon-

---

* **Going further.** Recent studies have slightly expanded our understanding of proton secretion. First, it appears that some H^+–ATPase pumps may be present in the *proximal* tubule, in addition to the predominant Na^+–H^+ exchangers. Second, in the distal tubule, it appears that some proton secretion may occur via an ATP-driven H^+–K^+ exchanger, which simultaneously secretes H^+ and reabsorbs K^+, in addition to the distal H^+–ATPase. These proximal H^+–ATPase and distal H^+–K^+–ATPase play a role in both bicarbonate reabsorption and titratable acid excretion.

ate, lowering plasma [HCO_3^-] and depleting the body's bicarbonate stores by an amount quantitatively equal to EAP.*

If plasma [HCO_3^-] is not to decline, the kidney must replace this lost bicarbonate. Since the kidney's net bicarbonate contribution is quantified as net acid excretion (NAE), we can say that for plasma [HCO_3^-] to remain constant, NAE must be matched to EAP. That is, at steady state:

$$NAE = EAP$$

This simple equation describes the kidney's major regulatory objective in bicarbonate handling. We can make the same point graphically, like this:

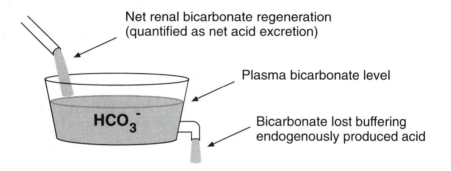

How does the kidney match NAE to EAP? Because EAP varies with diet, gut function, and other variables, net bicarbonate regeneration (and hence NAE) cannot simply occur at some preset rate. It must rise and fall as needed. Although the details are not known with certainty, NAE is probably matched to EAP by a feedback loop, like this: (1) an increase in EAP causes a slight fall in plasma [HCO_3^-]; (2) this fall is detected by the renal tubule, where it stimulates NAE; (3) increased NAE raises plasma [HCO_3^-] to normal, which (4) returns the NAE stimulus to normal levels. We can portray this sequence schematically, like this:

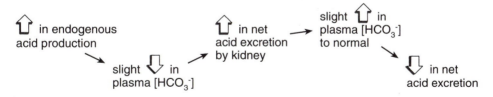

---

* **Going further.** Shouldn't the loss of bicarbonate be less than EAP, since some protons are buffered by hemoglobin and other non-bicarbonate buffers? No. During an acute acid load, the decline in pH is buffered by both bicarbonate and non-bicarbonate buffers, causing a fall in [HCO_3^-] and a partial conversion of non-bicarbonate buffers to the conjugate acid (i.e., HA) form. However, as the kidneys regenerate bicarbonate, which normalizes [HCO_3^-] and pH, non-bicarbonate buffers give up protons, which then combine with bicarbonate. Thus, non-bicarbonate buffers are restored to their original titration states and additional bicarbonate is lost. In terms of overall bicarbonate balance, it is as if non-bicarbonate buffers didn't even exist.

How does the change in plasma [HCO_3^-] cause a change in the rate of renal acid excretion? The mechanism is speculative, but changes in intracellular pH may play a key role. For example, a fall in ECF [HCO_3^-] creates a gradient for bicarbonate to leave the cell, slightly lowering cell [HCO_3^-] and pH. This pH change may stimulate NH_4^+ production and proton secretion. Whatever the exact mechanism, the matching of NAE to EAP is precise and relatively rapid. Therefore, in health, plasma [HCO_3^-] varies little from its normal set point.*

Summary

Net renal bicarbonate production can be quantified by measuring net acid excretion, defined as Urinary NH_4^+ + T.A. − HCO_3^-. Although bicarbonate regeneration, titratable acid excretion, and ammonium excretion are conceptually distinct, the three processes overlap mechanistically and are carried out by the same cell types. In the proximal tubule, protons are secreted by the Na^+–H^+ exchanger, irrespective of what substance ultimately buffers these protons in the lumen. NH_4^+ is secreted by this same exchanger, by substituting for protons. In the distal tubule, the H^+–ATPase ("proton pump") is responsible for proton secretion. For plasma [HCO_3^-] to remain constant, net acid excretion (and hence net bicarbonate regeneration) must be matched to endogenous acid production.

---

* **Clinical note.** During disease, several pathologic factors modify the rate of net acid excretion. For example, abnormal changes in plasma [K^+], [aldosterone], and extracellular volume can affect renal bicarbonate handling. We discuss these regulatory factors in the Pathophysiology section, when the diseases that bring them into play are described.

Concluding Overview 13

As we have seen, plasma pH is determined by the relative levels of PCO_2, which is regulated by the lung, and $[HCO_3^-]$, which is regulated by the kidney. When plasma $[HCO_3^-]$ is about 24 mmol/l and PCO_2 is about 40 mm Hg, arterial pH is normal, about 7.4. You can prove this with the Henderson-Hasselbalch equation:

$$pH = 6.1 + \log [HCO_3^-]/0.03PCO_2$$
$$pH = 6.1 + \log 24/(0.03 \times 40)$$
$$pH = 6.1 + \log 24/1.2$$
$$pH = 6.1 + \log 20$$
$$pH = 6.1 + 1.3$$
$$pH = 7.4$$

As this equation suggests, plasma pH is determined indirectly, via the maintenance of normal $[HCO_3^-]$ and PCO_2 levels. At the beginning of this section (Chapter 7), we portrayed this regulatory mechanism as a balance. We now return to that illustration, but add additional details:

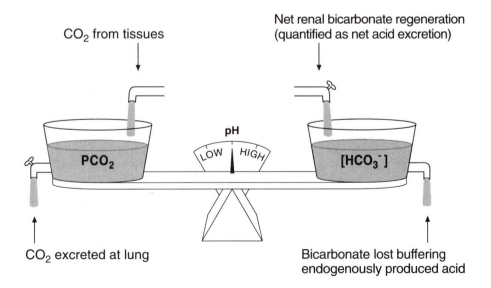

CO₂ from tissues

Net renal bicarbonate regeneration
(quantified as net acid excretion)

pH

LOW | HIGH

PCO₂

[HCO₃⁻]

CO₂ excreted at lung

Bicarbonate lost buffering
endogenously produced acid

This illustration is useful because it emphasizes two important points. First, as noted, plasma pH is a dependent variable, which is regulated indirectly via the body's control of PCO_2 and $[HCO_3^-]$. Second, PCO_2 and $[HCO_3^-]$ are regulated by the lung and kidney as steady-state functions, through the careful matching of input and output. As a final review of acid-base physiology, take a few moments to study this illustration.

This completes the Physiology section. Congratulations. You now possess a solid, conceptual foundation upon which to overlay your studies of acid-base pathophysiology, diagnosis, and treatment.*

---

* **Getting a preview.** For students reading this section as part of a physiology course: If you want a quick preview of pathophysiology, without yet studying it in depth, you can read the following parts of the next section: (1) Chapter 14, (2) the "Compensation" subsection of Chapter 15, and (3) the "Definitions" and "Introduction" subsections of Chapters 16 through 19.

Self-Assessment Quiz

This quiz tests your knowledge of core concepts and facts. More importantly, the process of taking and correcting the quiz will strengthen your understanding of the essentials. To get the most from this process, answer all questions in writing. Use a separate answer sheet if you wish. Take your time. When you finish, check your answers against the key. It doesn't matter whether you ace this quiz or fail it. The important thing is to grapple with the questions and then, for those that you miss, to study the correct answers carefully.

1. Extracellular pH can be considered a dependent variable; that is, dependent on $[HCO_3^-]$ and PCO_2. If $[HCO_3^-] = 24$ mmol/l and $PCO_2 = 40$ mm Hg, what will pH be?

2. In health, what is the PCO_2 of air in the alveoli?

3. List the PCO_2 values, in mm Hg, of blood in the following structures: pulmonary arteries, pulmonary veins, systemic arteries, systemic veins, the right ventricle, the left ventricle.

4. CO_2 diffuses from tissues to systemic capillary blood, which has a PCO_2 of about 45–46 mm Hg. What do you think tissue PCO_2 is?

5. Look at the illustration on page 72. For artistic reasons, an aspect of the shading was deliberately made inaccurate. What is the inaccuracy?

6. Assume a starting arterial PCO_2 of 40 mm Hg. If CO_2 production stays the same and alveolar ventilation is halved, PCO_2 will begin to rise. At what PCO_2 will the level stabilize?

7. Assume a starting arterial PCO_2 of 40 mm Hg. If both CO_2 production and alveolar ventilation fall by 50%, what will happen to PCO_2?

8. Assume a starting arterial PCO_2 of 40 mm Hg. If CO_2 production triples and alveolar ventilation doubles, what will the new steady-state arterial PCO_2 be?

9. Ventilatory rate is regulated by various control systems. Two important types are _____ and _____. In health, what is the major variable that is "fed back" into the feedback loop?

10. During bicarbonate reabsorption, what intracellular reaction produces the bicarbonate that is ultimately "reabsorbed"? Is this reaction the same in both proximal and distal nephron?

11. In the proximal tubule, what is the major proton-secreting mechanism? What is the minimum pH of luminal fluid in the proximal tubule?

12. In the collecting tubule (distal nephron), how are protons secreted? What is the minimum luminal pH?

13. Bicarbonate reabsorption is indirect. If filtered bicarbonate were directly reabsorbed via passage from lumen, through the cell, to blood, would it make any quantitative difference?

14. What does EAP stand for? What are its two components and their abbreviations?

15. For acid-base purposes, we can distinguish five main types of metabolic reactions. List them. Indicate which types liberate protons and which consume protons.

16. Proton-generating metabolic reactions are sometimes called "bicarbonate-consuming" reactions. By what reaction is the bicarbonate consumed?

17. Proton-consuming metabolic reactions are sometimes called "bicarbonate-producing" reactions. By what reaction is the bicarbonate produced?

18. If a quantity of protein contains 1 mmol sulfur, 1 meq cationic side groups, and 1 meq anionic side groups, does the oxidation of the protein lead to net proton liberation or net proton consumption? What quantity of protons is liberated/consumed?

19. If a urine sample contains high levels of organic anions, what can you infer about plasma $[HCO_3^-]$?

20. A patient's urine contains high levels of the sulfate ion (SO_4^{2-}). It might be reasonable to ask if this patient takes dietary supplements of which two amino acids? Would you expect urine pH to be high or low?

21. In the gastric epithelium, what reaction produces the H^+ that is secreted into the stomach lumen? What happens to the other ionic product of this reaction (i.e., the ionic species that is not secreted into the lumen)?

22. In the colonic epithelium, what reaction produces the HCO_3^- that is secreted into the colonic lumen? What happens to the other ionic product of this reaction (i.e., the ionic species that is not secreted into the lumen)?

23. Imagine a simplified gut consisting of only a stomach and colon. If the stomach secretes 18 mmol H^+ into the gut lumen, and the colon secretes 20 mmol HCO_3^- into the gut lumen, what is the net effect on ECF acid-base status? What is the net effect in the gut lumen?

24. Use the same, simplified gut as in the previous problem. If 5 mmol H^+ are secreted into the stomach and 5 mmol HCO_3^- are secreted into the

colon, what is the net effect on the body fluids? If any CO_2 is produced in the gut lumen, where do you think it goes?

25. A patient is undergoing intestinal surgery. A tube is inserted into the duct leading to the pancreas, and fluid is drained into a disposal bottle. If this fluid contains high concentrations of bicarbonate, will the blood be acidified or alkalinized?

26. Follow-up question. If $[HCO_3^-]$ in the drainage fluid is 75 mmol/l, and a total of 2 liters is drained, what is the total proton load that enters the extracellular fluid?

27. If a person drinks a lactate solution (e.g., sodium lactate), will urinary pH tend to rise or fall? Why?

28. Chloride (Cl^-), like lactate, is a monovalent anion. But ingesting chloride does not have the same acid-base effect as ingesting lactate. Why not?

29. What two processes are responsible for bicarbonate regeneration?

30. In titratable acid excretion, protons are secreted into the lumen of the nephron. What is the predominant proton-secreting mechanism in the proximal tubule? In the distal tubule?

31. In bicarbonate reabsorption and titratable acid excretion, the cellular processes are identical. The only difference occurs after the proton is secreted into the lumen. What is this difference?

32. During titratable acid excretion, what intracellular reaction produces the regenerated bicarbonate?

33. Titratable acid excretion is quantified by measuring the amount of NaOH that must be added to a urine sample to raise its pH to 7.4. Why is pH 7.4 used as the titration end point?

34. If 37 mmol NaOH is required to titrate a urine sample to pH 7.4, how many secreted protons were buffered by filtered non-bicarbonate buffers? In this example, what is titratable acid excretion? What is the main non-bicarbonate buffer in the filtrate?

35. During ammonium excretion, from what substance is most ammonium derived? How many ammonium ions can be extracted from it? What is the name of the structure that remains after all ammonium ions are extracted? What is its abbreviation? What is the charge of this residual structure?

36. For each molecule of glutamine that is metabolized in the proximal tubule, how many bicarbonates are regenerated? What intracellular reaction produces these new bicarbonates?

37. Follow-up question. The intracellular reaction just referred to also produces protons. What happens to these protons? As a shorthand, we can say that "_____ is metabolized to bicarbonate."

38. If ammonium enters the blood instead of being excreted in the urine, it is ultimately converted to _____. Where does this conversion take place? What is the effect of this conversion on plasma $[HCO_3^-]$?

39. When the body's need for bicarbonate regeneration rises sharply, the kidney can increase ammonium production and excretion. What is the approximate maximum mmols per day that can be excreted? About how many times above normal is this?

40. Titratable acid excretion does not usually increase markedly when the need for bicarbonate regeneration is high. What limits it?

41. Imagine that bicarbonate reabsorption remains normal but bicarbonate regeneration ceases entirely. What will happen to plasma $[HCO_3^-]$? Give two reasons.

42. Write the formula for net acid excretion (NAE).

43. During a 12-hour period, a person excretes 45 meq of net acid. How much net bicarbonate is added to the body fluids during that period?

44. A urine sample contains 10 meq titratable acid, 25 mmol NH_4^+, and 3 mmol HCO_3^-. What is NAE during the time this urine was produced? How much net bicarbonate is regenerated?

45. What is a typical range of NAE for an individual eating a Western diet? How much net bicarbonate does this regenerate?

46. Assume that endogenous acid production (EAP) is 40 meq during a 12-hour period. A urine sample collected during this time contains 30 mmol NH_4^+ and 15 meq titratable acid. If the body is in steady state for bicarbonate, how much bicarbonate must be in this urine sample?

47. For an individual to be in steady state for bicarbonate, the following must be true: _____ = _____.

48. Both $[HCO_3^-]$ and PCO_2 are regulated as steady-state functions; that is, by a matching of input and output. Are these steady states achieved by matching input to output, or output to input? Think about both $[HCO_3^-]$ and PCO_2 before answering.

   If you need a hint: Look at the illustration on p. 109. Do you notice any asymmetry in the buckets?

Answer Key

1. 7.4.

2. About 40 mm Hg.

3. 46, 40, 40, 46, 46, 40.

4. About 46; just slightly above capillary PCO_2.

5. Tissues are not shaded.

6. 80 mm Hg.

7. No change.

8. 60 mm Hg; i.e., $40 \times 3/2$.

9. Anticipatory, feedback. PCO_2.

10. $CO_2 + H_2O \rightarrow HCO_3^- + H^+$. Yes.

11. $Na^+ - H^+$ exchange. About 6.5.

12. H^+–ATPase. About 4.5.

13. No. Reabsorbed bicarbonate would still disappear from the lumen and appear in the blood. Unreabsorbed bicarbonate would still appear in the urine. The numerical relationships would be unchanged.

14. Endogenous acid production. Metabolic acid production, MAP; Gastrointestinal acid production, GAP.

15. Check your answer against the table on p. 85.

16. $HCO_3^- + H^+ \rightarrow CO_2 + H_2O$. The addition of protons drives the reaction.

17. $CO_2 + H_2O \rightarrow HCO_3^- + H^+$. The removal of protons draws the reaction to right, i.e., shifts the equilibrium point.

18. Liberation. 2 mmol. Remember: $S \rightarrow 2H^+$.

19. It is probably low. Organic acids have been produced; these liberate protons and consume bicarbonate; the anions have been spilled in the urine.

20. Methionine, Cysteine. Low. Increased EAP causes a slight fall in

plasma $[HCO_3^-]$ and pH. The kidney responds with increased proton secretion.

21. $CO_2 + H_2O \rightarrow HCO_3^- + H^+$. The HCO_3^- enters the blood.

22.   Same reaction as in 21. The H^+ enters the blood.

23.   2 mmol of net protons liberated into body fluids. 2 mmol net bicarbonate secreted.

24.   No acid-base effect. The protons and bicarbonate neutralize each other via the reaction $HCO_3^- + H^+ \rightarrow CO_2 + H_2O$. Most CO_2 is absorbed into blood and excreted at the lung.

25.   Acidified; pancreatic fluid is alkaline.

26.   150 mmol.

27.   Rise. Lactate is metabolized to bicarbonate; excess bicarbonate spills in urine.

28.   Only organic ions can be metabolized; no bicarbonate is produced.

29.   Titratable acid excretion, ammonium excretion.

30. Na^+-H^+ exchange. H^+–ATPase.

31.   The filtered luminal buffer. Bicarbonate reabsorption: bicarbonate. Titratable acid excretion: non-bicarbonate buffers.

32. $CO_2 + H_2O \rightarrow HCO_3^- + H^+$.

33.   7.4 is the pH of blood, and thus of glomerular filtrate before being acidified by secreted protons.

34.   37 mmol. 37 meq. Monoprotic phosphate, HPO_4^{2-}.

35.   Glutamine. Two. Alpha-ketoglutarate. AKG^{2-}. Minus two.

36.   Two. $CO_2 + H_2O \rightarrow HCO_3^- + H^+$.

37.   They are consumed during the metabolism of AKG^{2-} to $CO_2 + H_2O$ or glucose. AKG^{2-}.

38.   Urea. Liver. A reduction.

39.   Typically 300–500. Ten.

40.   Urinary phosphate excretion.

41. It will fall gradually. EAP consumes bicarbonate (both MAP and GAP). Reabsorption is never 100% efficient.

42. Urinary ammonium + Urinary titratable acid − Urinary bicarbonate.

43. 45 mmol.

44. 32 meq. 32 mmol.

45. 70–100 meq per day. 70–100 mmol per day.

46. 5 mmol.

47. NAE, EAP.

48. For $[HCO_3^-]$, input is matched to output; i.e., net acid excretion is regulated to match endogenous acid production. In contrast, for PCO_2, output is matched to input; i.e., alveolar ventilation is regulated to match CO_2 production. In the illustration, the faucets, which indicate regulatory control, are asymmetrical.

Section 3
Pathophysiology

Pathophysiology—which refers to the mechanisms of disease—is the transitional step from classroom to bedside. It is rooted in basic science and forms the essential foundation for clinical practice.

In the field of acid-base, pathophysiology deals with a category of clinical entities that are known as either "acid-base disturbances" or "acid-base disorders." These two terms are synonyms and can be used interchangeably. Thus, you can say that a patient has an acid-base disturbance, or you can say that the patient has an acid-base disorder.

This section has six chapters:

> The Language of Pathophysiology
> Homeostatic Responses to Acid-Base Disorders
> Metabolic Acidosis
> Metabolic Alkalosis
> Respiratory Acidosis
> Respiratory Alkalosis

In the first of these chapters, *The Language of Pathophysiology,* we introduce a number of specialized terms that are used when discussing acid-base disturbances. Although these terms are familiar even to premedical students, their precise meanings are often missed, and this sometimes leads to misunderstanding.

Next, in the chapter on *Homeostatic Responses to Acid-Base Disorders,* we look at mechanisms used by the body to lessen the harmful impact of acid-base disturbances. In some cases, these homeostatic mechanisms keep the patient alive while the physician repairs the underlying problem. In other cases, when the acid-base disorder is irreversible, the homeostatic response simply makes the disease more tolerable.

Finally, in the remaining chapters of the section, we explore in detail the four main types of acid-base disorders: metabolic acidosis, metabolic alkalosis, respiratory acidosis, and respiratory alkalosis. We devote a separate chapter to each of these disorders, exploring both general concepts and specific mechanisms.*

---

* **Hint for the reader.** This section presumes a basic knowledge of acid-base physiology. Readers who lack this knowledge are encouraged to review the Physiology section by reading the following: (1) Chapter 7, (2) the chapter summaries at the ends of Chapters 8–12, and (3) Chapter 13.

The Language of Pathophysiology 14

All discussion about acid-base pathophysiology depends on four pairs of terms:

Acidemia and Alkalemia
Acidosis and Alkalosis
Respiratory and Metabolic
Simple and Mixed

Understanding the precise meaning of these terms lets you communicate clearly and without ambiguity. It's like knowing a foreign language that has just eight words. In this chapter, we discuss these terms in detail.

Acidemia and Alkalemia ("-emia")

The "-emia" in acidemia and alkalemia is the same suffix (word ending) found in anemia and ischemia. It means "blood." Thus, based on word roots, acidemia means "acid blood" and alkalemia means "alkaline blood." More specifically, acidemia refers to a blood pH below normal (i.e., an increased $[H^+]$), whereas alkalemia refers to a blood pH above normal (i.e., a decreased $[H^+]$).

Some clinicians use these "-emia" terms to describe *any* deviation of pH from an individual's normal set point, even if this deviation is so small as to leave pH within the normal range of 7.35 to 7.45. Other clinicians use these terms only when pH is outside the normal range. Either way, the essence of the definition is the same: a change in blood pH.

It is important to note that the terms acidemia and alkalemia tell you absolutely nothing about the *cause* of the pH change: they tell you only that a change has occurred.

Acidosis and alkalosis ("-osis")

Acidosis and alkalosis refer to the processes that cause pH to change. Any disease process or condition that acts to lower pH is termed an acidosis, and any disease process or condition that acts to raise pH is termed an alkalosis.

123

Thus, acidosis is what causes acidemia, and alkalosis is what causes alkalemia. Note that the plural for acidosis is acidoses, and for alkalosis, alkaloses.

The definitions for acidosis and alkalosis are implicit in the word roots. The suffix "-osis" means "pathologic process or condition," as in thrombosis, psychosis, and halitosis. Therefore, acidosis means "pathologic acid process" and alkalosis means "pathologic alkaline process." It makes sense that acidemia is caused by a pathologic acid process, and that alkalemia is caused by a pathologic alkaline process.

Almost by definition, then, acidosis and alkalosis will affect blood pH. However, there is a special situation in which pH does not change. This "osis-without-emia" situation can occur if an acidosis and alkalosis exist together in the same patient: if the processes are of equal magnitudes, the effects on pH cancel. This situation can be likened to building a roaring fire, during the winter, in a room with an open window. The fire's heat and winter's cold balance each other, leaving the room temperature unchanged. We will say more about this special situation at the end of the chapter.

Respiratory and Metabolic

To understand how "respiratory" and "metabolic" are used in the field of acid-base, it is helpful to look at the bicarbonate buffer system, which is the most important buffer in the body:

$$CO_2 + H_2O \rightleftharpoons HCO_3^- + H^+$$

This equilibrium suggests two ways to alter [H^+]: change PCO_2 or change [HCO_3^-]. We can shift the equilibrium point to the right, thereby raising [H^+], by either increasing PCO_2 or lowering [HCO_3^-]. We can shift the equilibrium point to the left, thereby reducing [H^+], by either lowering PCO_2 or raising [HCO_3^-]. We can express this same idea by saying that since CO_2 acts as an acid (p. 45–46), increasing its concentration acidifies whereas decreasing its concentration alkalinizes. And since bicarbonate is a base, increasing its concentration alkalinizes whereas decreasing its concentration acidifies.*

This brings us to the main point: "respiratory" is used to indicate an acidosis or alkalosis caused by a pathologic change in PCO_2, whereas "metabolic" is used to indicate an acidosis or alkalosis caused by a pathologic change in [HCO_3^-]. Therefore,

---

* **Reminder.** Recall that CO_2 gas is dissolved in solution, just as it is in an unopened soda bottle, and that its concentration is quantified in terms of its partial pressure, symbolized PCO_2. If you need to review the bicarbonate buffer system or the concept of PCO_2, see Chapter 5.

When you see "respiratory", think PCO_2

and

When you see "metabolic", think $[HCO_3{}^-]$

All processes in the body that affect pH (i.e., all acidoses and alkaloses) are either "respiratory" or "metabolic". Thus, there are four general types of acid-base disturbances: respiratory acidosis, respiratory alkalosis, metabolic acidosis, and metabolic alkalosis. By definition, a pathologic rise in plasma PCO_2 is a respiratory acidosis, a pathologic fall in plasma PCO_2 is a respiratory alkalosis, a pathologic fall in plasma $[HCO_3{}^-]$ is a metabolic acidosis, and a pathologic rise in plasma $[HCO_3{}^-]$ is a metabolic alkalosis.

If we wish to describe the essence of these four disturbances concisely, we can say that respiratory acidosis is a hypercapnic acidosis (the word root *cap* refers to carbon dioxide), respiratory alkalosis is a hypocapnic alkalosis, metabolic acidosis is a hypobicarbonatemic acidosis (literally: low-blood-bicarbonate acidosis), and metabolic alkalosis is a hyperbicarbonatemic alkalosis. We can summarize these ideas in a table:

Name	Change	Description
Respiratory acidosis	↑ PCO_2	Hypercapnic acidosis
Respiratory alkalosis	↓ PCO_2	Hypocapnic alkalosis
Metabolic acidosis	↓ $[HCO_3{}^-]$	Hypobicarbonatemic acidosis
Metabolic alkalosis	↑ $[HCO_3{}^-]$	Hyperbicarbonatemic alkalosis

Here are some examples. If lung disease raises PCO_2 to 65 mm Hg (normal arterial PCO_2 is 40), a respiratory acidosis is present. If anxiety causes a patient to hyperventilate, lowering PCO_2 to 20 mm Hg, a respiratory alkalosis is present. If a defect in the kidneys leads to excess spillage of bicarbonate into the urine, lowering plasma $[HCO_3{}^-]$ to 16 mmol/l (normal is about 24), metabolic acidosis is present. Similarly, if a pathologic increase in endogenous acid production lowers $[HCO_3{}^-]$ to 12 mmol/l (the bicarbonate is consumed in buffering excess protons), metabolic acidosis is again present. If severe vomiting raises plasma $[HCO_3{}^-]$ to 37 mmol/l (we'll study the mechanism of this rise later), metabolic alkalosis is present.

Let's continue our discussion of respiratory and metabolic by making explicit something that has been implicit until now. The terms respiratory and metabolic are used in many areas of medicine and biology. In most contexts, respiratory refers to either cellular energy production or pulmonary gas exchange, and metabolic refers to the pathways of anabolism and catabolism. However, in the field of acid-base, respiratory and metabolic have specific meanings that <u>are not the same</u> as in other contexts.

Consider the term respiratory. In common usage, we refer to the activity of the lung as respiration. Since abnormalities in lung function affect PCO_2, it seems reasonable to use the term respiratory when speaking about acid-base disturbances that are caused by an abnormal PCO_2. Nonetheless, it is crucial to recognize that the defining characteristic of these disturbances is the abnormal PCO_2, *not* the fact that they are usually caused by abnormalities of the lung.

This distinction becomes clear when you recognize that respiratory disturbances can occur even when lung function is normal. For example, during hemodialysis, dissolved CO_2 diffuses from the blood, across the dialysis membrane, and into the fluid bath. This diffusion of CO_2 can transiently reduce the PCO_2 of the blood, thereby producing a respiratory alkalosis. Here we see a respiratory acid-base disturbance without any defect in "respiration." Similarly, if a healthy person breathes carbon dioxide gas, respiratory acidosis rapidly develops even though lung function is normal.

Now consider the term metabolic. Metabolic, as it is commonly used (i.e., anabolism and catabolism), has no necessary connection with plasma $[HCO_3^-]$. Thus, it is especially important to remember that "metabolic" has two entirely different meanings, only one of which applies specifically to acid-base disorders.

To end this part of our discussion, we present key concepts in visual form. Take a moment to study each disorder. Notice which variable ($[HCO_3^-]$ or PCO_2) is abnormal, whether this variable is high or low, and which way the balance tips.

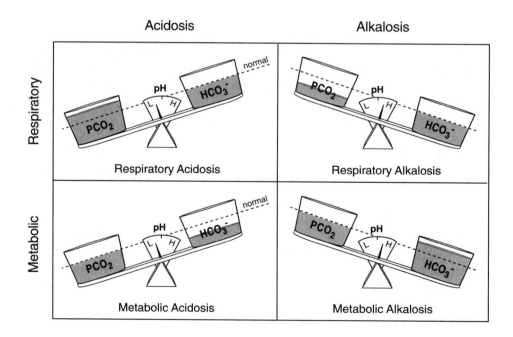

We now move on to our final pair of terms.*

Simple and Mixed

As we have just seen, there are four major types of acid-base disturbances (i.e., metabolic acidosis, metabolic alkalosis, etc.). These four are referred to as *primary* acid-base disturbances. A patient who has one of these primary disturbances is said to have a *simple* disturbance. Occasionally, a patient will have more than one primary disorder at the same time. Such a patient is said to have a *mixed* or *complex* disturbance (either term can be used). For example, if a patient has both respiratory acidosis (high PCO_2) and metabolic acidosis (low $[HCO_3^-]$), a mixed disturbance is present.

Mixed disturbances typically involve two primary disorders (although mixed disturbances consisting of three or even four primaries are possible). Two varieties of the same primary disturbance can also form a mixed disturbance, as in a mixed metabolic acidosis composed of two different pathologic conditions that act independently to lower plasma $[HCO_3^-]$.

When both disorders in a mixed disturbance are acidoses, or both are alkaloses, the pH changes are additive. The acidemia or alkalemia can be life threatening even if the component primary disorders are not by themselves severe. Conversely, when an acidosis and an alkalosis occur together, the pH change is "subtractive" and usually modest. The final pH can be either high or low, depending on which of the component disorders is dominant. Occasionally, the effects on pH exactly cancel and pH is normal.

The following sentence will let you test your understanding of the terms simple and mixed: "A patient who was initially thought to have a simple respiratory disturbance was later found to have a mixed disturbance consisting of three primary disorders: a respiratory alkalosis and two different types of metabolic acidosis." Be sure you understand what this sentence is saying.

---

* **Going further.** Although not illustrated, respiratory disturbances have a small, indirect effect on plasma $[HCO_3^-]$. During respiratory acidosis, the rise in PCO_2 pushes the equilibrium point of the $CO_2 + H_2O \rightleftharpoons HCO_3^- + H^+$ buffer system to the right, slightly raising $[HCO_3^-]$. During respiratory alkalosis, the fall in PCO_2 shifts the equilibrium to the left, slightly lowering $[HCO_3^-]$. These changes are so small that $[HCO_3^-]$ typically remains well within the normal range. For example, raising PCO_2 from 40 to 60 mm Hg increases plasma $[HCO_3^-]$ by only about 2 mmol/l. Although these equilibrium shifts produce or consume protons as well as bicarbonate, pH changes little because the protons are buffered by non-bicarbonate buffers such as hemoglobin. The changes in $[HCO_3^-]$ discussed here appear within seconds of the pathologic change in PCO_2. These small and nearly instantaneous changes in $[HCO_3^-]$ are distinct from, and should not be confused with, the much slower and larger "compensatory" changes in $[HCO_3^-]$, which we discuss in the next chapter.

Summary

Acidemia refers to a fall in blood pH. *Alkalemia* refers to a rise in blood pH. *Acidosis* and *alkalosis* refer, respectively, to pathologic processes that tend to lower or raise blood pH, i.e., to cause acidemia or alkalemia. *Respiratory* and *metabolic,* which are adjectives used to modify the terms acidosis and alkalosis, have specific meanings in the context of acid-base, which are not the same as in other contexts. *Respiratory* indicates a primary change in PCO_2, whereas *metabolic* indicates a primary change in plasma $[HCO_3^-]$. There are four "primary" acid-base disorders: metabolic acidosis, metabolic alkalosis, respiratory acidosis, respiratory alkalosis. A *simple* disturbance refers to the presence of one of these four primaries. A *mixed* or *complex* disturbance refers to the simultaneous presence of two or more primaries.

Homeostatic Responses to Acid-Base Disorders

15

Homeostasis (etymology: "same status") refers to the body's innate tendency to maintain the normal state of its internal environment. When diseases occur, automatic homeostatic mechanisms act to limit their impact. In military parlance, these mechanisms are "damage-control strategies." During acid-base disturbances, three major homeostatic processes come into play: buffering, compensation, and correction. Buffering occurs first, within minutes; compensation develops over a period of hours or days; correction, if it occurs, usually takes several days. In this chapter, we study each of these processes individually, beginning with buffering. We then conclude with an integrative example, which shows how the various homeostatic mechanisms occur in the same patient.

Buffering

Buffering occurs in three main body compartments: extracellular fluid (ECF), intracellular fluid (ICF), and bone. Let's look at how buffering occurs in each of these compartments.

Extracellular buffering

As described in the Chemistry section, there are four major ECF buffers: the bicarbonate system and three "non-bicarbonate" buffers (e.g., buffer sites on hemoglobin and plasma proteins).

During <u>metabolic</u> acid-base disturbances, all four buffers act to mitigate the pH change, but the bicarbonate system is quantitatively the most important. For example, between pH 7.2 and 7.6, bicarbonate accounts for more than 90% of the ECF's buffering capacity. When a strong acid is buffered by bicarbonate, carbon dioxide and small quantities of water are generated (because the added protons drive the $CO_2 + H_2O \rightleftharpoons HCO_3^- + H^+$ buffer equilibrium to the left). The CO_2 exits the body at the lung. The water enters the body fluids and is eventually excreted. Conversely, during metabolic alkalosis, small quantities of CO_2 and H_2O are consumed (because the fall in

[H$^+$], as might occur with the addition of NaOH, pulls the buffer equilibrium to the right).

During <u>respiratory</u> disturbances, the bicarbonate system plays no role in buffering. Only the non-bicarbonate buffers act to stabilize pH. Why? During respiratory acidosis, the rise in PCO$_2$ drives the CO$_2$ + H$_2$O $\rightleftharpoons$ HCO$_3^-$ + H$^+$ equilibrium to the right, liberating protons. These protons cannot be buffered by bicarbonate because this would require that the equilibrium simultaneously shift to the left. Conversely, during respiratory alkalosis, the equilibrium shifts left and cannot simultaneously shift right. Because the bicarbonate system is ineffective, buffering is less efficient in stabilizing pH during respiratory disturbances than during metabolic disturbances.

All ECF buffering occurs rapidly. The maximum effect on pH becomes apparent as soon as the buffer systems equilibrate, which occurs within a few minutes.

Intracellular buffering (a.k.a. "cell buffering")

Because cell membranes are semipermeable, pH changes in the ECF are gradually transmitted to the ICF. Intracellular buffers help minimize these changes. The major ICF buffers are proteins, organic phosphates, and bicarbonate. Because pH changes are transmitted into cells slowly, ICF buffering occurs gradually, over a period of several hours.

Bone buffering

About two thirds of bone mass consists of inorganic minerals, especially hydroxyapatite (Ca$_{10}$(PO$_4$)$_6$(OH)$_2$), but also brushite (CaHPO$_4$) and the Na$^+$, K$^+$, and Ca^{2+} salts of carbonate (CO$_3^{2-}$). When you mentally dissect these formulas, it becomes clear that bone contains a huge potential source of proton acceptors, including PO$_4^{3-}$, HPO$_4^{2-}$, OH$^-$, and CO$_3^{2-}$. Thus, bone dissolution can help mitigate a fall in pH.

During <u>acute</u> metabolic acidosis, carbonate on the bone surface acts as a proton acceptor. An important mechanism appears to be the chemical exchange of free protons for Ca^{2+}, Na$^+$, and K$^+$ bound to the carbonate. The buffering reaction is:

$$2H^+ + CO_3^{2-} \rightarrow CO_2 + H_2O$$

During <u>chronic</u> metabolic acidosis, such as occurs in renal failure, buffering takes place through a combination of (1) direct chemical exchange with bone cations, just as occurs during acute buffering, and (2) increased activity of osteoclast cells, which help mobilize additional bone mineral. Both acute and chronic bone buffering lead to the urinary excretion of bone calcium, which can reduce bone mass (osteopenia) and cause calcium stone formation in the kidneys. These stones, in turn, can lead to renal damage.

In which disturbances does bone buffering occur? It plays a clear role in metabolic acidosis, although its quantitative importance is not known with certainty. It plays no role in respiratory disturbances, and its role in metabolic alkalosis is uncertain.*

Relative importance of the buffering compartments

Data on the relative importance of ECF, ICF, and bone buffering are sparse. However, a few generalizations are possible. In metabolic disturbances, the ECF bicarbonate system plays a key role. In contrast, buffering during respiratory disturbances is mostly intracellular (because non-bicarbonate buffers have a high concentration in cells). Bone plays a clear role in metabolic acidosis, and might play some role in metabolic alkalosis. Quantitatively, it has been estimated that when an HCl load is infused into the blood of a mammal, about half of total-body buffering occurs in the ECF, with the remaining half taking place in cells and bone. This 50–50 breakdown is not absolute. The proportions vary with acid type, rate of acid infusion, and time elapsed since the infusion.

Compensation

In body fluids, $[H^+]$ is directly proportional to PCO_2 and inversely proportional to $[HCO_3^-]$:

$$[H^+] \propto PCO_2/[HCO_3^-]$$

This relationship means that it is neither $[HCO_3^-]$ alone, nor PCO_2 alone, that determines $[H^+]$. It is the ratio between them. For example, if $[HCO_3^-]$ doubles and PCO_2 is unchanged, $[H^+]$ will be halved. However, if both $[HCO_3^-]$ and PCO_2 double, or if both $[HCO_3^-]$ and PCO_2 are halved, $[H^+]$ (and pH) do not change at all.

The body makes use of these relationships in a protective strategy called "compensation." If pathologic changes in $[HCO_3^-]$ or PCO_2 occur, the body responds by bringing about a homeostatic change in the other variable. Thus, during metabolic acidosis (low $[HCO_3^-]$), the body responds by increasing alveolar ventilation and hence lowering PCO_2. Similarly, during

* **Food for thought.** Because bone buffering can cause permanent bone and kidney damage, you could reasonably argue that bone buffering is really a pathologic consequence of acid-base disturbances, not a true homeostatic mechanism.

respiratory acidosis (high PCO_2), the kidney acts to raise plasma $[HCO_3^-]$. In these examples, the original or pathologic change in either PCO_2 or HCO_3^- is referred to as "primary." The change that occurs in the other variable, which acts to keep pH constant, is referred to as either "secondary" or "compensatory," because it compensates for the pH change produced by the primary disturbance.*

The following chart shows the primary and secondary changes that occur in the four simple acid-base disturbances:

Disturbance	Primary change	Secondary change
Metabolic acidosis	$[HCO_3^-]$ down	PCO_2 down
Metabolic alkalosis	$[HCO_3^-]$ up	PCO_2 up
Respiratory acidosis	PCO_2 up	$[HCO_3^-]$ up
Respiratory alkalosis	PCO_2 down	$[HCO_3^-]$ down

Notice that in each case the compensatory change is in the same direction as the primary change (i.e., up yields up, down yields down). We can thus say that compensation follows the *same-direction rule*. This rule makes sense when you realize that only same-direction changes in the numerator and denominator of a fraction (in this case, $PCO_2/[HCO_3^-]$) will minimize the change in the fraction's value (and hence in $[H^+]$).

To develop a more visual, intuitive grasp of the compensatory process, do the following mental exercise. Look at the balance, below. Visualize what change in the bicarbonate bucket would occur during metabolic acidosis. Notice which way the balance tips and how it affects pH. Then visualize a same-directional, compensatory change in the other bucket. Notice how the balance tips back to the center. Repeat this mental exercise for metabolic alkalosis, respiratory acidosis, and respiratory alkalosis.

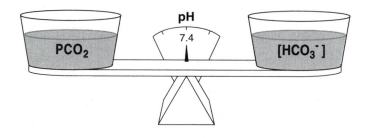

---

* **Terminology.** The terms *primary* and *secondary* are used in many areas of medicine, often in slightly different ways, but they always indicate a sequential, cause-and-effect relationship. The terms can describe normal physiologic sequence ("a primary increase in renin secretion leading to a secondary increase in aldosterone"), pathologic sequence ("hypoperfusion secondary to volume depletion"), or, as used here, homeostatic sequence ("secondary changes in the compensatory variable").

Terminology of compensation

What are the various compensatory responses called? Secondary changes in [HCO_3^-] are termed either "renal" (because they are orchestrated by the kidney) or "metabolic" (because they involve bicarbonate). For example, "renal compensation for respiratory acidosis" and "metabolic compensation for respiratory acidosis" both refer to a secondary rise in plasma [HCO_3^-]. Secondary changes in PCO_2 are always called "respiratory"; for example, "respiratory compensation for metabolic alkalosis." Compensation can also be referred to using succinct phrases like "compensatory hyperventilation," "secondary hypoventilation," and "compensatory hypobicarbonatemia." The term *Kussmaul's respiration* (named after the 19th century German physician, Adolph Kussmaul) also refers to hyperventilation.

Effectiveness of compensation

If compensatory changes completely matched primary changes (e.g., a 50% fall in PCO_2 matched by a 50% fall in [HCO_3^-]), pH would not change at all. In reality, compensation is not quite so efficient. Thus, it would be more typical to see a 50% primary change matched by a 40% secondary change. As a result, even compensated acid-base disturbances cause *some* change in pH, although the change is much less than would occur without compensation. The following graphic illustrates this point, using metabolic alkalosis as an example:

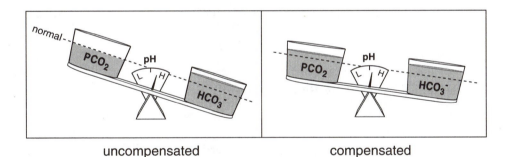

uncompensated   compensated

Not all compensations are equally effective. Renal (i.e., metabolic) compensation of respiratory disturbances is generally more efficient than respiratory compensation of metabolic disturbances. That is, the secondary change more closely matches the primary one. It makes sense that renal compensation is more complete, because changes in plasma [HCO_3^-] "cost" the body much less than changes in PCO_2. Altering [HCO_3^-] requires only a change in renal bicarbonate handling, whereas altering PCO_2 involves either intense muscular work (during hyperventilation) or the risk of hypoxemia and hypercapnia (during hypoventilation). The best-compensated primary disturbance is respiratory alkalosis. In this condition, the secondary fall in [HCO_3^-] so closely matches the primary fall in PCO_2 that pH may actually be in the normal range (even here, however, pH does not return to its original set point). In the other three primary acid-base disturbances, pH always remains outside the normal range.

Mechanism of compensation

Compensation occurs because the primary change in $[HCO_3^-]$ or PCO_2 affects the organ responsible for regulating the "other" variable. Thus, a primary change in PCO_2 affects the kidney, and a primary change in plasma $[HCO_3^-]$ affects the respiratory center in the brain. Here are the details . . .

During <u>metabolic</u> disturbances, the primary change in plasma $[HCO_3^-]$ causes a roughly parallel change in the $[HCO_3^-]$, and hence the pH, of the interstitial fluid that bathes the respiratory center in the medulla. Decreased interstitial pH stimulates the chemoreceptor and increases ventilation, whereas increased interstitial pH inhibits ventilation.* During metabolic acidosis, the sequence looks like this:

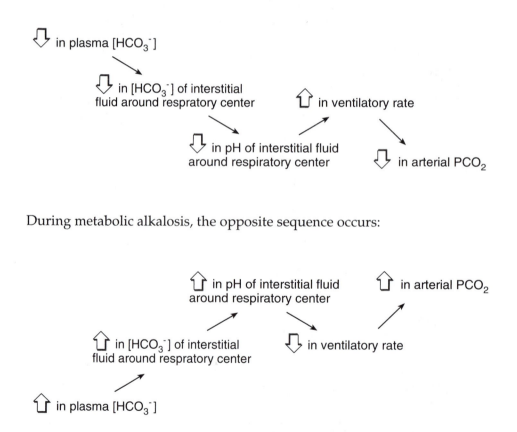

During metabolic alkalosis, the opposite sequence occurs:

* **Going further.** This same chemoreceptor modulates ventilation in response to changes in PCO_2. In fact, it is because PCO_2 affects the $CO_2 + H_2O \rightleftharpoons HCO_3^- + H^+$ equilibrium in the brain's interstitial fluid, and thus affects pH, that the chemoreceptor responds to PCO_2. For example, a rise in PCO_2 lowers interstitial pH, and this low pH stimulates ventilation.

During <u>respiratory</u> disturbances, the change in extracellular PCO_2 causes a roughly parallel change in the PCO_2 of renal tubular cells, and this change, in turn, causes an inverse change in cell pH. Consider respiratory acidosis first. The rise in PCO_2 causes cell pH to fall. Low intracellular pH increases the uptake and utilization of glutamine, which causes an increase in ammonium excretion, thus regenerating additional bicarbonate and raising plasma $[HCO_3^-]$. Low intracellular pH also augments tubular proton secretion, which increases the rate of bicarbonate reabsorption and thus raises the reabsorptive threshold for bicarbonate. This elevated threshold allows the new, higher $[HCO_3^-]$ to be maintained. We can schematize these steps like this:

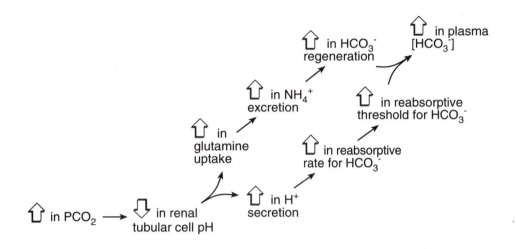

During respiratory alkalosis, proton secretion and hence bicarbonate reabsorption falls. Bicarbonate spills out in the urine and plasma $[HCO_3^-]$ falls. The schema looks like this:

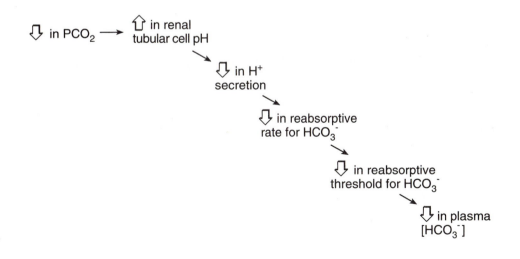

Time frame for compensation

During *metabolic* disturbances, changes in ventilatory rate develop quickly, and the new steady-state PCO_2 is usually reached within about 12 hours. During *respiratory* disturbances, compensation develops more slowly, over 2–5 days. Although the kidney begins to spill (in respiratory alkalosis) or regenerate (in respiratory acidosis) bicarbonate within hours, it takes time for these processes to reach peak levels. Additional time is then required for plasma $[HCO_3^-]$ to fall or rise to its new steady state level. Because increased ammonium excretion requires changes in proximal tubule enzymes, which occur gradually, compensation develops more slowly in respiratory acidosis than in respiratory alkalosis (3–5 days vs. 2–4 days are figures often cited).

Correction

During metabolic acidosis, the kidneys increase net acid excretion (NAE) and, hence, bicarbonate regeneration. This increase is homeostatic because it adds additional bicarbonate to the ECF, thereby helping keep plasma $[HCO_3^-]$ from falling as low as it would otherwise. This renal response occurs only during metabolic acidosis of *non-renal* origin. In contrast, in "nephrogenic" metabolic acidosis the kidney is itself disabled and is thus unable to markedly augment acid excretion.

This homeostatic response is called either "correction" or "restoration." Sometimes it is referred to as "increased bicarbonate regeneration secondary to metabolic acidosis," or other such phrases. The increase in NAE is due largely to a rise in ammonium excretion, which can take several days to fully develop but can be quite striking. For example, in metabolic acidosis due to uncontrolled diabetes ("diabetic ketoacidosis"), ammonium excretion can reach 300–500 mmol/day, ten times normal.

What mediates increased ammonium excretion? A fall in ECF $[HCO_3^-]$ creates a steeper gradient for bicarbonate to exit cells, thus lowering intracellular $[HCO_3^-]$. Since intracellular PCO_2 is unchanged, the intracellular $[HCO_3^-]/PCO_2$ ratio, and hence pH, falls as well. Low intracellular pH acts as a signal to increase ammonium excretion.

The term "correction" is sometimes used in another, less specific, way: to refer to the normalization of any acid-base disturbance. For example, when an asthma attack subsides, the accompanying abnormality in PCO_2 gradually "corrects." This "correction" is not really a homeostatic response, but an elimination of the underlying problem.

Integrative example

We conclude this chapter by seeing how the various homeostatic responses occur together in the same patient. As an example, we consider metabolic acidosis caused by an overproduction of lactic acid ("lactic acidosis"). We can distinguish four partially-overlapping stages:

1. *Disorder.* Lactic acid is released into the body fluids, where it dissociates into lactate anions and free protons.

2. *Buffering.* Dissociating protons immediately react with ECF bicarbonate ($H^+ + HCO_3^- \rightarrow CO_2 + H_2O$). This reaction consumes bicarbonate, thus lowering plasma $[HCO_3^-]$. The carbon dioxide that is produced is rapidly excreted at the lung, without raising plasma PCO_2. Non-bicarbonate buffers, such as hemoglobin, also act immediately to mitigate the fall in ECF pH. Over several hours, as the intracellular compartment equilibrates with the low $[HCO_3^-]$ and pH of the ECF, the pH of various body tissues declines. This fall in cell pH leads to buffering by intracellular proteins, organic phosphates, and bicarbonate. If metabolic acidosis persists, bone buffering may occur.

3. *Compensation.* The low plasma $[HCO_3^-]$ and pH are gradually transmitted to the brain interstitial fluid that bathes the respiratory center. Ventilation is stimulated. Arterial PCO_2 falls, reaching its new steady-state level within about 12 hours.

4. *Correction.* The kidneys gradually increase ammonium excretion and thus regenerate additional bicarbonate. The new bicarbonate helps mitigate the fall in plasma $[HCO_3^-]$. Bicarbonate regeneration does not peak for several days.

This sequence provides a model for thinking about patients with simple (i.e., not mixed) acid-base disturbances. In most patients with non-nephrogenic metabolic acidosis, all four steps occur. In most other patients, only the first three steps occur, although the nature of the buffering and compensatory responses vary, depending on which primary disturbance is present.

Summary

Three homeostatic responses minimize the changes in pH that occur during acid-base disturbances. Buffering, a nearly instantaneous chemical process, occurs in the ECF, ICF, and sometimes bone. Compensation, a slower, physiologic process, further mitigates pH changes through a same-direction change in the "other" variable (i.e., PCO_2 or $[HCO_3^-]$). For example, metabolic acidosis, a primary fall in $[HCO_3^-]$, is compensated by a secondary fall in PCO_2. This secondary change returns the ratio $PCO_2/[HCO_3^-]$, and hence pH, towards its normal value. Correction, in its specific and truly homeostatic sense, occurs only during metabolic acidosis of non-renal origin. It refers to the partial renal replacement of lost bicarbonate, which occurs primarily through a gradual but marked rise in ammonium excretion.

In this chapter and the previous one (Chapter 14), we've laid a foundation of terms and concepts that will let us develop a deep understanding of the four primary acid-base disturbances. We are now ready to focus on these disturbances individually, starting with metabolic acidosis.

Metabolic Acidosis

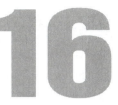

Definition

Metabolic acidosis is a disease process that causes an abnormal fall in plasma bicarbonate concentration, thereby producing acidemia. With the exception of renal compensation for respiratory alkalosis, all hypobicarbonatemia is abnormal. Thus, all non-compensatory hypobicarbonatemia is, by definition, metabolic acidosis. In patients with an intact ventilatory response, metabolic acidosis causes compensatory hyperventilation, which lowers arterial PCO_2 and mitigates the fall in plasma pH.

Introduction

Bicarbonate (HCO_3^-) is continually added to, and eliminated from, the extracellular fluid (ECF). That is, there is an "inflow" and "outflow" of bicarbonate to the ECF. The inflow consists of net bicarbonate added to blood by the kidney. The rate of this inflow can be quantified, indirectly, by measuring renal net acid excretion in the urine. The outflow consists of bicarbonate consumed in buffering endogenously produced strong acids, such as the sulfuric acid produced by the liver when dietary protein is metabolized. The protons from these acids react with bicarbonate via the reaction $H^+ + HCO_3^- \rightarrow CO_2 + H_2O$.

In health, renal net acid excretion, and hence the inflow of new bicarbonate from the kidney, exactly matches endogenous acid production. All lost bicarbonate is replaced, so plasma $[HCO_3^-]$ remains constant. That is, there is a steady state. Take a moment to look at the figure on page 107, which illustrates this point.

Disease can disrupt the bicarbonate steady state. If endogenous acid production rises sharply, and net acid excretion cannot keep pace, then bicarbonate lost in buffering is not replaced. Plasma $[HCO_3^-]$ falls; that is, metabolic acidosis develops. Similarly, if the kidney is damaged and unable to maintain its usual rate of net acid excretion, metabolic acidosis will result even if the rate of endogenous acid production remains normal. Put simply, metabolic acidosis develops whenever endogenous acid production exceeds renal net acid excretion.

In the clinical setting, there are four general mechanisms that cause metabolic acidosis. All involve either an increase in endogenous acid production or a fall in renal acid excretion:

1. Elevated acid production due to derangements in gut function.
2. Elevated acid production due to derangements in metabolism.
3. Elevated acid production due to exogenous intoxicants.
4. Reduced net acid excretion due to renal defects.

In a moment, we will study these mechanisms in detail. But first we briefly turn our attention to the word "metabolic." We do so because discussions of metabolic acidosis can easily lead to confusion about this word. Consider this sentence:

"Metabolic derangements can cause metabolic acidosis."

This sentence highlights the fact that "metabolic" has two distinct meanings (p. 124). The first "metabolic" in the sentence has the usual meaning; it refers to the pathways of catabolism and anabolism. The second "metabolic" is a usage specific to acid-base; it refers to a primary abnormality in plasma $[HCO_3^-]$. If we wanted to rewrite this sentence without using the word metabolic, it would read: "Derangements in the pathways of catabolism or anabolism can cause a pathologic fall in plasma $[HCO_3^-]$."

It is also important to see what this sentence does *not* say. It does not say that metabolic derangements are the only cause of metabolic acidosis. As noted above, metabolic acidosis can also be caused by derangements of the gut or kidney. And it does not say that metabolic derangements always result in metabolic acidosis. As we will see, only certain types of metabolic derangements cause metabolic acidosis.

With this background, we are now ready to explore the causes of metabolic acidosis in detail. The rest of this chapter consists of four subsections, which correspond to the four general mechanisms listed a few paragraphs above.

Gastrointestinal causes of metabolic acidosis

During normal digestion, many alimentary segments below the pylorus secrete bicarbonate into the gut lumen. The duodenum, ileum, pancreas, gall bladder, and, especially, the colon all secrete bicarbonate into the gut lumen. This bicarbonate is produced inside the secretory cells by the reaction $CO_2 + H_2O \rightarrow H^+ + HCO_3^-$. The protons produced by this reaction cross the basolateral cell membrane and enter the ECF. Thus, the alkalinization of the sub-pyloric lumen is matched by an equal and opposite acidification of the ECF. Take a moment to glance at the figure on page 92, which illustrates this concept.

In diarrheal states, secretion by the lower gut increases. This increase is largely due to increased stool volume. In addition, in some diseases (e.g., cholera), the infectious or toxic agent directly stimulates secretory activity. Thus, in patients with diarrhea, large quantities of bicarbonate enter the lower gut lumen, and large quantities of protons enter the body fluids. These protons are buffered by extracellular bicarbonate, causing plasma $[HCO_3^-]$ to fall. In severe diarrhea, profound metabolic acidosis can develop, with $[HCO_3^-]$ below 10 mmol/l.

There are other fluid and electrolyte consequences as well. Diarrhea fluid contains water, Na^+, Cl^-, and K^+. The loss of water and Na^+ lowers ECF volume. This decrease in ECF volume stimulates the renin-angiotensin-aldosterone axis. This stimulation is homeostatic because angiotensin II raises blood pressure, and aldosterone augments renal sodium reabsorption, which helps maintain ECF volume. However, aldosterone also stimulates potassium excretion by both kidney and colonic mucosa, exacerbating K^+ losses in urine and stool. As a result, metabolic acidosis caused by diarrhea presents with hypokalemia.

Like diarrhea itself, a number of "diarrhea equivalent" conditions can, by essentially the same mechanism, also lead to metabolic acidosis. These include laxative abuse and the drainage of intestinal fluids from anywhere below the pylorus.

Metabolic causes of metabolic acidosis

In health, the body constantly produces organic acids. For example, lactic acid is normally produced at a rate of over 1000 mmol per day. These acids dissociate, liberating protons and organic anions (e.g., lactate). Although the protons are buffered by, and thereby consume, bicarbonate, plasma $[HCO_3^-]$ does not fall because almost all the organic anions are themselves metabolized to bicarbonate (p. 86–87), which replaces the lost bicarbonate. This ongoing anion metabolism also keeps the plasma concentration of organic anions from rising. For example, plasma lactate levels usually do not exceed 2 mmol/l. This sequence of acid production followed by the metabolic consumption of the anion occurs for many organic acids.

In certain diseases, organic acid production can rise without a matching increase in anion metabolism. This imbalance has three consequences. First, lost bicarbonate is not adequately replaced, so plasma $[HCO_3^-]$ falls. That is, metabolic acidosis develops. Second, the plasma concentration of organic anions increases. For example, an imbalance in lactic acid metabolism might lower plasma $[HCO_3^-]$ to 11 mmol/l (from 24) and raise plasma lactate concentration to 15 mmol/l (from 2). Third, excess anions in the plasma may be spilled in the urine. Such spillage occurs if the quantity of anions filtered at the glomerulus exceeds the kidney's reabsorptive threshold. This spillage has important consequences: as long as the anions remain in the body, they can potentially be metabolized to bicarbonate at a later time, but once they are excreted in the urine, the "potential bicarbonate" they represent is lost.

There are two common clinical settings in which an imbalance between organic acid production and anion consumption causes metabolic acidosis: lactic acidosis and ketoacidosis. Let's look at these individually.

Lactic acidosis

Lactic acid is a three-carbon carboxylic acid, a slightly modified form of simple propionic acid (CH_3CH_2COOH). Its structure is shown on page 8. Take a moment to look at it.

Lactic acid is produced in many tissues, including skin, brain, muscle, and red blood cells. Because it is formed as a product of anaerobic metabolism, lactic acid production increases when tissue blood flow, or the delivery or utilization of oxygen, is impaired. Lactate is consumed primarily in the liver, and to a lesser extent in the renal cortex and elsewhere. In these organs, the lactate is either burned to carbon dioxide and water for energy (aerobic respiration) or built up into glucose for storage (gluconeogenesis). Both these routes require oxygen. Thus, a generalized decrease in either blood perfusion or oxygen carriage causes a rise in lactic acid production and, simultaneously, a fall in lactate consumption. "Lactic acidosis" refers to the metabolic acidosis caused by this imbalance.

The most common clinical cause of lactic acidosis is circulatory failure, especially that resulting from either acute heart failure ("cardiogenic shock") or severe sepsis ("septic shock"). These conditions cause lactic acidosis by reducing perfusion of many tissues, including muscle and liver. Many less common conditions cause lactic acidosis as well, and most involve decreased oxygen delivery. The following paragraph describes some of the less common causes that are nonetheless likely to be encountered clinically:

Severe acute hypoxemia; in contrast, chronic hypoxemia is usually well compensated by increases in cardiac output, hematocrit, and 2,3-diphosphoglycerate in red blood cells. Severe convulsions sharply increase muscle activity at a time when ventilatory arrest causes hypoxemia. Strenuous exercise, especially with concomitant dehydration. Exercise increases lactic acid production, and dehydration hinders lactate metabolism by (1) causing hypovolemia and hence generalized hypoperfusion and (2) inducing a shift in blood flow to non-splanchnic vascular beds, thereby additionally reducing hepatic perfusion. Carbon monoxide (CO) reduces the oxygen-carrying capacity of blood by occupying oxygen sites on hemoglobin. CO also raises the oxygen affinity of hemoglobin at those sites not occupied by CO, thereby inhibiting unloading of oxygen at the tissues. Severe anemia reduces the hemoglobin concentration, and hence the oxygen-carrying capacity, of blood. Iron-deficiency anemia additionally inhibits key iron-dependent steps in the oxidative phosphorylation chain. Malignancies, especially certain leukemias, lymphomas, and oat cell lung cancer, are metabolically active foci that can outstrip their blood supply, leading to localized anaerobic respiration. Acquired metabolic defects, metastatic invasion of the liver, and other, unidentified factors may also contribute to the acidosis. Diabetes mellitus most commonly causes ketoacidosis (discussed below), but it can occasionally also cause lactic acidosis, partly because uncontrolled diabetes may lead to hypovolemia with decreased tissue perfusion. Severe liver disease can inhibit hepatic lactate metabolism. Alcoholism, also, may impair the liver's capacity to metabolize lactate. However, the resulting acidosis is mild.

Ketoacidosis

Let's begin our discussion of ketoacidosis with terminology. "Ketoacid" refers to two related organic acids: acetoacetic acid and beta-hydroxybutyric acid. The name "ketoacid" is given because acetoacetic acid has a keto group, a fact suggested by the name ac_eto_acetic (the "k" is missing). Beta-hydroxybutyric acid contains not a keto group but, as its name indicates, a hydroxy group. It is therefore not a true ketoacid but the name is used nonetheless. Aside from the presence of a hydroxy group (and the opposing hydrogen atom) instead of a keto group, its structure is identical to acetoacetic acid:

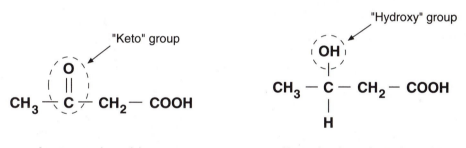

Acetoacetic acid   Beta-hydroxybutyric acid

Notice that both molecules are simply butyric acid ($CH_3CH_2CH_2COOH$), with modifications (hydroxy or keto) at the second carbon from the carboxyl group. Upon entering the body fluids, the ketoacids dissociate almost completely. Therefore, they exist almost entirely as the anions acetoacetate and beta-hydroxybutyrate.*

A related substance is acetone. It is also a ketone (ac_etone_) but it is not an acid and it has only three carbons:

---

* **Terminology.** In an organic acid chain, carbons are counted off using the letters of the Greek alphabet (alpha, beta, gamma, etc.). The counting starts with the carbon *next to* the carboxyl carbon. This explains the name beta-hydroxybutyric acid (sometimes written β-hydroxybutyric acid) and why acetoacetic acid is also called beta-ketobutyric acid. The name acetoacetic acid also describes the structure: an acetyl group, CH_3CO-, attached to an acetic acid molecule, CH_3COOH (the acetyl group replaces one of the acid's methyl hydrogens). Lactic acid, shown on page 8, is alpha-hydroxypropionic acid.

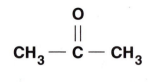

Acetone

"Ketone body" is the generic name given to acetone and the two ketoacids. Acetoacetic acid can be converted into the other two ketone bodies. When reduced (via the addition of hydrogen), it becomes beta-hydroxybutyric acid. When decarboxylated (i.e., removal of carbon dioxide), it becomes acetone. Because of these reactions, all three ketone bodies are present whenever acetoacetic acid is produced:

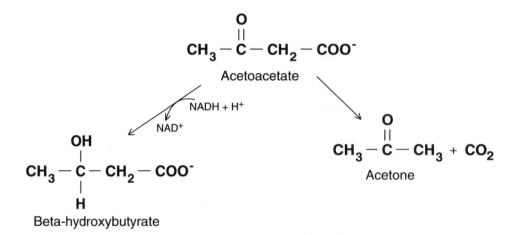

"Ketoacidosis" refers to the metabolic acidosis caused by the overproduction of ketoacids. Let's see how this condition arises. As part of normal metabolism, fat cells continually break down triglycerides into fatty acids and glycerol. The fatty acids enter the blood and are transported to the liver, where they are metabolized in three ways: (1) re-synthesized into triglycerides (three fatty acids are linked to a molecule of glycerol), (2) burned for energy, by beta oxidation, into carbon dioxide and water, and (3) sections of the carbon chain are broken off and converted into ketoacids. This last pathway is called ketogenic ("ketone producing"). In health, the three pathways are carefully regulated. In ketoacidosis, regulation is altered and the ketogenic pathway becomes overly active.

Ketoacidosis is caused by an abnormal hormonal milieu consisting of low levels of insulin and high levels of glucagon. Insulin promotes growth via the cellular uptake of foodstuffs. Thus, a fall in insulin causes fat cells to liberate fatty acids, which flood the hepatocytes. Simultaneously, high glucagon levels promote entry of fatty acids into the ketogenic pathway. There are three clinical situations that cause this abnormal hormonal milieu and thus result in ketoacidosis. Let's look at each briefly:

Diabetic ketoacidosis. The classic cause of ketoacidosis is uncontrolled diabetes mellitus. This form of ketoacidosis is called diabetic ketoacidosis or, simply, "DKA." DKA is frequently encountered clinically. It can cause a severe, life-threatening fall in plasma [HCO_3^-].

Starvation ketoacidosis. The body responds to starvation by mobilizing cellular foodstuffs, the homeostatic goal being to prevent or repair hypoglycemia. It accomplishes this mobilization by lowering insulin and raising glucagon levels. Although this hormonal profile is ketogenic, the hypobicarbonatemia is relatively mild, for three reasons: (1) the hormonal changes are less pronounced than in uncontrolled diabetes; (2) the metabolism of ketoacid anions to bicarbonate is more efficient than in DKA; and (3) starvation and hence ketogenesis develops gradually, which, in contrast to the rapid onset of DKA, allows renal bicarbonate regeneration to become fully active. This mild form of metabolic acidosis is called starvation ketoacidosis. It is of little importance clinically.

Alcoholic ketoacidosis. When an alcoholic has an acute drinking-vomiting binge, decreased food intake coupled with vomiting (which empties residual food from the stomach) effectively produces starvation, with accompanying ketoacidosis. High levels of plasma catecholamines, a response to volume depletion (from vomiting) and alcohol withdrawal, augment the liberation of free fatty acids and further intensifies ketogenesis. The combined effect of starvation and catecholamine excess can cause rapid ketogenesis and hypobicarbonatemia. This form of metabolic acidosis is called alcoholic ketoacidosis. It is relatively common clinically.*

In all three types of ketoacidosis, plasma levels of ketoacid anions and acetone rise, and large amounts of the anions are spilled into the urine. These anions, and the cations (usually Na^+) that are excreted with them to maintain electroneutrality, are osmotically active and thus can drag a large volume of water into the urine ("osmotic diuresis"). In diabetic ketoacidosis, urinary glucose spillage has the same osmotic effect, compounding fluid losses. As a result, volume depletion is frequently severe in DKA.

Note: Acetone has a characteristic smell. This smell is similar to nail polish remover (acetone is the primary solvent in nail polish removers) and is sometimes described as "fruity." Because acetone is volatile (i.e., it readily converts from liquid to gas), it is excreted largely via the lung. Thus, acetone on the breath of a diabetic suggests ketoacidosis.

---

* **Terminology.** Alcoholic ketoacidosis is sometimes called by the more general name "alcoholic acidosis" because, in addition to ketoacids, lactic acid and acetic acid, a product of ethanol metabolism, may also be present.

Exogenous causes of metabolic acidosis

Many drugs and toxins can cause lactic acidosis. This lactic acidosis is most commonly secondary to cardiovascular collapse, ventilatory suppression, or seizures, which can be produced by the drugs. In addition, three widely available substances can cause metabolic acidosis by unique mechanisms, in which lactic acidosis plays at most a contributory role. These substances are methanol, ethylene glycol, and salicylates. These three substances account for most ingestion-associated metabolic acidosis, so we will study them in detail.

Methanol and ethylene glycol

Methanol (methyl alcohol, "wood alcohol") is widely used as an industrial solvent and as an ingredient in windshield washing solutions. Ethylene glycol, another organic solvent, is a major ingredient of most radiator antifreeze solutions. Because ethylene glycol is odorless and tastes sweet, it is sometimes illegally used to sweeten wine. Methanol and ethylene glycol are not acids, and neither is directly toxic. However, both are metabolized to toxic acids and other products that can cause severe acidosis and other lethal effects. As little as 30 ml of either methanol or ethylene glycol can be lethal in an adult (one tablespoon equals 15 ml). Chemically, both have structures similar to ethanol (ethyl alcohol, "drinking alcohol"):

$$CH_3 - CH_2 - OH \qquad \text{Ethanol}$$

$$CH_3 - OH \qquad \text{Methanol}$$

$$HO - CH_2 - CH_2 - OH \qquad \text{Ethylene glycol}$$

The metabolism of methanol and ethylene glycol can best be understood by studying ethanol metabolism. Ethanol is metabolized in two steps. First, in a reaction catalyzed by the enzyme alcohol dehydrogenase, ethanol is converted to acetaldehyde. Second, in a reaction catalyzed by aldehyde dehydrogenase, it is converted to acetic acid. (Acetic acid does not accumulate, or cause metabolic acidosis, because it is readily oxidized to carbon dioxide and water.) The process is shown here:

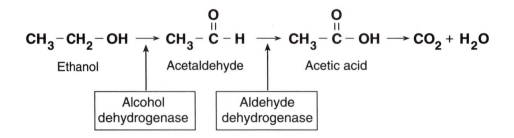

The essential feature of this process is this progression: alcohol → aldehyde → carboxylic acid. These same steps occur for methanol and ethylene glycol, with the same enzymes acting as catalysts. For methanol, the toxic end product is formic acid, which is not readily metabolized and, therefore, accumulates in the ECF. For ethylene glycol, the primary acid product is glycolic acid, which is further metabolized to other toxic products, including oxalic acid. The pathways look like this:

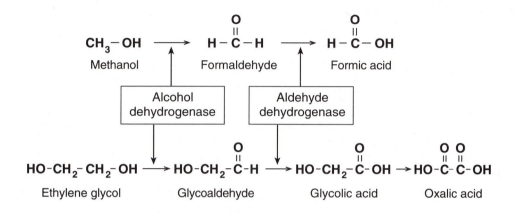

These acids all dissociate in body fluids, thereby consuming bicarbonate.

Salicylates

Salicylate intoxication causes metabolic acidosis *and* respiratory alkalosis. Respiratory alkalosis usually develops first and occurs in almost all patients. A superimposed metabolic acidosis then develops in some patients, especially those with more severe intoxication. In children under ten, the respiratory alkalosis is often mild, so the metabolic acidosis tends to predominate, resulting in a low plasma pH. In patients over ten, there is a greater tendency for the two disorders to be coequal, resulting in an approximately normal pH, or for the respiratory alkalosis to predominate, causing alkalemia. Salicylates are usually ingested as acetylsalicylic acid (plain "aspirin"). This compound rapidly dissociates to acetylsalicylate, which is metabolized in the liver to salicylate (by removal of the acetyl group). It is salicylate that causes the acid-base disturbances.

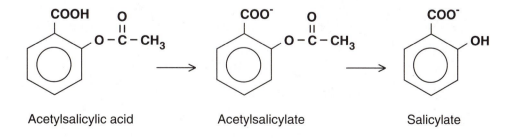

Salicylate interferes with various enzymes, leading to increased production of organic acids, especially keto and lactic acids. These acids cause the metabolic acidosis. (Protons liberated during the dissociation of acetylsalicylic acid do consume bicarbonate, but the amount of aspirin typically ingested is too small to substantially lower [HCO_3^-] by this mechanism.) Salicylate also directly stimulates the medullary respiratory center, causing hyperventilation and respiratory alkalosis.

Renal causes of metabolic acidosis

The kidney carries out two different processes involving bicarbonate: reabsorption and regeneration. If either process is impaired, metabolic acidosis results. If bicarbonate reabsorption fails, filtered HCO_3^- is lost in the urine. At normal glomerular filtration rate (GFR) and plasma [HCO_3^-], a 15% inefficiency in reabsorption means bicarbonate is lost at almost 30 mmol per hour. If bicarbonate regeneration is impaired, the HCO_3^- consumed buffering endogenously produced acids is not adequately replaced. If regeneration fails entirely, HCO_3^- is lost at a rate equal to endogenous acid production.

There are two major conditions that impair the kidney's handling of bicarbonate: renal failure and renal tubular acidosis. Both involve a defect in the renal tubule, and (because both bicarbonate reabsorption and regeneration are tubular functions) it is this tubular defect that causes metabolic acidosis. In addition, renal failure also involves a marked defect in glomerular filtration. We will now study these two conditions individually, starting with renal failure.

Renal failure

Renal failure, both chronic and acute, is characterized by injury to both the glomerulus, which results in low GFR and high plasma levels of nitrogenous waste, and the tubule. High blood levels of nitrogenous waste is referred to as azotemia ("azote," from the French, means nitrogen). Urea (usually measured as Blood Urea Nitrogen, BUN) and creatinine are the nitrogenous wastes most commonly measured. Therefore, urea and creatinine serve as laboratory markers for azotemia. In chronic renal failure, creatinine levels of 10 mg/dl or higher are common (normal is around 1 mg/dl). Plasma levels of several nonnitrogenous anions (including sulfate, phosphate, and various organic anions) also frequently rise. Because these anions are not measured on routine lab tests, they are called "unmeasured anions."*

How does renal failure cause metabolic acidosis? The primary mechanism is a *decrease in ammonium excretion* by the tubule, which is the major route for regenerating bicarbonate. During severe renal failure, daily ammonium ex-

---

* **Terminology.** The concentration of unmeasured anions in blood is assessed by calculating the "anion gap," a concept we discuss in detail in the Diagnosis section, in Chapter 21.

cretion falls to between 0.5 and 15 mmol. When you consider that these levels occur during metabolic acidosis, which normally stimulates a homeostatic increase in ammonium excretion (e.g., during ketoacidosis, daily ammonium excretion can reach 300–500 mmol), the extent of the decline becomes apparent.

What causes this decline? The major mechanism is a reduction in the total number of functioning nephrons. This loss of nephrons is often referred to as "nephronal dropout." Because this dropout involves the entire nephron, it affects both glomerular filtration and tubular function. The rise in plasma waste products (BUN, creatinine, unmeasured anions) is due mainly to the reduction in glomerular filtration. As described, the fall in $[HCO_3^-]$ is due to the tubular defect.

At what point in the progression of renal failure does metabolic acidosis (i.e., hypobicarbonatemia) occur? It is often said that by the time GFR falls to one-fourth its normal level (indicated by an approximately four-fold rise in plasma creatinine), metabolic acidosis will be present. This statement is a good rule of thumb. However, the appearance of acidosis is variable; it can set in earlier, later, or not at all.

Two main factors account for this variability in the onset of hypobicarbonatemia. First, residual functioning nephrons can homeostatically increase ammonium excretion by up to four times, but this response is inconsistent. Second, although nephronal dropout affects both glomerulus and tubule, it does not always affect them at the same rate. If tubular failure is more pronounced, metabolic acidosis tends to occur early; if tubular failure is less pronounced, acidosis occurs later.

Renal Tubular Acidosis

The name Renal Tubular Acidosis (RTA) conveys the essence of the disease:

Renal: the problem is in the kidney.
Tubular: the specific defect is in the tubules.
Acidosis: it causes acidosis.

Therefore, RTA is a *kidney disorder that affects the tubules and causes acidosis.* As the "T" in RTA implies, glomerular defects are not central to the disease. In many RTA patients, glomerular function, and hence plasma [creatinine], are completely normal. In other patients, glomerular function is impaired, but not to the extent found in severe renal failure, so plasma [creatinine] is slightly elevated (2 mg/dl is a typical value). The total or relative preservation of glomerular function in RTA is the main difference between RTA and renal failure. Recall that the essential feature of renal failure is a major defect in glomerular function, with a consequent marked elevation in [creatinine], often to 10 mg/dl or higher.

How is the acidosis of RTA caused? The tubule handles bicarbonate at several locations (proximal, distal, even the loop of Henle) and in different ways (reabsorption, regeneration). A defect in any of these locations or processes fulfills the criteria imposed by the name Renal Tubular Acidosis. Therefore, it should not be surprising that RTA is not really a single disease, but is a general term applied to perhaps a dozen different entities, all of which are renal, tubular, and acidosis-causing. Some of these entities are primarily proximal whereas others are distal. Some affect reabsorption whereas others affect ammonium excretion. And some affect the same locations and processes but do so by different mechanisms.

When an RTA is encountered clinically, it can be difficult to determine the specific pathophysiologic defect. Therefore, it has been traditional to subdivide the RTAs into three broad groups, called "types," and to limit the initial diagnosis to differentiating among these. The types are numbered 1, 2, and 4.* Before discussing the three types in detail, we will first summarize their essential features in tabular form. Take a moment to familiarize yourself with these features.

Key Characteristics of Renal Tubular Acidosis

	Type 1	**Type 2**	**Type 4**
Also called	Distal RTA	Proximal RTA	Hyperkalemic RTA
Defect	Defect in distal tubule lowers capacity to concentrate $[H^+]$ in distal luminal fluid	Defect in proximal tubule lowers capacity to reabsorb HCO_3^- from proximal luminal fluid	Usually caused by reduced aldosterone secretion. This causes acidosis by inhibiting NH_4^+ production
Urine pH	Above 5.5 even though acidemia stimulates proton secretion	Biphasic. Above 5.5 as acidosis develops. Below 5.5 once acidosis is fully established	Usually below 5.5
Plasma $[K^+]$	Usually low (but may be normal)	Usually low (but may be normal)	High
Glomerular function	Relatively normal	Relatively normal	Modest impairment
Plasma $[HCO_3^-]$	Often below 10 mmol/l	Typically 15–20 mmol/l	Typically 15–20 mmol/l
Epidemiology	Rare in both children and adults	Most common RTA in children	Most common RTA in adults

---

* **Terminology.** There is no Type 3. There used to be, but it is now considered a variant of Type 1.

This chart suggests several key differences in clinical presentation:

1.   Types 1 and 2 present with low or normal plasma [K$^+$], whereas Type 4 presents with high [K$^+$] (hence the name "Hyperkalemic RTA").

2.   Types 1 and 2 have relatively normal glomerular function, so plasma BUN and creatinine are essentially normal. In contrast, Type 4 typically has modest glomerular impairment, which raises BUN and creatinine slightly (creatinine levels around 2 mg/dl, about twice normal, are typical).

3.   Type 2 ("Proximal RTA") can cause substantial bicarbonaturia (i.e., urinary bicarbonate spillage), because most reabsorption occurs proximally. Types 1 and 4 do not.

4.   Types 2 and 4 cause moderate hypobicarbonatemia. Type 1 can cause severe hypobicarbonatemia.

We now examine the three types individually. As you read, don't worry about remembering all the details. Just be sure to follow the progression of ideas. Following this progression will help you master the main concepts. Note: those studying acid-base pathophysiology for the first time may wish to skip these detailed discussions of RTA. If an in-depth understanding of RTA is not currently important to you, simply scan the table once more, and then move directly to the chapter summary. You can always review later, when the need arises.

Type 1: Distal RTA

Type 1 is characterized by a reduced capacity of the distal nephron (specifically, the collecting tubule) to lower luminal fluid pH. The defect is in either proton secretion or in the retention of protons in the lumen. The result is high urinary pH and reduced excretion of titratable acid and ammonium. Because a small amount of bicarbonate is reabsorbed distally, Type 1 also causes mild bicarbonaturia, usually just a few percent of the filtered load.*

The reduced excretion of titratable acid and ammonium, coupled with the slight increase in bicarbonate spillage, means that net acid excretion, and

---

* **Going further.** It is obvious why a defect in proton secretion impairs distal bicarbonate reabsorption and titratable acid excretion. But why should ammonium excretion also be impaired? The usual explanation is as follows. Secreted ammonium in the luminal fluid exists in equilibrium with ammonia: $NH_4^+ \rightleftharpoons NH_3 + H^+$. High luminal pH shifts the equilibrium to the right, raising luminal [NH_3]. Since NH_3 is more permeant across biologic membranes than NH_4^+, more total ammonia (i.e., $NH_3 + NH_4^+$) diffuses out of the nephron lumen into peritubular blood, thereby reducing urinary ammonium excretion. Readers with an interest in the more esoteric aspects of ammonium excretion will find a detailed discussion in appendix topic B.

hence net bicarbonate regeneration, falls sharply. As a result, bicarbonate that is lost buffering endogenously produced acid is not fully replaced, and plasma $[HCO_3^-]$ falls. The decline in $[HCO_3^-]$ is gradual, with the rate of decline being (at least initially) roughly proportional to the rate of endogenous acid production. Plasma $[HCO_3^-]$ before treatment is often below 10 mmol/l.

A fully functioning distal nephron can lower urinary pH to between 4.5 and 5.0. In distal RTA, urinary pH does not fall below about 5.5. This inability to fully lower urinary pH, not withstanding the powerful stimulus for proton secretion provided by acidemia, is *the* hallmark of Type 1. In contrast, patients with Types 2 and 4 can usually lower urine pH to below 5.5.

Mechanisms.   Three different mechanisms have been proposed to cause distal RTA. One or more may be present in any given patient. (1) *Permeability defect.* A defect in the epithelial barrier of the distal nephron results in the diffusion (or "back leak") of protons out of the lumen. (2) *Pump defect.* The luminal membrane of the distal nephron secretes protons via an H^+–ATPase ("proton pump"). A defect in this pump impairs proton secretion. (3) H^+-K^+ *defect.* Recent evidence suggests that, in addition to the H^+–ATPase, there is an ATP-driven H^+-K^+ exchanger in the luminal membrane of the distal nephron. This exchanger actively secretes H^+ and reabsorbs K^+. A defect in this exchanger would impair proton secretion (and account for the hypokalemia as well). The following schematic illustrates these three mechanisms:

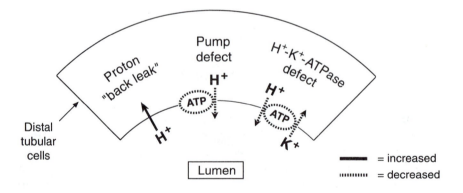

Etiology.   In adults, Distal RTA is often associated with autoimmune diseases (e.g., Sjogren's syndrome, rheumatoid arthritis). Many other causes exist, including nephrocalcinosis, the sniffing of toluene (found in varnish, paint, and airplane glue), and amphotericin B administration. Severe volume depletion can induce a reversible form of Type 1 RTA. In children, Distal RTA is usually hereditary.

Type 2: Proximal RTA

In Type 2 RTA, the renal "threshold" for bicarbonate reabsorption is reduced from its normal range of about 26–28 mmol/l to a pathologically low level, usually somewhere between 14–20 mmol/l. When plasma $[HCO_3^-]$

exceeds the threshold, reabsorption is incomplete and as much as 20% of filtered HCO_3^- is spilled into the urine, causing plasma $[HCO_3^-]$ to fall. This heavy bicarbonate spillage is *the* hallmark of Type 2 RTA. However, once $[HCO_3^-]$ drops to the threshold level, reabsorption rises, bicarbonaturia ceases, and plasma $[HCO_3^-]$ stabilizes. The situation is analogous to a bucket of water that has a small hole in the side; the water drops to the level of the hole and then stabilizes, as illustrated here:

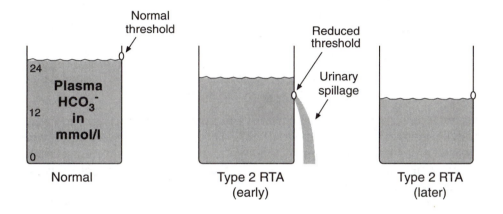

This bucket analogy explains the biphasic urine pH typical of Type 2: while HCO_3^- is being spilled, urine pH is high (because the urine's HCO_3^-/PCO_2 ratio is high), but when the spillage ceases, urine pH falls, typically to 4.5–5.0. Stable plasma $[HCO_3^-]$ before treatment is usually around 15 mmol/l.

Cellular mechanisms. The specific cellular causes of Proximal RTA are not known. A defect in one or more of the following mechanisms may be involved: Na^+-H^+ exchange, ATP-driven Na^+-K^+ exchange (which provides the driving force for Na^+-H^+ exchange), or carbonic anhydrase function (either intracellular or luminal). These possible defects are indicated by bold arrows:

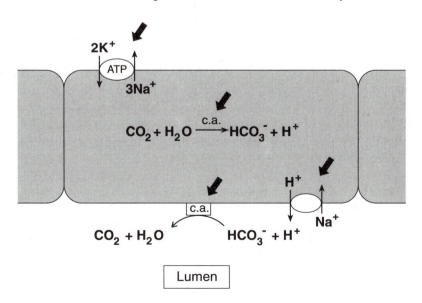

Patients with Type 2 RTA typically have impaired reabsorption (with resulting urinary spillage) of not only bicarbonate but also of other substances, including glucose, phosphate, urate, citrate, and amino acids. The constellation of multiple proximal reabsorptive defects is called the *Fanconi syndrome*.

Etiology.   In adults, proximal RTA is most commonly caused by carbonic anhydrase inhibitors (usually Diamox given for glaucoma; this RTA self-corrects when the drug is stopped) or multiple myeloma. Among children, where the disorder is more common, proximal RTA is usually either idiopathic or due to cystinosis (a hereditary disease of cystine metabolism).

Type 4: Hyperkalemic RTA

Type 4 is generally defined by clinical criteria: it is typically diagnosed when an RTA is associated with hyperkalemia. The causative defect is usually decreased aldosterone secretion, often secondary to low renal renin secretion ("hyporeninemic hypoaldosteronism"). A defect in the distal nephron's aldosterone receptor ("aldosterone resistance") may also be present. In some cases, a receptor defect is the sole cause. Plasma $[HCO_3^-]$ before treatment is typically 15–20 mmol/l.

Mechanisms.   In health, aldosterone has several effects on the distal tubule: (1) it directly stimulates the proton pump; (2) it promotes Na^+ reabsorption in the collecting duct, leaving the distal luminal fluid with a slight negative charge, which in turn facilitates the secretion of K^+ and H^+ (because the luminal negative charge attracts cations); and (3) it increases the K^+ permeability of the luminal membrane, further enhancing K^+ secretion. Based on these effects, a pathologic fall in aldosterone would be expected to suppress proton secretion and (by slowing K^+ excretion) raise plasma $[K^+]$. In Type 4, both these effects are observed.

Perhaps surprisingly, the main cause of hypobicarbonatemia is *not* the decrease in proton secretion (which is mild) but the hyperkalemia, which acts to directly suppress ammonium production. One mechanism of ammoniogenesis suppression is as follows: As plasma $[K^+]$ rises, a gradient is created for entry of K^+ into proximal renal tubular cells. The influx of (cationic) K^+ causes, by electrical attraction, an influx of (anionic) bicarbonate, thereby raising intracellular pH. The cells "perceive" alkalemia and respond as if it were due to generalized extracellular alkalosis: by slowing ammonium excretion and, hence, bicarbonate regeneration.

Etiology.   Type 4 is the most common adult RTA. It is often found in diabetics, with hyporeninemic hypoaldosteronism being the usual cause. Primary disorders of the adrenal cortex that reduce aldosterone secretion may also be responsible; in some cases, cortisol secretion is decreased as well (e.g., Addison's disease, AIDS-associated adrenal disease). Almost all of these conditions cause some reduction in glomerular filtration rate, resulting in a modest rise in plasma levels of nitrogenous wastes.

Type 4 and Chronic Renal Failure. Type 4 RTA has much in common with chronic renal failure (CRF). Focusing on these similarities can help you better appreciate the essential features of the two conditions. There are four major similarities between Type 4 and CRF:

1. Both present with elevated creatinine and urea. However, the glomerular defect is relatively mild in Type 4 and severe in CRF. Thus, Type 4 patients typically present with relatively small elevations in creatinine and BUN. As noted above, the metabolic acidosis of CRF often presents with creatinine above 10 mg/dl, whereas a typical value for Type 4 is around 2 mg/dl. Also, because glomerular defects elevate "unmeasured anions" only if GFR is severely depressed, Type 4 patients do not present with an increased level of unmeasured anions, whereas patients with renal failure frequently do.

2. Both cause hyperkalemia. However, whereas Type 4 typically *presents* with hyperkalemia, CRF usually does not cause frank hyperkalemia until GFR falls to about 10 ml/minute (which corresponds to a creatinine of about 10 mg/dl), unless the patient is subjected to an abnormal potassium load (e.g., potassium supplement, rhabdomyolysis). In this case, hyperkalemia may appear acutely, but it is usually transient because the excess K^+ is gradually excreted by the residual functioning nephrons.

3. Both cause metabolic acidosis (i.e., hypobicarbonatemia) primarily via decreased ammonium excretion. However, in Type 4 the decrease is caused by hyperkalemia and is reversible (ammonium excretion rises almost to normal if hyperkalemia is corrected), whereas in CRF the reduction is primarily due to irreversible nephronal "drop-out," although hyperkalemia may also play a small role.

4. Both have appropriately low urine pH. In Type 4, pH is almost always less than 5.5. In CRF, pH is consistently less than 6.0 and is usually near 5.0.

To consolidate your grasp of the essential features of the RTAs, take a moment to reread the table at the beginning of this discussion (p. 150).

Summary

Metabolic acidosis, a disease process that causes an abnormal fall in plasma $[HCO_3^-]$, is compensated by a fall in PCO_2. Metabolic acidosis occurs when

ECF bicarbonate losses exceed net renal bicarbonate production. Put differently, metabolic acidosis occurs when endogenous acid production exceeds renal net acid excretion. There are four general causes of metabolic acidosis: (1) increased endogenous acid production due to sub-pyloric G.I. derangements, such as diarrhea or lower G.I. drainage; (2) increased endogenous acid production due to derangements of metabolism, especially lactic acidosis or ketoacidosis; (3) increased endogenous acid production due to ingestion of exogenous intoxicants such as methanol, ethylene glycol, or salicylates (salicylates also cause respiratory alkalosis); and (4) decreased renal net acid excretion due to either renal failure or renal tubular acidosis.

Metabolic Alkalosis

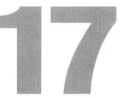

Definition

Metabolic alkalosis is a disease process that causes an abnormal rise in plasma bicarbonate concentration, thereby producing alkalemia. With the exception of renal compensation for respiratory acidosis, all hyperbicarbonatemia is abnormal. Thus, all non-compensatory hyperbicarbonatemia is, by definition, metabolic alkalosis. In patients with an intact ventilatory response, metabolic alkalosis causes compensatory hypoventilation, which raises arterial PCO_2 and mitigates the rise in plasma pH.

Introduction

The kidney has a functional reabsorptive "threshold" for bicarbonate of about 26–28 mmol per liter. If plasma $[HCO_3^-]$ exceeds this level, the fraction of filtered bicarbonate that is reabsorbed decreases, and unreabsorbed HCO_3^- is spilled into the urine. This homeostatic spillage is highly efficient and keeps plasma $[HCO_3^-]$ at the threshold level. For example, normal subjects can be given 1000 mmol of bicarbonate per day for two weeks without plasma $[HCO_3^-]$ rising substantially.

This raises a question: If excess bicarbonate is excreted so efficiently, how can the hyperbicarbonatemia of metabolic alkalosis occur? The answer is that many of the clinical conditions that act to increase plasma $[HCO_3^-]$ *have the additional effect* of raising the reabsorptive threshold for bicarbonate. As a result, reabsorption is complete, and little or no urinary bicarbonate spillage occurs, even when plasma $[HCO_3^-]$ is markedly elevated.

Thus, understanding metabolic alkalosis requires a knowledge of two sets of processes: (1) those that act to raise $[HCO_3^-]$ and (2) those that raise the reabsorptive threshold. The first process is called "generation" of the alkalosis. The second is called "maintenance" of the alkalosis. It is natural to assume that generation precedes maintenance but, in reality, both must occur simultaneously. If they did not, $[HCO_3^-]$ could not rise in the first place and there would be nothing to "maintain." Put simply, Generation + Maintenance = Metabolic Alkalosis.

To better understand these concepts, take a moment to scan this illustration, then read the paragraph that follows, referring back to the illustration as you read:

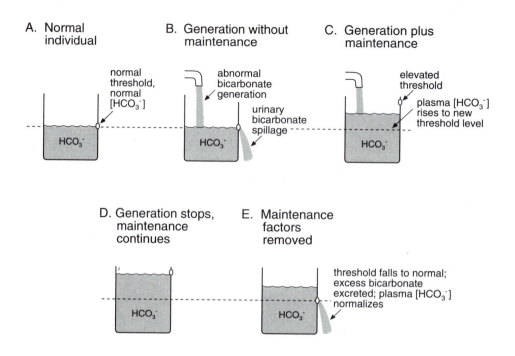

Bucket A represents a normal individual. There is no abnormal bicarbonate generation and the reabsorptive threshold is normal. Bucket B represents generation without maintenance. Excess bicarbonate is produced but the threshold is normal, so the bicarbonate spills into the urine without raising plasma [HCO_3^-]. Bucket C represents generation plus maintenance. Excess bicarbonate is produced and retained, thus raising [HCO_3^-]. No bicarbonate spills unless [HCO_3^-] reaches the new threshold level. This patient has metabolic alkalosis. Bucket D shows what happens to Bucket C if generation stops but the factors maintaining the abnormal threshold remain. Plasma [HCO_3^-] stays high. That is, metabolic alkalosis persists. Only after the reabsorptive threshold falls can the kidney excrete the excess bicarbonate, as shown in Bucket E.

The above discussion gives a broad overview of metabolic alkalosis. The rest of the chapter, which consists of two sections, looks at the details. The first section describes the factors that raise the reabsorptive threshold; i.e., maintain alkalosis. Understanding these factors provides the background for the second section, in which we look at the specific disease states associated with metabolic alkalosis.

Maintenance of metabolic alkalosis

Three main factors are responsible for maintaining metabolic alkalosis. In any given patient with metabolic alkalosis, at least one, and usually several, of these factors will be present. The three factors are:

Volume depletion
Hypokalemia
Aldosterone excess

How do these factors maintain metabolic alkalosis? We can answer this question with a general answer and a specific answer. The general answer we already know: the factors maintain alkalosis by raising the renal threshold for bicarbonate reabsorption, thereby inhibiting the excretion of excess bicarbonate. For most clinical situations, this general answer is all you need to know.

The specific answer focuses on the cellular processes that cause the threshold to rise. Our current understanding of these processes is incomplete, and many details may be modified as research continues. Therefore, as you read the details below, don't waste time memorizing. Just try to get a broad sense of the kinds of mechanisms involved.

Of the three maintenance factors, volume depletion is the most important. However, as we will see, the effects of volume depletion are partly mediated by hypokalemia and elevated aldosterone levels. We therefore discuss hypokalemia and aldosterone first, to lay a foundation for our discussion of volume depletion. An additional benefit of presenting the material in this order (Hypokalemia, Aldosterone, Volume) is that it suggests a simple mnemonic, the acronym HAV: "It's all you HAV to remember."

Hypokalemia

As noted, hypokalemia (i.e., low plasma $[K^+]$) can raise the threshold for bicarbonate reabsorption. One or more of the following mechanisms are thought to explain this effect:

1. Intracellular acidosis

Low plasma $[K^+]$ creates a cell-to-ECF diffusion gradient for K^+, and some K^+ leaves cells. To maintain electroneutrality, some intracellular bicarbonate may exit with the K^+. Intracellular $[HCO_3^-]$ falls, causing an intracellular metabolic acidosis. Inside renal tubular cells, this acidosis is "interpreted" as being due to generalized extracellular acidosis, and the renal cells react "homeostatically" by conserving extracellular bicarbonate via increased reabsorption. We can schematize the sequence in four steps, like this:

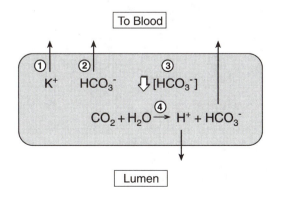

2. Increased H^+-K^+ exchange

In the distal nephron, there appears to be a population of luminal ATP-driven H^+-K^+ exchangers (in addition to the H^+–ATPase). When active, these exchangers lead to the simultaneous reabsorption of K^+ and bicarbonate. Hypokalemia may cause a homeostatic increase in the number of these exchangers. These additional exchangers apparently help conserve K^+ but also raise bicarbonate reabsorption:

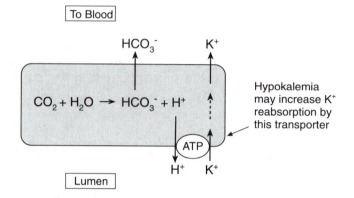

3. Reduced filtration rate

In some settings, hypokalemia may reduce glomerular filtration rate (GFR) via a vasoconstrictive effect on renal arterioles. A fall in GFR reduces the amount of bicarbonate that is filtered. If the absolute rate of bicarbonate reabsorption does not change (reabsorption is a tubular function, so it is not necessarily affected by GFR), the reabsorptive fraction increases.

4. Ammonium excretion

The above three mechanisms increase bicarbonate reabsorption. In addition, hypokalemia can stimulate ammonium excretion in the proximal tubule, thus increasing bicarbonate regeneration and, hence, raising plasma $[HCO_3^-]$. How? The mechanism described above (number 1), by which HCO_3^- follows K^+ out of renal cells, causes a fall in cell pH. Low cell pH appears to stimulate ammonium production and excretion. We can schematize the sequence in five steps, like this:

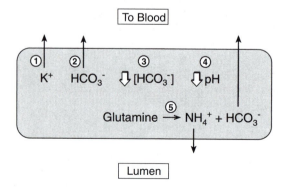

Aldosterone excess

High plasma levels of aldosterone, either secondary to volume depletion or primary (as occurs with aldosterone-secreting tumors), increase bicarbonate reabsorption. One or both of the following mechanisms are thought to mediate this increase:

1. Proton pump stimulation

By an unknown mechanism, aldosterone directly stimulates the H^+–ATPase in the collecting tubule. Increased H^+–ATPase action raises distal bicarbonate reabsorption.

2. Voltage-dependent stimulation

Aldosterone also stimulates proton secretion indirectly, via its effects on sodium and potassium. Aldosterone stimulates distal Na^+ reabsorption. The removal of Na^+ from the lumen leaves the tubular fluid with a slight negative charge, which facilitates secretion of (positive) H^+. Because this facilitation is mediated by the negative electrical charge in the lumen, it is said to be "voltage-dependent." This same luminal negative charge also facilitates secretion of (positive) K^+, promoting hypokalemia. As described above, hypokalemia both maintains metabolic alkalosis and stimulates bicarbonate regeneration.* We can illustrate these processes like this:

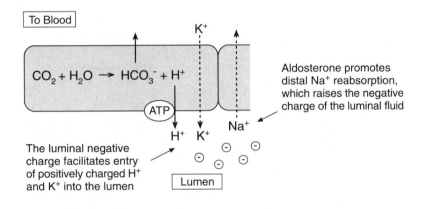

Volume depletion

Patients who lose extracellular fluid volume tend to maintain metabolic alkalosis. It appears this effect is mediated by a reduction in the amount of cir-

---

* **Going further.** What accounts for the effects of aldosterone on Na^+ and K^+? Aldosterone stimulates the basolateral Na^+–K^+–ATPase while simultaneously increasing the permeability of the luminal membrane to Na^+ and K^+. The Na^+–K^+–ATPase lowers $[Na^+]$ and raises $[K^+]$ in cells, producing a steep gradient for the reabsorption of Na^+ and the secretion of K^+. Both Na^+ reabsorption and K^+ secretion are facilitated by the increased permeability of the luminal membrane. In addition, the increased reabsorption of Na^+ increases luminal negativity, which further promotes secretion of K^+ (as well as protons).

culating blood that stimulates sensors in the vasculature (e.g., in the carotid sinuses, aortic arch, pulmonary blood vessels, and afferent glomerular arterioles). This conclusion is supported by the finding that, so long as tissue perfusion is decreased, alkalosis can be maintained even if ECF volume is normal or high.

For example, metabolic alkalosis may be maintained in patients with ascites from liver cirrhosis, or systemic edema from congestive heart failure, even though total ECF water and sodium are increased. The key factor in these cases is that much of the volume is "third spaced" (i.e., localized in the peritoneal cavity or subcutaneous tissues) and therefore does not circulate. As a result, the volume sensors "perceive" volume depletion.

It is therefore the circulatory correlates of ECF volume depletion, not ECF volume depletion itself, that maintains metabolic alkalosis. To express this idea, the phrase "effective circulating volume depletion" (or just "effective volume depletion") was coined. Using this terminology, we can say that effective circulating volume depletion maintains metabolic alkalosis. However, for the sake of brevity, the less precise term "volume depletion" is often used. This less precise usage is generally acceptable because, in most cases, ECF volume depletion and effective circulating volume depletion occur together.

With this background, we can now ask: How does effective volume depletion maintain metabolic alkalosis? Here are some likely possibilities:

1. Aldosterone excess

In response to volume depletion, the kidneys release renin, which results in high plasma levels of aldosterone (via the renin-angiotensin-aldosterone axis). As described above, high plasma [aldosterone] maintains metabolic alkalosis both directly and, by promoting hypokalemia, indirectly.

2. Angiotensin II production

The renin-angiotensin-aldosterone axis also results in high plasma levels of angiotensin II (some angiotensin II may also be produced locally, inside the kidney). Angiotensin II stimulates Na^+-H^+ exchange, and hence bicarbonate reabsorption, in the proximal tubule.

3. Adrenergic stimulation

The nervous system responds to hypovolemia by increasing alpha-adrenergic output to the kidney. By an unknown mechanism, this adrenergic stimulation increases Na^+-H^+ exchange in the proximal tubule.

4. Reduced filtration rate

Volume depletion can sometimes decrease renal blood flow, lowering filtration pressure and, hence, GFR. As discussed for hypokalemia, reduced GFR can increase reabsorptive efficiency.

5. Chloride effects

It has recently been proposed that much of the alkalosis-maintaining effect of volume depletion is mediated by the chloride ion. Specifically, the key mediating event may be a decrease in the flow of Cl^- into the lumen of the distal nephron. Note that it is not simply a low $[Cl^-]$ in the ECF or blood plasma that is proposed to maintain alkalosis; it is a deficit in the distal luminal fluid. This distinction will become clear in a moment.

The possible role of chloride is suggested by studies in which hypovolemia is treated with infusions of albumin solution. These solutions, which restore intravascular volume without raising either body stores or distal delivery of chloride, only partially correct metabolic alkalosis. However, when chloride delivery is increased, even without fully repairing the volume deficit, the alkalosis is corrected.

What causes a reduction in distal chloride delivery? Two factors act together. First, metabolic alkalosis is always accompanied by hypochloremia (i.e., low plasma $[Cl^-]$), because the excess HCO_3^- displaces Cl^- in the ECF.* Because plasma $[Cl^-]$ is low, glomerular Cl^- filtration falls, so delivery of Cl^- to all parts of the nephron is reduced. Second, volume depletion causes a homeostatic increase in Na^+ reabsorption in the proximal nephron. To maintain electroneutrality, proximal Cl^- reabsorption also increases. As more Cl^- is removed proximally, less Cl^- remains in the lumen for delivery to the distal nephron.

How does a fall in distal chloride delivery act to raise bicarbonate reabsorption? There are several possible mechanisms:

a. Renin release. The macula densa, which is located at the beginning of the distal convoluted tubule, helps sense tubular fluid flow by a mechanism dependent on Cl^- in the luminal fluid. Thus, the kidney interprets a decrease in distal Cl^- delivery as a sign of low tubular flow, and it responds as if the decreased tubular flow were caused by ECF volume depletion, with renin release. As described above, stimulation of the renin-angiotensin-aldosterone axis increases bicarbonate reabsorption.

b. Electroneutral facilitation. Low luminal $[Cl^-]$ causes a steeper gradient for the passive flux of Cl^- from interstitial fluid, across tubular cells, into the lumen. This flux of negative charges facilitates proton secretion, and the accompanying bicarbonate reabsorption, by keeping positive charges from the secreted protons from building up in the lumen. The process "looks" like this:

---

* **Going further.** For example, in metabolic alkalosis caused by gastric fluid losses, protons are secreted into the stomach along with Cl^- from the ECF, and the lost Cl^- is replaced by HCO_3^-.

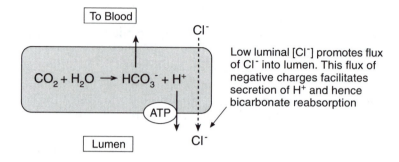

c. Decreased bicarbonate secretion.   When plasma [HCO_3^-] exceeds the renal reabsorptive threshold, most urinary spillage occurs because filtered bicarbonate remains in the lumen, unreabsorbed. In addition, recent evidence suggests that a fraction of spilled bicarbonate may enter the lumen by secretion, across the luminal membrane, in exchange for chloride. Low luminal [Cl^-] inhibits this exchange:

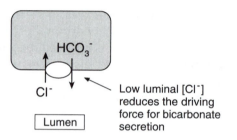

Essential facts about alkalosis maintenance

As noted previously, many of the above mechanisms are speculative and not important to remember. What is essential can be summarized in three sentences:

1. Three key factors maintain metabolic alkalosis: volume depletion (actual or effective), hypokalemia, and aldosterone excess.

2. These three factors act via various mechanisms, but all have the same effect: they raise the renal threshold for bicarbonate reabsorption, thereby inhibiting the spillage of excess bicarbonate into the urine.

3. In addition, some of the maintenance factors stimulate ammonium excretion and, hence, bicarbonate regeneration; thus, some of these factors actually can contribute to the generation of alkalosis, as well as maintenance.

We are now ready to discuss specific diseases responsible for metabolic alkalosis.

Specific disease states

Metabolic alkalosis develops in four main clinical settings: (1) loss of gastric fluid from vomiting or nasogastric drainage, (2) diuretic therapy, especially for edema, (3) mechanical ventilation of patients with COPD, and (4) a group of clinical entities known as volume-resistant metabolic alkalosis. We will now discuss each of these, focusing on how the metabolic alkalosis is generated, and on which maintenance factors come into play.

Loss of gastric fluid

During normal digestion, parietal cells in the stomach wall secrete protons into the gastric lumen, acidifying the gastric contents. These protons are produced inside the parietal cells by the reaction $CO_2 + H_2O \rightarrow H^+ + HCO_3^-$. The bicarbonate produced by this reaction crosses the basolateral cell membrane and enters the ECF. Thus, the acidification of the gastric lumen is matched by an equal and opposite alkalinization of the ECF. The figure on page 92 illustrates this concept. Take a moment to study it.

When gastric fluids are lost due to vomiting or nasogastric drainage, the stomach increases its secretory activity, the "goal" being to restore the normal fluid environment in the lumen. Thus, proton secretion into the lumen, and bicarbonate secretion into the ECF, increases. This increase persists for as long as gastric fluids are being lost. Therefore, vomiting and nasogastric drainage lead to the addition of large quantities of bicarbonate to blood.

This addition of bicarbonate to blood represents the *generation* of metabolic alkalosis during vomiting and nasogastric drainage. To understand how this alkalosis is *maintained*, it is useful to consider gastric fluid loss as a three-step process.

> *Step 1.* Gastric fluid contains Na^+, water, and K^+ ([K^+] is 5–10 mmol/l, slightly higher than in the ECF). Gastric losses thus cause ECF volume depletion and hypokalemia. However, both are initially mild and therefore do not substantially impede the urinary spillage of excess HCO_3^-. Thus, early gastric losses result in the formation *and excretion* of excess HCO_3^-.

> *Step 2.* To maintain electroneutrality, HCO_3^- spilled into the urine must be accompanied by a cation. Na^+ and K^+ serve as the accompanying cations because they are the major cations in luminal fluid. Thus, Na^+ and K^+ are now lost in both urine and gastric fluid. This exacerbates volume depletion and hypokalemia.

> *Step 3.* Worsening volume depletion leads to renal release of renin, which stimulates aldosterone secretion. Aldosterone is itself a maintenance factor, and it also increases K^+ excretion, exacerbating hypokalemia further. At this point, significant hypokalemia, aldos-

terone excess, and volume depletion (i.e., all three major maintenance factors) are present. Urinary bicarbonate spillage ceases.

Several points implicit in these steps are worth emphasizing. First, urine is initially alkaline (i.e., high pH) as HCO_3^- is spilled, but it gradually becomes acidic as the maintenance factors intensify and HCO_3^- reabsorption rises. Second, because gastric fluid $[K^+]$ is relatively low, most K^+ losses occur via the urine, stimulated by high plasma [aldosterone]. Third, once metabolic alkalosis is established, it is maintained even if gastric fluid losses cease. Only repair of volume depletion and hypokalemia will ameliorate the alkalosis (the aldosterone excess will self-correct when volume deficits are replaced).

Diuretic use

The treatment of edema (e.g., in cirrhosis, heart failure, or nephrotic syndrome) with thiazide or loop diuretics is the most common cause of metabolic alkalosis. These agents cause a saline diuresis by inhibiting the reabsorption of Na^+ and Cl^- from the luminal fluid. Because thiazide and loop agents cause metabolic alkalosis by similar mechanisms, we will discuss them together. The following can all play a role in the generation and maintenance of the alkalosis.

Contraction alkalosis

In patients who have edema or ascites, diuretics can reduce ECF volume by five or more liters. Because diuretics lead to the excretion of a low-bicarbonate saline, virtually all bicarbonate contained in the edema fluid is retained in the body. This retained bicarbonate raises extracellular $[HCO_3^-]$. For example, in a patient with a plasma $[HCO_3^-]$ of 24 mmol/l, the excretion of 5 liters of bicarbonate-free urine would add 120 mmol (i.e., 5×24) of HCO_3^- to the remaining ECF. This process is called contraction alkalosis because the rise in $[HCO_3^-]$ is caused by the "contraction" of the extracellular compartment around a fixed amount of bicarbonate. The process can be pictured like this:

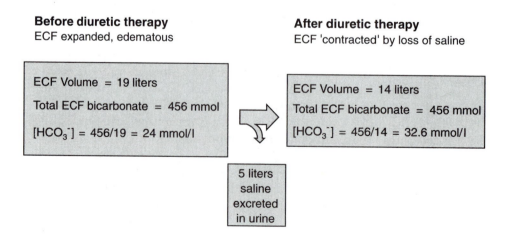

Before diuretic therapy
ECF expanded, edematous

ECF Volume = 19 liters

Total ECF bicarbonate = 456 mmol

$[HCO_3^-]$ = 456/19 = 24 mmol/l

After diuretic therapy
ECF 'contracted' by loss of saline

ECF Volume = 14 liters

Total ECF bicarbonate = 456 mmol

$[HCO_3^-]$ = 456/14 = 32.6 mmol/l

5 liters
saline
excreted
in urine

Volume depletion

In edematous states, the ECF is expanded but a substantial portion is "third spaced." Thus, most edematous patients have a degree of preexisting effective circulating volume depletion, which is further aggravated by diuretic therapy. Note: volume depletion is often confused with ECF contraction, but the two are not the same. Specifically, contraction generates alkalosis whereas volume depletion maintains it.

Aldosterone excess and hypokalemia

By a variety of mechanisms, diuretics lead to aldosterone excess and hypokalemia. First, diuretic-induced volume depletion causes a secondary increase in plasma [aldosterone], which, in turn, stimulates K^+ excretion, contributing to hypokalemia. Second, the saline diuresis caused by diuretics augments delivery of luminal Na^+ to the collecting tubule. The increased availability of Na^+ in this segment, especially in the context of elevated plasma [aldosterone], augments Na^+ reabsorption, thereby raising luminal negativity. This high luminal negativity promotes secretion of cations, especially H^+, which raises bicarbonate reabsorption, and K^+, which exacerbates the hypokalemia. Third, the saline diuresis increases fluid flow through the distal nephron. Rapid fluid flow keeps luminal $[K^+]$ low by quickly carrying away, and thus preventing the accumulation of, any K^+ that enters the lumen. The low luminal $[K^+]$ causes a steep, downhill gradient for cell-to-lumen K^+ diffusion, which results in additional K^+ losses.*

Post-hypercapnic metabolic alkalosis

The compensation for respiratory acidosis is an elevated plasma $[HCO_3^-]$. If a patient with chronic respiratory acidosis is mechanically ventilated, and PCO_2 is rapidly reduced to normal (or near-normal), there is no immediate effect on $[HCO_3^-]$, which remains elevated. The patient now has high $[HCO_3^-]$ and normal PCO_2; by definition, the patient has metabolic alkalosis. For obvious reasons, this condition is called post-hypercapnic metabolic alkalosis. It occurs most commonly when a patient with hypercapnic COPD

---

* **Clinical note.** The other two categories of diuretics, potassium-sparing and carbonic anhydrase inhibitors, do not cause metabolic alkalosis. Potassium-sparing agents (e.g., spironolactone) are mild diuretics, do not produce severe volume depletion or hypokalemia, and therefore do not, by themselves, cause metabolic alkalosis. However, because K^+-sparing agents may cause hyperkalemia, which can result in intracellular alkalosis, and hence in decreased ammonium production and proton secretion, they occasionally cause a metabolic *acidosis* characterized by hyperkalemia. Carbonic anhydrase inhibitors (e.g., acetazolamide) inhibit renal carbonic anhydrase, which is essential for efficient bicarbonate reabsorption, and therefore cause a (reversible) condition similar to Type 2 RTA.

(a disease discussed next chapter) decompensates acutely and is mechanically ventilated. We can schematize the sequence like this:

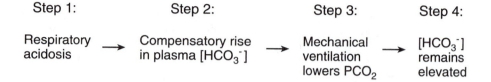

Step 1:   Step 2:   Step 3:   Step 4:

Respiratory → Compensatory rise → Mechanical → [HCO$_3^-$]
acidosis   in plasma [HCO$_3^-$]   ventilation   remains
                                                   lowers PCO$_2$ elevated

Two factors act to maintain the high [HCO$_3^-$]. First, renal compensation occurs because high PCO$_2$ in renal tubular cells causes a transient increase in bicarbonate regeneration (which adds HCO$_3^-$ to the ECF) and a sustained increase in reabsorption (which keeps [HCO$_3^-$] at its new, higher level). Although the fall in PCO$_2$ removes the stimulus for continued high rates of reabsorption, there appears to be a "memory" effect whereby reabsorption remains high for another 24 hours or so, during which time alkalosis is maintained.

Second, patients with chronic lung disease often have other diseases (e.g., cor pulmonale, hypertension) that are treated with low-salt diets and diuretics, which cause volume depletion. In these patients, metabolic alkalosis can be maintained indefinitely, until the volume (and possibly also K$^+$) deficits are replaced.

Volume-resistant metabolic alkalosis

The three causes of metabolic alkalosis discussed so far (i.e., gastric fluid loss, diuretics, and post-hypercapnic mechanical ventilation) all are associated with, and maintained by, large losses of volume and potassium. They can therefore be treated by replacing volume and potassium (via the administration of NaCl solutions and KCl). For this reason, these forms of metabolic alkalosis are often called either "volume responsive" (i.e., they "respond" to volume therapy) or "volume sensitive." In contrast, there exists a group of uncommon entities that are not maintained by volume loss and cannot be repaired by giving volume. These are called "volume resistant."

The classic example of volume-resistant metabolic alkalosis is primary hyperaldosteronism, a condition in which an intrinsic adrenal defect, such as an adrenal adenoma or adrenal hyperplasia, leads to the oversecretion of aldosterone. The elevated plasma [aldosterone] leads to urinary potassium losses and hypokalemia. The combination of aldosterone excess and hypokalemia is responsible for both generating and maintaining the metabolic alkalosis.

In all, there are over a dozen volume-resistant causes of metabolic alkalosis, most of which are quite rare. The majority are pathophysiologically similar to primary hyperaldosteronism in that an excess of aldosterone (or some other endogenous steroid with mineralocorticoid activity) causes hypokalemia and metabolic alkalosis. For example, Cushing's syndrome can cause volume-resistant metabolic alkalosis because excess cortisol and associated steroids (e.g., deoxycorticosterone) act as partial aldosterone agonists. However, several of the volume-resistant entities cause metabolic alkalosis by pathophysiologic mechanisms unrelated to aldosterone. For example, there is a rare clinical entity called Bartter's syndrome (pronounced "barters") in which the primary defect is intrinsic to the kidney.

As a memory device, you may find it helpful to recognize that the volume-resistant causes occupy a niche among the metabolic alkaloses that is somewhat analogous to the niche occupied by renal tubular acidosis (RTA) among the metabolic acidoses. Both volume-resistant metabolic alkalosis and RTA are umbrella terms. Both designate groups of distinct but related pathophysiologic entities. And both occupy a small but interesting corner of their respective primary disorder.

Taken together, the volume-resistant causes account for only about 5% of cases of metabolic alkalosis. The other 95% are volume-responsive. Thus, it is not essential to remember the individual volume-resistant entities, only the category. When you finally do encounter a volume-resistant cause, you can worry about the details then (appendix Topic K, "Rare causes of acid-base disorders," gives additional details).*

Summary

Metabolic alkalosis, a disease process that causes an abnormal rise in plasma $[HCO_3^-]$, is compensated by a rise in PCO_2. Because the kidneys normally spill excess bicarbonate into the urine, metabolic alkalosis requires the presence of one or more "maintenance" factors, which raise the renal reabsorptive threshold for filtered bicarbonate. Key maintenance factors are volume depletion, hypokalemia, and aldosterone excess. There are four major clinical causes of metabolic alkalosis: (1) loss of gastric fluid, such as occurs with vomiting or upper G.I. drainage; (2) thiazide or loop diuretics, especially for the treatment of edema; (3) post-hypercapnic metabolic alkalosis, which can occur when patients with compensated hypercapnia experience an acute fall in PCO_2. These three causes produce a metabolic alkalosis that can be repaired with volume (i.e., saline) and potassium and are therefore called "volume-responsive." In contrast, the last cause, (4), which is known as volume-resistant metabolic alkalosis, is a group of relatively rare entities that do not "respond" to volume therapy. About 95% of metabolic alkalosis cases are volume-responsive; only 5% are volume-resistant.

---

* **Terminology.** Instead of "volume responsive" and "volume resistant," some texts and clinicians use the terms "saline responsive" and "saline resistant," or (because of the proposed role of chloride in mediating the effects of volume depletion) "chloride responsive" and "chloride resistant." These pairs of terms have essentially the same meanings and can be used interchangeably.

Respiratory Acidosis

18

Definition

Respiratory acidosis is a disease process that causes an abnormal rise in arterial PCO_2, thereby producing acidemia. With the exception of respiratory compensation for metabolic alkalosis, all hypercapnia is abnormal. Thus, all non-compensatory hypercapnia is, by definition, respiratory acidosis. In patients with an intact renal response, respiratory acidosis causes a compensatory rise in plasma $[HCO_3^-]$, which mitigates the fall in plasma pH. This renal (or "metabolic") compensation takes several days to develop fully.

Patients with respiratory acidosis are sometimes said to be "retaining carbon dioxide." This phrase can give the false impression that the rate of CO_2 production exceeds that of CO_2 excretion, with the difference being "retained" in the body. In reality, there is usually a steady state for CO_2, in which CO_2 production equals CO_2 excretion, although the *level* of the steady state is abnormally high. We can illustrate this point as follows:

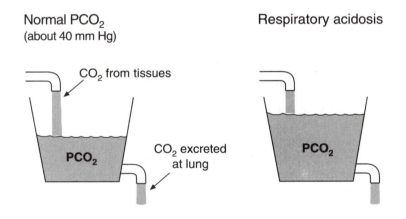

Normal PCO_2
(about 40 mm Hg)

CO_2 from tissues

PCO_2

CO_2 excreted
at lung

Respiratory acidosis

PCO_2

In contrast, during the very early stages of respiratory acidosis, for the brief period when PCO_2 is actually *rising* from its normal steady-state level to its new, higher steady-state level, CO_2 production does outpace excretion, and CO_2 actually is being retained. Thus, although the term "retaining CO_2" is commonly used as a synonym for respiratory acidosis, it is only during the early part of the process that net CO_2 is actually retained.

This chapter has four main parts. In the first part, we focus on fundamental pathophysiologic concepts. In the second part, we use these concepts to analyze the major types of problems that occur during respiratory disease. In the third part, we look at how respiratory disorders increase the amount of work that the body must do to ventilate adequately. In the last part, we look at clinical causes of respiratory acidosis.

Fundamental concepts

Arterial blood PCO_2 is directly proportional to the rate of carbon dioxide production, and inversely proportional to the rate of alveolar ventilation. That is,

$$PCO_2 \propto CO_2 \text{ Production} / \text{Alveolar ventilation}$$

This formula tells us many things. Here are some examples. If CO_2 production rises, and alveolar ventilation is constant, arterial PCO_2 rises. If alveolar ventilation falls, and CO_2 production is constant, PCO_2 rises. If alveolar ventilation rises, and CO_2 production is constant, PCO_2 falls.

Based on this formula, we might expect that respiratory acidosis can be caused by either an increase in CO_2 production or a decrease in alveolar ventilation. However, because the body can normally raise ventilatory rate to match almost any increase in CO_2 production, elevated CO_2 production does not usually affect PCO_2 unless alveolar ventilation is severely limited (e.g., due to pulmonary disease or a fixed rate of mechanical ventilation).*

In order to move forward from here, we need to review some basic respiratory concepts. Actually, we're going to start at the beginning. This will let us build on a solid foundation.

The broadest measure of ventilation is *total ventilation*. This term refers to the total amount of air that moves in and out of the respiratory tree (i.e., past the opening of the trachea) in a given amount of time. In a healthy adult of average size, total ventilation at rest is about 7.5 liters per minute. This rate is determined by both the respiratory rate (i.e., the number of breaths per minute) and the size of each breath (i.e., the *tidal volume*). The same total ventilation can be achieved by various combinations of respiratory rate and tidal volume. One typical combination is a respiratory rate of 15 and a tidal volume of 500 ml.

A term related to total ventilation is *minute ventilation*. Minute ventilation refers to the total ventilation that occurs in one minute. If you breathe normally for one minute, but exhale each breath into a large empty plastic bag, the volume of the bag is your minute ventilation. Minute ventilation = respirations per minute $\times$ average tidal volume. Because the typical adult total ventilation

---

* **Hint for the reader.** Think of how your body responds when you are doing exercise: CO_2 production increases, but ventilation increases at the same time, so arterial PCO_2 stays about the same.

is about 7.5 liters per minute, the typical adult minute ventilation is about 7.5 liters. (Notice that we don't have to say 7.5 liters *per minute*, because the time is already included in the name, *minute* ventilation.)

The respiratory system consists of conducting airways and gas exchange areas. The conducting airways comprise (in order) the trachea, mainstem bronchi, and the many branching levels of bronchioles down to the terminal bronchioles, which are the smallest bronchioles without any alveoli attached. Then the gas exchange area begins. This area comprises the next few levels of bronchioles, which are known as respiratory bronchioles because they have some alveoli attached. Then, at the very end, come the alveolar ducts and sacs—which are the passageways (ducts) and blind alleys (sacs) that are totally lined with alveoli. These ducts and sacs are where the vast majority of the alveoli are located. Although there are a few alveoli attached to the respiratory bronchioles, we will simplify and say that the lower respiratory tree consists of two distinct parts: bronchioles (which conduct air) and alveoli (which exchange gases with blood). We will disregard the respiratory bronchioles, which form the transition between these two parts.

The total volume of conducting airways (trachea and all bronchioles) is about 150 ml. That is, these airways contain about 150 ml of air. Thus, of the normal tidal volume of 500 ml, only about 350 ml ventilate the alveoli and participate in gas exchange. The other 150 ml just move in and out of the conducting airways. If we multiply a respiratory rate of 15 by 350 ml, we see that alveolar ventilation is normally about 5 liters per minute. (We are rounding off to keep the numbers simple.) Since the conducting airways don't contribute to gas exchange, they are considered "dead space." Thus, normal "dead space ventilation" is about 15×150 ml, or about 2.5 liters per minute. Since this dead space (the conducting airways) is a normal part of the body's anatomy, it is sometimes called *anatomic* dead space. The word anatomic emphasizes the fact that even though the space is "dead," it is still normal. If we add the 5 liters per minute of alveolar ventilation to the 2.5 liters per minute of anatomic dead space ventilation, we get 7.5 liters per minute of total ventilation, which is where we started.

We can now construct an equation. Minute ventilation = Alveolar ventilation + Dead space ventilation. To write this equation compactly, we can use "V" for ventilation, and the subscripts "A" for alveolar, "D" for dead space, and "E" for minute ("E" is used because minute ventilation is quantified by measuring the total amount of exhaled air). The abbreviated equation is: $V_E = V_A + V_D$. If we plug the numbers we've been using into this equation, we get $7.5 = 5.0 + 2.5$. Let's now rearrange this equation to: Alveolar ventilation = Minute ventilation − Dead space ventilation. Using symbols, this becomes: $V_A = V_E - V_D$. If we plug our working numbers into this rearranged equation, we get $5.0 = 7.5 - 2.5$.

At this point, pause for a moment to review anything that isn't clear. Don't worry about memorizing. The important thing is to follow each step of the presentation, so that things really make sense as you read them. When you are ready, keep going.

What is dead space, really? As the word space indicates, dead space is empty. It is not filled with anything except air. It is simply space. Thus, dead space refers to a part of the air cavity of the lung. It does not refer to the parenchyma of the lung. What about dead? What we mean by dead is that it is functionally dead—that is, it doesn't participate in gas exchange. Why doesn't it participate in gas exchange? Because there is no gas exchange surface. And why is there no gas exchange surface? Because there is no blood perfusing the lung surface that surrounds the air space. Thus, dead space is surrounded by a non-exchange surface of the lung, such as the conducting airways. In contrast, normal alveoli are surrounded by a continuous network of superficial capillaries, making a huge surface where air and blood are right next to each other. In this sense, alveoli form live space—functionally alive, that is. So it all comes down to this: dead space is that part of the air cavity of the lung which is ventilated but not perfused.

Let's keep going. In the normal lung, virtually all the dead space is in the conducting airways. All the rest of the air is in functioning alveoli. In the diseased lung, however, blood flow can get interrupted, so that some of the alveoli lose their perfusion. Although these alveoli may be surrounded by capillaries, and could be "alive" if the blood flow started again, they are for the moment dead. Air moves in and out of them, just like normal, but no gas exchange occurs. Thus, diseased lungs can sometimes have additional dead space—that is, normal anatomic dead space plus abnormal dead space created by unperfused alveoli. To differentiate this abnormal dead space from anatomic dead space, these unperfused alveoli are called either *alveolar* dead space or *physiologic* dead space.*

Now think back to the equation $V_E = V_A + V_D$, and to the rearranged version, $V_A = V_E - V_D$. Using the rearranged equation, notice that if lung disease impairs blood flow to some alveoli, thereby increasing dead space (V_D), alveolar ventilation (V_A) will tend to fall. As a result, PCO_2 will rise. Similarly, if dead space increases, and we want to keep V_A (and hence PCO_2) constant, we have to increase V_E. We can express this idea by saying that, when dead space increases, our "minute ventilation requirement" rises—that is, there is a rise in the V_E needed to keep PCO_2 constant. If the new, higher minute ventilation requirement is not met, PCO_2 will increase. The term *minute ventilation requirement* is important, so we'll define it explicitly: it is the level of minute ventilation needed, in any given circumstance, to keep PCO_2 constant. By definition, if minute ventilation (V_E) is less than the minute ventilation requirement, PCO_2 will rise. Pause to be sure you clearly understand this paragraph, and the term minute ventilation requirement, before going on.

---

* **Terminology.** Physiologic dead space ventilation is sometimes referred to as "wasted ventilation," since it serves no useful purpose but still requires ventilatory effort by the body.

We are now ready to look again at the "PCO_2 formula" we presented earlier:

$$PCO_2 \propto CO_2 \text{ Production} / \text{Alveolar ventilation}$$

We can also write this formula with symbols. CO_2 production can be symbolized VCO_2. (The "V" indicates "volume produced.") Using this symbol, and the symbol for alveolar ventilation, V_A, we can write the formula like this:

$$PCO_2 \propto VCO_2/V_A$$

To repeat, this is the same "PCO_2 formula" presented just above, but it is written using symbols. As we have seen, Alveolar ventilation = Minute ventilation − Dead space ventilation ($V_A = V_E - V_D$). We can use this fact to modify the PCO_2 formula slightly. Specifically, since V_A equals $V_E - V_D$, we can replace the V_A in the formula with $V_E - V_D$, like this:

$$PCO_2 \propto VCO_2/(V_E - V_D)$$

Once again, pause to be sure this formula really makes sense to you. Review the abbreviations if you need to. Be sure you see where the denominator ($V_E - V_D$) comes from. When you're ready, keep reading.

This formula tells us many things. Specifically, it lets us see how PCO_2 is affected by changes in CO_2 production, minute ventilation, and dead space ventilation. As you read the numbered points that follow, keep referring to the formula so that you see where the statements come from: (1) If CO_2 production increases, PCO_2 will rise if all else stays the same. (2) If CO_2 production increases, and dead space remains constant, the minute ventilation requirement increases; that is, we can keep PCO_2 constant by increasing minute ventilation. (3) If dead space increases, and everything else stays the same, PCO_2 will increase. (4) If dead space increases, and we want to keep PCO_2 constant, we can raise minute ventilation. (5) If CO_2 production and dead space remain constant, and we increase minute ventilation, PCO_2 will fall.

This concludes the first part of the chapter. The concepts we've just studied form the necessary foundation for all that follows. Therefore, if you are unclear on anything you have just read, spend a moment reviewing before you continue. The rest of this chapter is less dense than the above, and most readers will find it relatively easy going.*

---

* **Technical note.** In this presentation of fundamental concepts, we used standard respiratory physiology symbols, but in slightly simplified form. V_A, V_E, V_D, and VCO_2 are, formally, written with dots above the V, like this: $\dot{V}_A$, $\dot{V}_E$, $\dot{V}_D$, $\dot{V}CO_2$. In all these symbols, the V stands for "volume," but the dot indicates that we are discussing volume *per time* (or volume *per minute*) and not simply volume. Thus, using the fully elaborated symbols, V_D (no dot) indicates the actual volume of dead space in the lung (e.g., 150 ml) whereas $\dot{V}_D$ (dot) indicates dead space ventilation (e.g., 2.5 liters per minute). Although minute ventilation has no time units, it is nonetheless, by convention, often written with a dot, $\dot{V}_E$.

The nature of respiratory disease

So far, we have discussed concepts that help us understand the effect of respiratory diseases on PCO_2. We now look at the specific types of problems that occur in patients with respiratory disease—and use the concepts to help us see what is happening. The three types of problems we look at here are: neuromuscular chain defects, pulmonary disease, and increased CO_2 production. We start with . . .

Neuromuscular chain defects

Ventilation refers to the movement of air into and out of the lung. Normal ventilation requires an intact neuromuscular "chain." The chain looks like this:

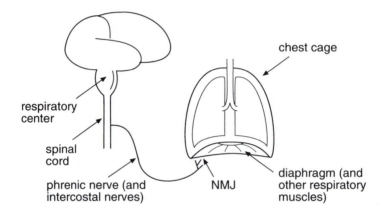

The "links" of this chain can be remembered by thinking of the steps involved in normal inspiration: the <u>respiratory center</u> initiates the neural impulse. The impulse travels down the cervical <u>spinal cord</u> and <u>phrenic nerves</u> (and intercostal nerves), then across the <u>neuromuscular junction</u> (NMJ). The respiratory <u>muscles</u>, especially the diaphragm, are stimulated and contract. These muscular contractions cause the diaphragm to flatten and the chest cage to expand, which lowers intrapleural pressure and causes the lungs to expand. Because these links are arranged in series (i.e., one after the other), normal ventilation requires that every link be intact.

When a link in the neuromuscular chain fails, minute ventilation decreases. This decrease may occur via a fall in either tidal volume or respiratory rate, or both. When minute ventilation decreases, alveolar ventilation decreases with it. The fall in alveolar ventilation causes arterial PCO_2 to rise, resulting in hypercapnia. Thus, in brief, neuromuscular chain defects reduce minute ventilation, thereby reducing alveolar ventilation, raising PCO_2 and causing hypercapnia.

One final point. A few pages ago, we saw that *minute ventilation requirement* is defined as the minute ventilation needed to keep PCO_2 constant. For example, we saw that if dead space increases, the minute ventilation requirement rises—and that if a patient can't meet this increased ventilatory requirement, hypercapnia results. The neuromuscular chain plays a key role in determining whether a person can meet their minute ventilation requirement. If the function of any part of the chain is impaired, even slightly, it may be impossible to raise minute ventilation enough to match a rising ventilatory requirement.

Pulmonary disease

The neuromuscular chain is like a machine whose job is to ventilate the lung. This machine-like task is reflected in the informal names "bellows" and "air pump," which are sometimes used to describe the final links of the ventilatory chain. Defects in this chain do not imply a defect in the lung itself, which may be normal. In contrast, the term "pulmonary disease" (or "lung disease") refers specifically to defects in the lung itself, not in the ventilatory chain—a fact that is sometimes emphasized by saying "intrinsic" pulmonary disease. Since the lung is primarily a gas exchange surface, you can think of lung disease as a gas exchange defect, in contrast to the *ventilatory* defect caused by neuromuscular chain lesions. Intrinsic pulmonary diseases typically affect the lung with uneven severity, so some areas are damaged and others are relatively normal.

What are the specific pulmonary defects that constitute pulmonary disease? The following illustration shows, in schematic form, the five major types of defects that occur in the lung. In many situations, these defects are not totally distinct from one another, but in this discussion, for clarity, we focus on their "pure" forms. First, scan the illustration. Then, as you read the text that follows, refer to the figures for visual reference:

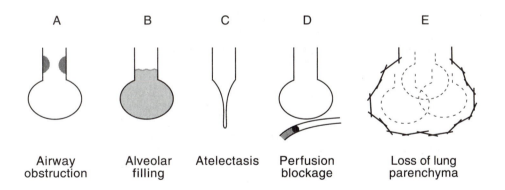

A	B	C	D	E
Airway obstruction	Alveolar filling	Atelectasis	Perfusion blockage	Loss of lung parenchyma

Figure A shows narrowing of the airway that supplies one region of alveoli. Narrowing may occur because of blockage in the lumen, thickening of the airway wall, or from contraction of smooth muscle in the airway walls. Airway narrowing reduces the amount of fresh air that reaches the alveoli. For this reason, airway narrowing can be thought of as causing "localized hypoventilation." Examples of diseases in which airways are narrowed are asthma and chronic bronchitis. Figure B shows alveoli filled with liquid or semi-liquid material. Air is entirely prevented from reaching the alveolar surface, so blood that perfuses affected alveoli does not participate in gas exchange. The blood vessels therefore act as a "shunt," effectively bypassing the lung and carrying venous blood directly into the arterial circulation. This defect is an extreme form of the localized hypoventilation seen in Figure A (because ventilation effectively falls to zero). Examples of alveolar filling and shunting occur in severe pulmonary edema, in which the alveoli fill with edema fluid, and severe pneumonia, in which alveoli fill with pus. Figure C shows the collapse of air spaces, a process known as atelectasis. If collapse is partial, ventilation is reduced, similar to Figure A. If collapse is total, ventilation is eliminated and the area acts like a shunt, as in Figure B.

Figure D shows a perfusion (i.e., blood flow) blockage. Ventilation is normal, but the loss of blood flow makes the alveoli completely ineffective as a gas exchange surface. In other words, perfusion blockage turns alveoli into dead space. An example is pulmonary thromboembolism, which occurs when a blood clot, or thrombus, lodges in the pulmonary arterial circulation. Figure E shows the loss of alveolar walls and capillaries, as happens in emphysema. This wall loss greatly reduces the area of the lung's gas exchange surface, creating abnormally large air spaces in the lung. (This process is analogous to knocking down the inside walls of a large building, which turns ordinary apartments into huge, wide-open lofts.) To the extent that ventilation is normal, this process turns normal alveoli into dead space.

What general statements can we make about these five defects? First, notice that the defects fall into two general categories. A, B, and C all decrease ventilation of the gas-exchange surface. Specifically, they directly lower alveolar ventilation, V_A. In the most extreme form (shunt), ventilation is eliminated entirely. D and E also decrease alveolar ventilation. However, they do so not by lowering alveolar ventilation per se, but by turning the alveoli into dead space, thereby increasing dead space ventilation. Since minute ventilation minus dead space ventilation equals alveolar ventilation ($V_E - V_D = V_A$), this rise in dead space effectively lowers alveolar ventilation.

Thus, by differing mechanisms, all the defects (A, B, C, D, and E), reduce alveolar ventilation, which means that the patient's minute ventilation requirement increases. That is, the presence of any of these defects means that minute ventilation, V_E, must rise if PCO_2 is to stay constant. If the new minute ventilation requirement is met, PCO_2 is stable. If the requirement is not met, hypercapnia sets in. If, for some reason, the minute ventilation requirement is *more* than met (i.e., if minute ventilation rises out of proportion to the fall in alveolar ventilation), PCO_2 falls and hypocapnia develops.

Let's look at three examples. (1) If lung disease halves alveolar ventilation (V_A), the minute ventilation requirement doubles; however, if minute ventilation (V_E) does not change, PCO_2 will double (i.e., hypercapnia). (2) If lung disease halves V_A, doubling the ventilation requirement, and V_E doubles as well, PCO_2 will remain stable (i.e., normocapnia). (3) If lung disease halves V_A, doubling the minute ventilation requirement, but for some reason V_E goes up by a factor of four, PCO_2 will fall to about half its previous level (i.e., hypocapnia).

So what happens to PCO_2 in "real life" when lung disease is present? In some cases, V_E rises proportionally to the fall in V_A, so PCO_2 is stable. In other cases, V_E doesn't increase enough, so respiratory acidosis results. In yet other cases, V_E increases disproportionately, driving PCO_2 into the hypocapnic range. Notwithstanding these different outcomes, V_E usually rises to some extent during lung disease, at least during the early stages of the disease. That is, V_E usually rises somewhat, even if it doesn't rise to the same extent as the minute ventilation requirement.

What accounts for this rise in minute ventilation? Put differently, what signals the neuromuscular chain to increase output? Several mechanisms are involved. First, lung disease directly activates pulmonary sense receptors (the disease process "tickles the lung"). This "tickling" acts as a ventilatory stimulus, increasing ventilatory drive. Second, hypoxemia, if it occurs, further increases ventilatory drive, via its effects on central and peripheral chemoreceptors. Third, to the extent that PCO_2 is elevated, hypercapnia acts as a strong ventilatory stimulus. Any or all of these mechanisms can increase central drive and hence raise V_E.

In summary, although intrinsic lung disease itself tends to reduce V_A and thus to raise arterial PCO_2, the central (i.e., ventilatory center) response is usually to increase V_E. In other words, lung disease raises the minute ventilation requirement, and the body usually responds by increasing ventilation to some degree. Depending on the magnitude of the lung defect (and hence the minute ventilation requirement), and the intensity of the ventilatory response, patients with intrinsic lung disease may present with hypercapnia, normocapnia, or hypocapnia. In general, patients with mild or moderately severe disease tend to present with hypocapnia. In contrast, patients with the most severe disease, or those who have some underlying defect in the neuromuscular chain, tend to present with hypercapnia. For example, a patient with mild pneumonia is likely to present with respiratory alkalosis. In contrast, a patient with severe pneumonia, whose respiratory muscles are failing due to overwork, may not be able to raise V_E and is likely to present with hypercapnia.

Increased carbon dioxide production

As CO_2 production increases, minute ventilation (V_E) must increase if PCO_2 is to remain constant. We can thus say that increased CO_2 production, like intrinsic lung disease, raises the patient's V_E requirement. In a patient with relatively healthy lungs, and an intact ventilatory chain, a high V_E requirement due to increased CO_2 production can easily be met. However, in patients with a defect in the ventilatory chain, or an already elevated V_E requirement due to severe lung disease, it may be impossible to raise V_E further. In these patients, increased CO_2 production can contribute to, or even precipitate, hypercapnia.

Common causes of increased CO_2 production in hospitalized patients include fever (which raises VCO_2 by about 13% per °C elevation), physical activity, anxiety, hyperthyroidism, and overfeeding with too many calories. In addition, patients with lung disease often have an elevated minute ventilation requirement, and thus may produce more CO_2 due to respiratory muscle exertion. (Like other muscles, the respiratory muscles produce more CO_2 when they do more work.) Thus, the very act of trying to meet an elevated V_E requirement can increase the V_E requirement further.

Before continuing, pause for a moment to be sure you have a "feel" for the three types of problems that can occur during respiratory disease: neuromuscular chain defects, pulmonary disease, and increased CO_2 production.

The work of breathing

Until now, we have said little about how much *work* is required to carry out ventilation during respiratory disease. For example, we described a situation where the minute ventilation requirement doubled, but we did not emphasize the extra work needed to meet this requirement. In this part of the chapter, we look at the subject of work in detail. As we will see, the work of breathing—and the patient's capacity to perform this work—are crucial determinants of whether an elevated minute ventilation requirement can be met (and, therefore, whether or not hypercapnia will develop).

The concept of respiratory load

For breathing to occur, the ventilatory muscles, especially the diaphragm, must overcome various forces. Taken together, these forces make up the respiratory "load." The higher the load, the more effort that is required, and the greater the work of breathing; the lower the load, the less effort that is required, and the lower the work of breathing. There are three main components of load:

1. *Resistance to airflow.* Airflow resistance is a function of the diameter of the airways. This resistance roughly follows Poiseuille's law, which tells us that resistance increases to the fourth power as the airway diameter decreases. Thus, if the airway diameter is halved, resistance increases about 16 times. Diseases that cause marked increases in airflow resistance are often described as "obstructive," because airways and airflow are obstructed. Asthma and chronic obstructive pulmonary disease (COPD) are classic examples of obstructive disease.

2. *Lung stiffness or elasticity.* These terms refer to the mechanical properties of the lung or chest wall that oppose expansion. A stiff or highly elastic lung is relatively non-compliant and non-deformable. More force is required to increase its volume. Diseases that cause marked increases in lung or chest wall stiffness are of-

ten described as "restrictive," because lung expansion is restricted. Pulmonary fibrosis is the classic example of a restrictive disease, although many other diseases also increase lung stiffness (e.g., atelectasis, pulmonary edema). Diseases of, or damage to, the spine or chest cage, such as kyphoscoliosis or broken ribs, can also restrict expansion, increasing work load.

3. *Ventilatory requirement.* Because ventilation requires work to overcome normal airflow resistance and lung stiffness, high minute ventilation requires more work than low minute ventilation. In many lung diseases, the minute ventilation requirement increases markedly. Similarly, high CO_2 production increases the minute ventilation requirement. Thus, many lung diseases, as well as a high CO_2 production from any cause, increases the respiratory load. Note that in the italicized heading of this paragraph we wrote "Ventilatory requirement" instead of "Minute ventilation requirement." We did so for brevity; the two terms are synonyms and can be used interchangeably.

The same disease process can affect two or even all three components of respiratory load. For example, it is common for lung diseases that increase airflow resistance or elasticity (stiffness) to also increase minute ventilation. These various components of load act together to greatly increase the work of breathing during lung disease.

The balance between load and strength

As we have seen, ventilation requires work against a load. We can describe the capacity of the neuromuscular chain to perform this work as its "strength." In health, strength is well matched to load, so the ventilatory apparatus can maintain an adequate minute ventilation with ease. In respiratory disease, however, load may exceed strength. When this happens, the neuromuscular chain cannot maintain output at a level that meets the increased ventilatory requirement. As a result, PCO_2 rises. Using these ideas, we can formulate a general explanation for hypercapnia: it occurs whenever respiratory load exceeds respiratory strength. We can portray this point visually:

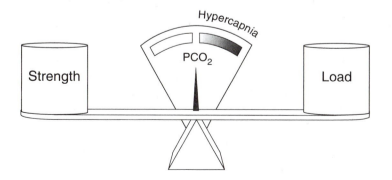

Anything that causes this "balance" to tip to the right causes hypercapnia. This rightward tip can occur in two general ways. First, if strength is impaired, hypercapnia can develop even if the load is normal. This strength impairment can occur at any point in the neuromuscular chain, from the brain to the respiratory muscles. For example, a narcotic overdose can suppress the respiratory center, causing hypercapnia. Second, if load increases, hypercapnia can occur even if respiratory strength is normal. For example, in a patient with severe asthma, the high work of breathing may overwhelm the capacity of the respiratory muscles to maintain an adequate minute ventilation. As minute ventilation falls, PCO_2 rises, even though the neuromuscular chain is essentially normal and the drive to breathe is strong.*

To emphasize the underlying physiology, we can redraw the load-strength balance as follows:

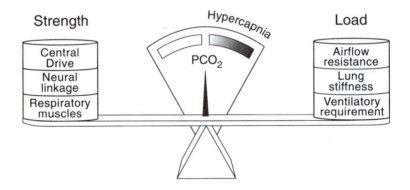

First, notice that the essential features of the balance are unchanged: the left side indicates strength, the right side indicates load, and hypercapnia results when load exceeds strength. Second, notice that the strength side of the balance comprises the neuromuscular chain which, for clarity, is broken into three segments: central drive, neural linkage, and respiratory muscles. By "neural linkage" we mean everything between the respiratory center and the respiratory muscles. Third, load is dissected into the three components discussed previously: airflow resistance, lung stiffness ("non-compliance"), and ventilatory requirement (i.e., minute ventilation requirement).

The effect of excess load on respiratory muscle function

Earlier, we hinted at the possibility that the respiratory muscles can fail when subject to excessive loads. This failure causes minute ventilation to fall and arterial PCO_2 to rise. Put differently, muscle failure reduces the patient's ability to meet the minute ventilation requirement. With this fact in mind, we can ask, *Exactly what causes muscle failure when load increases?* The

---

* **Hint for the reader.** Earlier in this book (e.g., p. 67) we used a similar balance figure to show the dependence of pH on the ratio of $[HCO_3^-]$ to PCO_2. Please don't confuse these two types of balance figures; they illustrate very different concepts.

complete answer is not known for sure, but it is useful to be aware of three different explanations that have been proposed.

First, we can see muscle failure as an expression of muscle fatigue—in the same way that, after pushing yourself to the limit and doing 30 bench presses, you might not even be able to raise your arms. Further muscle output is absolutely prevented by factors such as depletion of muscle glycogen or phosphate (required for reforming ATP), muscle injury from oxygen free radicals, accumulation of lactate or H^+, or inadequate delivery of oxygen and other substrates. The only solution for muscle fatigue is rest—that is, relief from the respiratory load that lasts long enough for the body to repair the damage and clear toxic metabolites.

Second, we can see muscle failure as resulting from a simple inability to meet the excess demand. If you try to lift your car, you probably won't succeed—not because your muscles are fatigued (although they may fatigue eventually), but simply because the car weighs too much. Similarly, some respiratory loads may simply exceed what, in engineering terms, might be called the design specifications of the respiratory muscles. In this case, since fatigue is not the problem, rest is not especially needed. What is needed is a reduction of the respiratory load to a more normal level.

Third, we can see muscle failure as resulting from a fall in central drive. In some patients, high respiratory load can lead to a decrease in central drive, thereby slowing minute ventilation. Central drive remains far above normal, but it is reduced from its previous, near-maximal level. This decrease can be conceptualized as a negative feedback of respiratory load on central drive. The process is poorly understood, but some have speculated that it may play a protective role. According to this view, the respiratory center lowers ventilatory drive to reduce the work of breathing, the goal being to prolong muscle function and delay fatigue or even ventilatory arrest (i.e., complete ventilatory standstill). The hypercapnia that may result from this reduction in central drive is seen as part of a quasi-homeostatic, muscle-protective response.*

As noted, the actual reasons why muscle function may decline when faced with excess respiratory loads is not known with certainty. All three models presented here may play some role, with one or the other of the models being most important in particular subsets of patients. It appears that the *duration* of the lung disease is one determinant of which model is most applicable. In general, muscle failure and hypercapnia are more ominous when they are of acute onset, and less ominous when they are part of a stable, chronic lung disease. We

---

* **Going further.** During stable hypercapnia, a CO_2 steady state (i.e., when CO_2 production = CO_2 excretion) is maintained at lower levels of minute ventilation and muscle output. For example, if CO_2 production and tidal volume remain constant, but PCO_2 rises from 40 mm Hg to 80 mm Hg, the CO_2 steady state can be maintained at half the minute ventilation. How is this possible? Alveolar PCO_2 equals arterial PCO_2, so each volume of exhaled air contains twice as much CO_2. Clearly, letting steady-state PCO_2 rise does result in a lower work load, even if the body is not "trying" to do this.

will say more about this difference during our discussion of specific disease entities, below. For now, the important thing is that you have a way to think about how excess load might impact (or feed back) on neuromuscular strength.

Let's summarize. Minute ventilation requirement is determined by several factors, including the possible presence of lung disease and the level of CO_2 production. If the minute ventilation requirement is met, PCO_2 is stable; if not, PCO_2 rises. The load-strength balance helps explain the factors that determine whether the minute ventilation requirement can be met. It shows that when load exceeds strength, minute ventilation requirement will not be met and PCO_2 will rise. This balance model is especially useful because it emphasizes the fact that it is the *relative* values of strength and load, not their individual values, that is important. For example, one patient (with low strength) may become hypercapnic with a low respiratory load, whereas another patient (with high strength) may maintain normocapnia even when load is very high.

Clinical causes of respiratory acidosis

We have now laid the foundation for understanding the clinical causes of respiratory acidosis—which are the focus of this last part of the chapter. In thinking about the origins of clinical hypercapnia, it is especially useful to emphasize the load-strength model presented above. That is, hypercapnia is said to develop whenever respiratory load exceeds neuromuscular strength.

The clinical causes of respiratory acidosis can be divided into two main categories: pulmonary and non-pulmonary. Pulmonary causes involve intrinsic lung disease whereas non-pulmonary causes do not. We discuss these two categories separately. In presenting the pulmonary causes, we make a further distinction between acute and chronic lung disease. We start our discussion with...

Non-pulmonary causes

Most non-pulmonary causes of respiratory acidosis involve defects in the neuromuscular chain—that is, on the "strength" side of the balance. We can discuss these defects using the same three divisions shown in the balance illustration: central drive, neural linkage, and respiratory muscles. We look at these individually.

Central drive

The most common cause of decreased central drive is drugs. Overdose with drugs that suppress ventilation can cause hypercapnia. Examples include heroin, morphine, barbiturates, "sleeping pills," and methaqualone. In patients with preexisting lung disease, therapeutic levels of medications with ventilatory suppressant effects can raise PCO_2. Examples include barbiturates, benzodiazepines, and narcotic analgesics. Less common causes of depressed central drive include lesions of the respiratory center due to stroke, trauma, tumors, or infection; and certain forms of sleep apnea.

Neural linkage

Damage or neurologic disease that affects the nerves running between the respiratory center and the respiratory muscles can cause hypercapnia. Examples include spinal cord damage above C5 (the phrenic nerves form from spinal roots at C3–C5), damage to the phrenic nerves, and diseases or other defects of nerve function or neurotransmission (e.g., poliomyelitis, amyotrophic lateral sclerosis, multiple sclerosis, Guillain-Barré syndrome, botulism, and myasthenia gravis). It is worth noting that aminoglycoside antibiotics can cause a myasthenia-like effect on neurotransmission.

Respiratory muscles

Muscle "weakness" refers to a reduction of contractile force per given level of neural stimulation. "Fatigue" is a particular type of weakness that is brought on by overwork and is relieved by muscle rest. Muscle weakness sometimes causes hypercapnia by itself, but even mild weakness can lower the threshold for muscle failure when respiratory load is increased. One common cause of muscle weakness is electrolyte depletion, especially low plasma levels of potassium or phosphate. By the time plasma $[K^+]$ falls below about 2.5 mmol/l or [phosphate] falls below about 1 mg/dl (about 0.3 mmol/l), severe muscle weakness may be present. Other important causes of muscle weakness include malnutrition, corticosteroid use, hypothyroidism, the residual effects of muscle-paralyzing drugs used in surgery, and primary muscle disease (e.g., Duchenne muscular dystrophy).*

Pulmonary causes

Pulmonary diseases (or simply "lung disease"), both acute and chronic, sometimes cause respiratory acidosis. Lung diseases almost always increase the respiratory load (via airflow resistance, lung stiffness, and/or increased ventilatory requirement). In addition, patients with lung disease may also have defects in neuromuscular strength. This strength defect may be secondary to the excess load (e.g., respiratory muscle fatigue) or it may be independent of it (e.g., respiratory muscle weakness from hypokalemia or underlying neuromuscular diseases). Let's consider acute lung diseases first.

Acute lung disease

"Acute" refers to processes that have a rapid onset and limited duration. Examples of acute lung disease include pneumonia, pulmonary edema, pul-

---

* **Going further.** The non-pulmonary causes of hypercapnia listed in the text all involve defects in the ventilatory chain, which impair respiratory strength. However, a few non-pulmonary causes produce hypercapnia by increasing respiratory load. In these cases, the high load has its origin outside the lung. Examples include disorders that restrict chest wall expansion (e.g., rib fracture, kyphoscoliosis); press upward on the diaphragm and thus impair its ability to flatten during contraction (e.g., severe abdominal obesity, ascites); and obstruct the upper airway (e.g., blockage of pharynx, larynx, or trachea).

monary embolus, and acute asthmatic episodes. In mild or moderately severe cases, acute lung diseases frequently present with hypocapnia—that is, respiratory alkalosis. The explanation, which was hinted at earlier in the chapter, can be restated as follows:

As lung disease evolves, load increases through obstruction, restriction, and/or increased minute ventilation requirement. At the same time, central drive increases, due to the stimulation of lung sense receptors and/or hypoxemia. The high central drive, acting through an intact neural linkage and a non-fatigued diaphragm, more than balances the high load. Minute ventilation exceeds the increased ventilatory requirement produced by the lung disease. As a result, PCO_2 falls into the hypocapnic range.

In many patients, this hypocapnia persists until the underlying lung disease improves, at which point PCO_2 gradually rises to normal. However, in some patients, especially those with the most severe lung disease, the very high respiratory load eventuates in respiratory muscle failure. If muscles fail, output decreases, minute ventilation falls, CO_2 is retained, and hypercapnia sets in. In other words, the load-strength balance tips to the right. If hypercapnia does develop, it usually indicates severe disease and an increased risk of respiratory collapse. It should be stressed, however, that severe or life-threatening lung disease does not always present with hypercapnia; some unstable patients may present with hypocapnia, and not develop hypercapnia until moments before ventilatory arrest (complete cessation of breathing).

When hypercapnia develops in acute lung disease, severe acidemia may be present. The reason is that the renal (or "metabolic") compensation, which raises plasma $[HCO_3{}^-]$ and thus helps return pH toward normal, takes several days to develop fully. In the interim, pH may be quite low.*

Chronic lung disease

"Chronic" refers to diseases that develop slowly and last for a long time, often years, and sometimes until the end of the patient's life. The end stage (i.e., advanced, severe, or near-terminal phase) of any chronic lung disease can cause hypercapnia. The most common example, largely because of the popularity of cigarette smoking, is chronic obstructive pulmonary disease (COPD). Because COPD is so common, we will emphasize it in this discussion.

The term "chronic obstructive pulmonary disease" refers to two overlapping disease entities: emphysema and chronic bronchitis. Emphysema is characterized by extensive destruction of lung tissue, especially the walls of distal airways and air spaces. Chronic bronchitis, in contrast, is characterized by inflammation of the airways and excess mucous production. In some patients,

---

* **Hint for the reader.** Because acute lung diseases frequently present with respiratory alkalosis, we devote more detailed attention to these diseases in Chapter 19, *Respiratory Alkalosis.*

both emphysema and chronic bronchitis play important roles. In others, one of the conditions clearly dominates the clinical picture. The adjectives "chronic" and "obstructive" are appropriate because emphysema and chronic bronchitis both cause persistent airflow obstruction that is largely incurable.

In general, hypercapnia is most common among patients with a chronic bronchitic (inflammatory, mucous-producing) pattern of disease, although even among these patients only some develop hypercapnia. Hypercapnia is much less common in patients with the emphysematous (tissue destruction) pattern of disease. If hypercapnia appears at all in emphysematous patients, it usually does so quite late in the course of the disease.

Unlike in acute lung disease, where hypercapnia often indicates severe respiratory failure (and, in some patients, may even signal the need for mechanical ventilation), patients with chronic hypercapnia may remain relatively stable for long periods. In fact, COPD patients may have stable hypercapnia for *years*. Some researchers have theorized that, in COPD patients, hypercapnia may be partly due to a muscle-protective decrease in central drive, as described earlier in the chapter.

In contrast to patients with acute hypercapnia, those with chronic stable hypercapnia have plenty of time for renal compensation to raise plasma $[HCO_3^-]$, so acidemia is mild. However, although these chronic patients are relatively stable and not seriously acidemic, they nonetheless remain in a precarious position. They "live on the edge of a precipice." Any acute medical stress can rapidly raise PCO_2 to a higher level, and severe acidemia can develop. Such acutely-worsened patients are said to have "acute-on-chronic hypercapnia" or "acute-on-chronic ventilatory failure." Examples of stresses that can precipitate this acute rise in PCO_2 include: worsening of the underlying lung disease, a superimposed lung infection, the onset of congestive heart failure with pulmonary edema, sedation with drugs that lower central drive, and sepsis.

Summary

Respiratory acidosis is defined as an abnormal rise in arterial PCO_2. The minute ventilation requirement, defined as the minute ventilation needed to keep PCO_2 stable, rises with lung disease and with increased CO_2 production. The work of breathing, and the body's ability to do this work, determine whether minute ventilation can match ventilatory requirement. If strength matches load, minute ventilation keeps pace with the ventilatory requirement, and PCO_2 is stable. If load exceeds strength, minute ventilation cannot keep pace with ventilatory requirement, and PCO_2 rises. Strength is a function of the neuromuscular chain, which runs from the brain to the respiratory muscles. Load is a function of airflow resistance, lung or chest wall stiffness, and minute ventilation requirement. Clinical causes of hypercapnia are either non-pulmonary or pulmonary. Non-pulmonary causes include defects in any "link" of the neuromuscular chain. Pulmonary causes may be acute or chronic. Acute pulmonary disease often presents with hypocapnia, but PCO_2 may rise with severe disease or failing respiratory muscles. Patients with chronic hypercapnia from lung disease are relatively stable and well compensated, but are at constant risk for an acute rise in PCO_2, with severe acidemia, due to many pathologic stresses. Chronic bronchitic COPD is the most common cause of chronic hypercapnia.

Respiratory Alkalosis

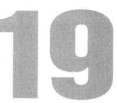

Definition

Respiratory alkalosis is a disease process that causes an abnormal fall in arterial PCO_2, thereby producing alkalemia. With the exception of respiratory compensation for metabolic acidosis, all hypocapnia is abnormal. Thus, all non-compensatory hypocapnia is, by definition, respiratory alkalosis. In patients with an intact renal response, respiratory alkalosis causes a compensatory fall in plasma $[HCO_3^-]$, which mitigates the rise in plasma pH. This renal (or "metabolic") compensation takes several days to become fully apparent.*

Hyperventilating patients are sometimes said to be "blowing off carbon dioxide." This phrase can give the false impression that CO_2 excretion is outpacing CO_2 production, with the difference being "blown off." In reality, there is usually a steady state for CO_2, although the *level* of the steady state is abnormally low. It is only during the very early stages of hyperventilation, for the brief period when PCO_2 is actually *falling* from its normal steady-state level to its new, reduced steady-state level, that CO_2 excretion outpaces production. Thus, both normal individuals and patients with respiratory alkalosis are generally in steady state for CO_2. We saw this same concept (in reverse) when we studied respiratory acidosis. The following illustration makes this point:

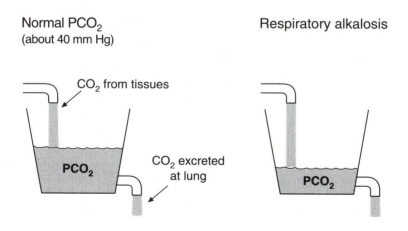

Normal PCO_2
(about 40 mm Hg)

CO_2 from tissues

PCO_2

CO_2 excreted
at lung

Respiratory alkalosis

PCO_2

---

* **Important note.** This chapter builds on concepts presented in Chapter 18, *Respiratory Acidosis*. Readers who have not already done so should read that chapter first.

Introduction

As we saw in the previous chapter (Chapter 18), arterial PCO_2 is directly proportional to CO_2 production, and inversely proportional to alveolar ventilation:

$$PCO_2 \propto CO_2 \text{ Production}/\text{Alveolar ventilation}$$

In theory, then, respiratory alkalosis can result from either a fall in CO_2 production or a rise in alveolar ventilation. However, in health, the body slows minute ventilation, and hence alveolar ventilation, to match almost any decrease in CO_2 production, thereby keeping PCO_2 constant. (Think of how your breathing slows down when you are sitting quietly.) Therefore, respiratory alkalosis is caused by a level of alveolar ventilation that is inappropriately high for the level of carbon dioxide production, a relationship sometimes called "relative hyperventilation."

This abnormally high ventilatory level occurs when some pathologic factor acts, directly or indirectly, as a stimulus to the respiratory center. In contrast to respiratory acidosis, which can be caused by a defect anywhere along the neuromuscular chain, respiratory alkalosis can occur only if (1) the entire neuromuscular chain is intact and (2) the respiratory center is pacing the chain to produce a high minute ventilation. In other words, respiratory alkalosis is caused by an increase in central drive.

The rest of this chapter has three parts. The first examines pathologic factors that can increase central drive, thereby stimulating ventilation and contributing to respiratory alkalosis. The second part "revisits" the load-strength balance, as well as some basic pathophysiologic concepts. The third part focuses on clinical disorders that cause respiratory alkalosis.

Abnormal stimuli for ventilation

Four conditions can act as abnormal ventilatory stimuli, increasing central drive: (1) arterial hypoxemia or tissue hypoxia, (2) direct stimulation of pulmonary sense receptors by a disease process in the lung, (3) chemical or physical factors that directly affect the medullary respiratory center, and (4) psychologic factors. The role of hypoxemia and lung disease in stimulating ventilation were already mentioned in the previous chapter, but we discuss them here in more detail.

Hypoxemia and tissue hypoxia

Arterial hypoxemia is sensed by chemoreceptors in the aortic arch ("aortic bodies") and at the bifurcation of the carotid arteries ("carotid bodies"). These receptors signal the medullary respiratory center, via neural impulses, to increase ventilatory drive. The increased ventilation homeostatically raises arterial PO_2 but, in the process, lowers PCO_2.

The hypoxemic stimulation to ventilation increases linearly as arterial oxygen saturation falls. Thus, any fall in O_2 saturation causes an increase in ventilatory drive. Because of the "sigmoidal" shape of the hemoglobin saturation curve, most patients have adequate saturation (i.e., above 90%) as long as PO_2 is above 60 mm Hg. Once PO_2 falls below about 60 mm Hg, saturation declines markedly and hypoxemic drive becomes increasingly strong.

The effect of hypoxemia on central drive is modified by several factors. For example, hypoxemic drive is potentiated by hypercapnia. That is, hypoxemic drive is stronger when PCO_2 is high and weaker when PCO_2 is low. This makes sense when you realize that hypercapnia is itself a strong ventilatory stimulus. Therefore, in a patient with respiratory alkalosis, hypoxemic drive is stronger when hypocapnia is mild, and weaker when hypocapnia is severe, all else being equal. (In patients with respiratory acidosis, PCO_2 is frankly elevated, so the potentiation of hypoxemic drive is very strong.) Hypoxemic drive also tends to be stronger when hypoxemia is acute. The reason why chronic hypoxemia is a weaker ventilatory stimulus is not well understood. It is possibly related to the fact that, when hypoxemia is chronic, the body has time to effect homeostatic changes that increase oxygen delivery and unloading (e.g., hematocrit rises, red cell [2,3-DPG] increases).

Certain conditions cause tissue hypoxia even without producing arterial hypoxemia. (Recall that hypoxemia refers to low oxygen levels *in blood*, whereas hypoxia refers to decreased tissue oxygenation from any cause.) These hypoxic conditions also raise ventilatory drive. Examples include severe anemia, severe hypotension, and carbon monoxide poisoning. Although arterial PO_2 is normal, these conditions cause hypoxia because less oxygen is delivered to, or unloaded at, the tissues.

Stimulation of pulmonary sense receptors

The walls of alveoli and conducting airways contain specialized sense receptors, including stretch receptors ("mechanoreceptors") and irritant receptors (i.e., chemoreceptors). When stimulated by lung disease, these receptors increase their neural output to the respiratory center, which can cause hyperventilation. For example, edema fluid in either the lung interstitium or airspaces can stimulate the stretch receptors, and purulent debris from a bacterial pneumonia can stimulate the irritant receptors. These sense receptors can cause hyperventilation even if PO_2 and oxygen delivery are normal.

Direct stimulation of the respiratory center

Various toxic, pharmacologic, mechanical, and physical insults to the medullary respiratory center can cause hyperventilation. These insults include normal physiologic factors (e.g., elevated progesterone during pregnancy), endogenous pathologic factors (e.g., un-detoxified waste products in liver disease), and exogenous agents (e.g., salicylates). Sepsis, fever, and trauma can also act to stimulate ventilation.

Psychologic factors

A variety of cortical and, possibly, subcortical influences can produce hyperventilation. These include anxiety, stress, fear, and pain. Although this hyperventilation can often be temporarily overridden by conscious effort, the pathways mediating hyperventilation are largely involuntary. The ability of the cortex to transiently affect ventilation is clearly seen when an individual voluntarily hyperventilates or breath-holds.

In summary, respiratory alkalosis is caused by an abnormal level of respiratory center stimulation. Four main factors are responsible: arterial hypoxemia or tissue hypoxia, stimulation of lung sense receptors by pulmonary disease, direct simulation of the respiratory center by physical or chemical factors, and psychologic factors. These stimuli can occur individually or in combination. For example, in bacterial pneumonia, all of the following may stimulate ventilation: hypoxemia, hypoxia, stretch and irritant receptors in the lung, fever, and anxiety.

The load-strength balance revisited

In the previous chapter (Chapter 18), we presented the concept of the load-strength balance. To illustrate the load-strength concept, we used a figure similar to the following. Scan this figure briefly, then keep reading:

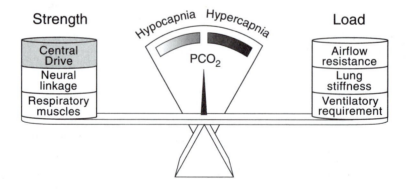

This balance is the same as the one presented in the last chapter, but we've added a region labeled "hypocapnia." In the last chapter, we saw that if load exceeds strength, PCO_2 rises. This is still true. But the converse is also true: if neuromuscular output (strength) exceeds load, minute ventilation will increase excessively and PCO_2 will fall into the hypocapnic range. Notice also that we have shaded the "central drive" component of strength. We did this to emphasize the crucial role of central drive in respiratory alkalosis—specifically, to indicate that abnormal increases in neuromuscular output occur only when central drive is elevated. Take a moment to study the balance figure, so you see clearly how the load-strength model can help explain either hypercapnia or hypocapnia.

In the last chapter, we explained how a patient with lung disease may present with respiratory alkalosis, develop respiratory muscle failure, and then become hypercapnic. We can now visualize this process. Refer to the balance illustration as you read. In lung disease, central drive may be elevated to the point that neuromuscular output exceeds load, which tips the balance left and causes hypocapnia. This leftward tip of the balance indicates a condition in which minute ventilation exceeds the minute ventilation requirement or, put differently, in which alveolar ventilation is higher than is appropriate for the level of CO_2 production. However, if load increases, or muscle strength decreases, to the point where load exceeds strength, then minute ventilation falls, the balance tips to the right, and PCO_2 rises—first to a normal (or normal-appearing) PCO_2, then to frank hypercapnia. This rightward tip of the balance indicates that the minute ventilation requirement is no longer being met.

To summarize, the load-strength balance model can be used to explain any level of PCO_2, or any change in this level. The balance model treats arterial PCO_2 as a dependent variable, which can be altered by a change in either (or both) of two independent variables, neuromuscular strength and respiratory load. When strength exceeds load, minute ventilation rises and arterial PCO_2 falls. When load exceeds strength, minute ventilation falls and PCO_2 rises. When strength is well-matched to load, minute ventilation (and hence alveolar ventilation) is appropriate for the level of CO_2 production, so arterial PCO_2 remains stable in the normocapnic range.

Clinical causes of respiratory alkalosis

The clinical conditions that cause respiratory alkalosis fall into two groups: those that involve intrinsic lung abnormalities ("pulmonary causes") and those that do not ("non-pulmonary causes"). These same two categories are distinguished in respiratory acidosis. We look at pulmonary causes first.

Pulmonary causes

Many pulmonary diseases can cause respiratory alkalosis. Examples include pneumonia, pulmonary embolus, interstitial fibrosis, asthma, and pulmonary edema. Not only *can* most lung diseases cause respiratory alkalosis, they often do. The following paragraphs describe the mechanisms that account for hyperventilation.

Pneumonia

Respiratory alkalosis is common in patients with pneumonia. In mild pneumonia, or early in the progression of more severe cases, PO_2 may be normal or only slightly low. However, hyperventilation with hypocapnia may nonetheless be present because of stimulation of pulmonary sense receptors by inflammatory debris in alveoli and airways. In severe cases, significant hypoxemia can develop and play an important role in mediating hyperventilation. Fever also stimulates ventilation.

Pulmonary edema

Pulmonary edema may be either cardiogenic or non-cardiogenic. In both cases, a major stimulus to ventilation is the presence of edema fluid in the interstitium ("interstitial edema") and, in more advanced cases, alveolar air spaces ("alveolar edema"). Hypoxemia also plays an important role in increasing respiratory drive.*

Pulmonary embolus

Pulmonary embolism causes hyperventilation by a variety of mechanisms, including stimulation of pulmonary sense receptors, hypoxemia, and sometimes pain.

Interstitial fibrosis

Interstitial fibrosis is a type of diffuse lung disease ("diffuse" means not localized, affecting the whole lung) in which alveolar walls are thickened, in part due to infiltration of the walls with fibroblasts and the subsequent deposition of thick collagen bundles. This condition can lead to hyperventilation by inducing hypoxemia and/or stimulating sense receptors in the lung parenchyma.

Asthma

During an acute asthmatic episode, hypertrophied smooth muscle in the walls of small airways contracts, narrowing the lumina and increasing resistance to air flow. Luminal narrowing is further aggravated by thickening of the airway walls due to intramural edema, inflammatory cell infiltration, and mucous gland hypertrophy. In addition, viscous mucus may obstruct the lumina ("mucous plugging"). Patients with acute asthma often present with respiratory alkalosis, caused by a combination of hypoxemia, stimulation of pulmonary sense receptors, and anxiety.

The progression to respiratory acidosis

As we have just seen, in many lung diseases, increased ventilatory drive due to stimulation of pulmonary sense receptors, hypoxemia, fever, pain, anxiety, and other factors leads to hyperventilation and respiratory alkalosis. Thus, hypocapnia (i.e., respiratory alkalosis) is present in many patients with lung disease.

However, it is essential to recognize that in patients with more severe lung disease, PCO_2 may rise and hypercapnia (i.e., respiratory acidosis) may su-

---

* **Terminology.** Cardiogenic (etymology: heart-caused) pulmonary edema is caused by increased pulmonary vascular back-pressure secondary to impaired left heart function (e.g., CHF). Other names for this entity are "cardiac," "high-pressure," or "hydrostatic" pulmonary edema. Non-cardiogenic (not heart-caused) pulmonary edema is caused by abnormal capillary permeability; vascular pressure is normal. Other names for non-cardiogenic pulmonary edema are "non-cardiac," "low-pressure," or "capillary leak" pulmonary edema. ARDS, an acronym for acute respiratory distress syndrome, also refers to non-cardiogenic pulmonary edema.

pervene. The rise in PCO_2 can result from a combination of factors, which raise the minute ventilation requirement and, simultaneously, impair the ventilatory system's capacity to meet that high requirement. For example, severe intrinsic lung disease and high CO_2 production (from vigorous respiratory muscle activity) both raise the minute ventilation requirement. Simultaneously, increased respiratory load from high airflow resistance or lung stiffness can cause the respiratory muscles to fail, impairing minute ventilation. In short, the very same diseases that can cause respiratory alkalosis can also cause respiratory acidosis. For example, pneumonia, pulmonary edema, pulmonary embolus, and asthma all can present with either respiratory alkalosis or acidosis.

Thus, although hypocapnia is quite common in acute lung disease, hypercapnia is not rare, and it may indicate an especially urgent clinical situation. For example, a patient with pneumonia who presents to the emergency department with respiratory alkalosis but progresses to respiratory acidosis may be in danger of ventilatory collapse. In fact, in a patient with respiratory alkalosis, *any* marked rise in PCO_2 not attributable to improvement of the underlying lung disease may signal muscle failure. Thus, a rise in PCO_2 from 25 to 35 mm Hg, or the onset of normocapnia, without significant underlying improvement, may represent a medical emergency. Similarly, if a patient with severe acute lung disease (hypoxemia, clinical distress, etc.) presents with a "normal" PCO_2, it may indicate that the patient passed through the respiratory alkalosis phase before presentation and is now decompensating.

Non-pulmonary causes

Sepsis

Sepsis, septic syndrome, and septicemia all refer to the entrance into the blood steam of pathogenic microorganisms—or of toxic byproducts from the microorganisms or host cells—leading to systemic (i.e., body-wide) clinical manifestations. Hyperventilation with respiratory alkalosis is common in these patients. Causes include gram-negative, gram-positive, and fungal organisms. Several mechanisms may mediate the hyperventilation, including stimulation of respiratory chemoreceptors by cytokines and other toxic byproducts.

Liver disease

Respiratory alkalosis can develop with all types of serious, chronic liver disease. With moderate hepatic dysfunction, a fall in PCO_2 of between 5 and 10 mm Hg is typical. With severe dysfunction accompanied by encephalopathy, PCO_2 may fall to below 30 mm Hg. Three hypotheses proposed to account for the hyperventilation are: an increase in plasma progesterone and estradiol; an increase in plasma nitrogenous waste products (which are usually deaminated by the liver); and hypoxemia secondary to intrapulmonary right-to-left shunting from anastomotic vascular dilatations in the lung (these vascular dilatations are analogous, and may be pathophysiologically related, to the "spider nevi" that appear on the skin in patients with liver disease).

Salicylate intoxication

Salicylate intoxication causes both respiratory alkalosis and metabolic acidosis. It is discussed in Chapter 16, *Metabolic Acidosis* (p. 147).

Hemodialysis

Patients frequently develop mild respiratory alkalosis and hypoxemia during dialysis sessions. The hypocapnia may result partly from diffusion of dissolved CO_2 from blood into the dialysis bath. It has been hypothesized that the body responds homeostatically to this fall in PCO_2 by slowing ventilation, thereby causing mild hypoxemia. This hypoxemia may drive ventilation enough to prevent full normalization of PCO_2. Another hypothesis is that, when dialysis membranes are incompletely biocompatible, aggregates of leukocytes form on the dialysis membrane and embolize into the pulmonary microcirculation. There, the aggregates may inhibit pulmonary oxygen uptake, leading to mild hypoxemia and hence hyperventilation.

Brain lesions

Cerebrovascular accidents (i.e., stroke), and brain trauma, tumors, infections, and inflammation can cause either hyper- or hypoventilation. The hyperventilatory syndromes have two general forms: (1) Midbrain lesions (especially strokes) can cause *central hyperventilation*, which is characterized by constant, rapid, deep breathing. (2) Diffuse injuries (often secondary to trauma, hemorrhage, or chronic hypoxia) can cause *Cheyne-Stokes respiration* (pronounced "chain-stokes," sometimes called periodic respiration), which is characterized by alternating periods of hyperventilation and apnea.

Cyanotic heart disease

Any cardiac disorder that causes right-to-left shunting (e.g., septal defects or patent ductus arteriosus with reversal of flow) can lead to hypoxemia with secondary hyperventilation and respiratory alkalosis.

Pregnancy

Respiratory alkalosis is a normal part of pregnancy and is not pathologic. Stimulation of the respiratory center by progesterone is the probable mechanism. Hyperventilation begins early in pregnancy, becomes maximal by the end of the first trimester (13 weeks), and continues unabated until after parturition (i.e., birth), when plasma progesterone falls to prepregnancy levels. On average, PCO_2 during pregnancy falls to approximately 30 mm Hg (i.e., a 10 mm decrease). Renal compensation lowers plasma $[HCO_3^-]$ to 18–20 mmol/l. Plasma pH is high-normal, averaging 7.44. An awareness of these laboratory values is important if one is to avoid mistakenly diagnosing a pathologic acid-base disorder. Because

$[HCO_3^-]$ and hence "buffer reserve" is low, pregnant women are relatively susceptible to significant hypobicarbonatemia if they develop metabolic acidosis. The hyperventilation of pregnancy may be associated with a sense of mild dyspnea.*

Psychogenic hyperventilation

Some people hyperventilate in response to psychologic stimuli such as anxiety, stress, fear, anger, or pain. Individuals of both sexes and all ages are affected. In these patients, the abnormal sensations produced by hypocapnia and alkalemia add to the underlying anxiety, contributing to a vicious cycle of continued hyperventilation. Two patient groups are recognized. One comprises patients who experience the acute onset of a single or occasional episode of hyperventilation. The other group comprises patients who chronically hyperventilate via increases in either respiratory rate or depth (sometimes manifested by frequent sighs, which represent increased tidal volume). These latter patients may show a degree of chronic hypobicarbonatemia (several mmol/l below normal) due to renal compensation, and they can rapidly become symptomatic if psychologic factors produce a small, additional fall in PCO_2. Psychogenic hyperventilation is sometimes called "primary hyperventilation," "anxiety-hyperventilation syndrome," or simply "hyperventilation syndrome." In some patients, psychogenic hyperventilation may represent a panic attack, with repeat episodes being an expression of panic disorder.

High altitude

Arterial PO_2 can never exceed atmospheric PO_2 unless supplemental oxygen is given. Atmospheric PO_2 at sea level is about 160 mm Hg (i.e., 760 mm Hg $\times$ 21% O_2 = 160 mm Hg). With increasing altitude, atmospheric pressure falls, and atmospheric PO_2 decreases proportionately. For example, at 4500 meters elevation, atmospheric PO_2 is about 80 mm Hg. At altitudes that cause alveolar PO_2 to approach 65 mm Hg, hypoxemia-induced hyperventilation is prominent. Extreme example: a climber at the peak of Mt. Everest (8848 m) had an arterial PO_2 of 29 mm Hg and a PCO_2 of 8 mm Hg.

Clinicians sometimes encounter this type of respiratory alkalosis in patients who take ski vacations at high altitudes. Individuals living at high altitudes may also experience respiratory alkalosis, but hypocapnia is less severe because chronic hypoxia leads to homeostatic physiological changes (p. 191).

---

* **Clinical note.** During childbirth, stress and pain cause hyperventilation to intensify further. During the luteal phase of the menstrual cycle, plasma progesterone levels are also elevated somewhat, resulting in mild hyperventilation and a modest fall in PCO_2.

Patients with lung disease who travel to high altitudes experience more profound hypoxemia than people with normal lungs.*

Summary

Respiratory alkalosis is defined as an abnormal fall in arterial PCO_2. Respiratory alkalosis is caused by an abnormal stimulus to ventilation, especially hypoxemia or tissue hypoxia, stimulation of lung sense receptors by pulmonary disease, chemical or physical factors that directly affect the respiratory center, and psychologic factors. Clinical causes are pulmonary or non-pulmonary. Pulmonary causes include most of the common pulmonary diseases. These pulmonary diseases most typically cause respiratory alkalosis but may eventuate in respiratory acidosis if they are very severe or associated with respiratory muscle failure. Non-pulmonary causes include sepsis, liver disease, salicylate intoxication, brain lesions, cyanotic heart disease, pregnancy, and psychogenic hyperventilation. Patients with acute respiratory alkalosis have relatively severe alkalemia, because the renal compensatory response (a fall in plasma HCO_3^-]), which mitigates the rise in pH, takes several days to develop. Patients with well-compensated, chronic respiratory alkalosis have relatively mild alkalemia.

---

* **Frequent flyers.** Modern commercial jets are pressurized, not to sea level pressure, but to an equivalent ("cabin altitude") of about 8000 feet. The reduced PO_2 lowers the arterial oxygen saturation (SaO_2) of passengers and crew. Even healthy individuals may transiently experience SaO_2s below 90% (some may even nadir at 80–82%). These levels may be dangerous to patients with unstable angina or severe CHF. Recent cigarette smoking or lung disease, including severe COPD, lowers SaO_2 still further. The major U.S. airlines can provide, with advance notice and physician confirmation, in-flight supplemental oxygen to ill passengers.

Self-Assessment Quiz

This quiz tests your knowledge of core concepts and facts. More importantly, the process of taking and correcting the quiz will strengthen your understanding of the essentials. To get the most from this process, answer all questions in writing. Use a separate answer sheet if you wish. Take your time. When you finish, check your answers against the key. It doesn't matter whether you ace this quiz or fail it. The important thing is to grapple with the questions and then, for those that you miss, to study the correct answers carefully.

1. Match the members of these two columns:

metabolic acidosis	high blood pH
metabolic alkalosis	hypercapnic acidosis
acidemia	hypobicarbonatemic acidosis
respiratory acidosis	hyperbicarbonatemic alkalosis
alkalemia	low blood pH
respiratory alkalosis	hypocapnic alkalosis

2. Can acidemia exist without acidosis? If so, how?

3. Can acidosis exist without acidemia? If so, how?

4. Simple acid-base disturbances are those that involve only one _____ disturbance.

5. Mixed disturbances are also called _____ disturbances. These involve _____ or more _____ disturbances. List the four primary disturbances.

6. Compensation follows the "_____-_____ rule."

7. Which disturbances are generally better compensated: metabolic or respiratory?

8. Compensation stabilizes pH most effectively during which primary disturbance? This is the one disturbance in which pH may actually be in the _____ _____.

9. Respiratory compensation is relatively rapid. PCO_2 will usually reach its new, _____-_____ level within about _____ hours.

10. Metabolic compensation is relatively slow. It will generally require at least two days for plasma _____ to approach its new steady-state level. The usual time required is _____-_____ days for respiratory alkalosis, and _____-_____ days for respiratory acidosis.

11. Bone buffering can occur during metabolic acidosis. When it does, urinary excretion of which ion will rise markedly?

12. Metabolic acidosis can be grouped into four general categories: derangements of _____, _____, and _____, plus exogenous _____.

13. The major gastrointestinal cause of metabolic acidosis is _____. It produces acidosis because it increases secretion by the gut, especially by the colon, of _____ into the extracellular fluid. This secretion matches, 1:1, the secretion of _____ into the gut lumen.

14. Severe diarrhea lowers plasma $[HCO_3^-]$ and causes acidemia. Name two other major fluid and electrolyte effects of diarrhea.

15. Consider the sentence, "Metabolic disturbances can cause metabolic acidosis." The first "metabolic" refers to the pathways of _____ and _____ (sometimes called _____ metabolism). The second "metabolic" indicates a process that alters _____ _____.

16. The production of organic acids does not necessarily cause plasma $[HCO_3^-]$ to fall. Plasma $[HCO_3^-]$ can be stable because acid _____ may be matched by the metabolic consumption of the organic _____. This metabolic consumption generates _____.

17. The two most common clinical causes of lactic acidosis are forms of shock. They are _____ shock and _____ shock.

18. Most forms of lactic acidosis, including the two forms of shock just mentioned, involve, as part of their pathophysiology, decreased delivery of _____ to the tissues.

19. In lactic acidosis and ketoacidosis, organic anions that are not spilled in the urine can ultimately be metabolized to _____. Once these anions are lost in urine, new bicarbonate must be produced by the _____.

20. Draw the structures of acetone, lactic acid, acetoacetic acid, and beta-hydroxybutyric acid. Do as complete a job as you can by memory. When you have gone as far as you can, read the following hints, one sentence at a time, and make as many modifications as you can based on each hint.

Hints: The three acids are carboxylic acids. Acetone and lactic acid have three carbons. Acetone is a ketone. Lactic acid is alpha-hydroxypropionic acid. Acetoacetic and beta-hydroxybutyric acids are both modified butyric acid. Butyric acid is straight-chain and has four carbons. Beta-hydroxybutyric acid, while considered a "ketone body," is not a true ketone. Another name for acetoacetic acid is beta-ketobutyric acid. Carbons are counted by Greek letter from the acid group to the tail, starting with the carbon adjacent to the carboxyl carbon.

21. You smell acetone on the breath of a comatose child. What is the most likely cause? If you could give this child one substance in an intravenous solution, what would it be? Can you name an additional cause of acetone-breath that is common in adults?

22. Draw the structure for ethanol (ethyl alcohol). Two substances with similar chemical structures can cause severe metabolic acidosis if ingested. Name them and draw their structures.

23. Follow-up question. During the metabolism of the two toxic substances just discussed, the alcohol groups are sequentially converted into _____ groups and then _____ groups. These last groups liberate _____ because their pK is much lower/higher (choose one) than the pH of extracellular fluid.

24. Follow-up question. These two sequential conversions are carried out by enzymes. Name the two enzymes.

25. Salicylate intoxication can cause a mixed acid-base disturbance. The two primary disturbances are _____ and _____. In young children, [HCO_3^-] and pH both tend to be _____. In adults, it is not unusual to find a _____ PCO_2 and a high pH.

26. The two general types of "nephrogenic" (i.e., kidney-caused) metabolic acidosis are _____ and _____. In both, the acidosis is caused by a defect in the renal _____. The additional defect present in renal failure is in the _____, which causes a marked reduction in _____ and, hence, a rise in the nitrogenous waste products _____ and _____. In addition, during renal failure, the plasma concentration of "unmeasured _____" may rise as well.

27. In chronic renal failure, the major defect that causes the acidosis is a decrease in the production and excretion of _____. This decrease is due to a fall in the number of functioning nephrons, a phenomenon sometimes called nephronal _____. Is this phenomenon reversible?

Note: Questions 28, 29, and 30 pertain to renal tubular acidosis. If you did not read the text discussion of this topic, you may wish to skip these questions.

28. There are three RTA Types: 1, 2, and 4. For each Type, make a list consisting of one entry from each of these six categories:

Mechanism | Plasma [HCO_3^-]
Reabsorptive defect | Typically 15–20 mmol/l
Distal proton defect | Sometimes below 10 mmol/l
Defect in aldosterone function |

Urine pH	Epidemiology
Below 5.5	Relatively common in children
Biphasic: first high, then low	Relatively common in adults
Above 5.5	Relatively rare in children and adults

Plasma [creatinine]	Plasma [K$^+$]
Slightly elevated	Hypokalemia or normokalemia
Normal	Hyperkalemia

29. A urine pH above 5.5 is often considered *the* defining characteristic of Type 1 RTA. However, healthy individuals may also have a urine pH above 5.5, or even above 7.0. Why is a urine pH above 5.5 in RTA patients diagnostically significant?

30. A patient has an RTA of unknown Type. If you give the patient an infusion of sodium bicarbonate, and the [HCO$_3^-$] and pH of urine increase rapidly, which Type of RTA is likely?

31. This question, which involves some repetition, will help you consolidate your knowledge of the causes of metabolic acidosis. List the following ten items: the major gastrointestinal cause of metabolic acidosis, the two most common causes of lactic acidosis, the two most important forms of ketoacidosis, the three exogenous intoxicants most commonly associated with metabolic acidosis, and the two renal causes of metabolic acidosis.

32. Name the three most common causes of metabolic alkalosis. The fourth most important form of metabolic alkalosis is actually a group of related clinical entities, known as _____. Taken together, this last group comprises about _____% of all cases of metabolic alkalosis.

33. The three most common causes of metabolic alkalosis will generally improve with an intravenous saline infusion. These are classified as _____-_____ metabolic alkalosis. The fourth will not improve with saline. Try to name two examples of this fourth group.

34. In metabolic alkalosis, a distinction is often made between *generation* and *maintenance*. Generation refers to mechanisms that either add additional bicarbonate to the ECF or concentrate existing bicarbonate. Maintenance refers to mechanisms that explain why excess bicarbonate is not _____ in the _____.

35. The major maintenance factors for metabolic alkalosis are _____, _____, and _____. A three-letter mnemonic for these factors is _____. In general, the most important of these factors is _____, which often plays a central role in producing the other two maintenance factors.

36. The maintenance factors act via incompletely understood mechanisms. However, the "bottom line" is clear: all maintain the alkalosis by causing an abnormal _____ in the renal reabsorptive threshold for bicar-

bonate. Another way to say the same thing is: They inhibit the urinary
_____ of _____ bicarbonate.

37. Vomiting and nasogastric drainage can cause hypokalemia. Perhaps surprisingly, most K^+ losses in these conditions occur via the _____. These losses are high because plasma _____ is elevated secondary to _____.

38. In discussions about metabolic alkalosis, "volume depletion" and "contraction alkalosis" are sometimes used interchangeably. This usage is a mistake. Which term pertains to generation of the alkalosis and which pertains to maintenance?

39. Two categories of diuretics are especially likely to cause metabolic alkalosis. Name them.

40. A patient has hypercapnia that is not the result of compensation for metabolic alkalosis. Is this hypercapnia, by definition, respiratory acidosis?

41. A patient has hypocapnia that is not the result of compensation for metabolic acidosis. Is this hypocapnia, by definition, respiratory alkalosis?

42. Patients with respiratory acidosis are sometimes said to be "_____ CO_2." Patients with respiratory alkalosis are sometimes said to be "_____ _____ CO_2." In general, are these patients in steady state for CO_2? When steady state does *not* exist, PCO_2 will be _____.

43. Dead space refers to air spaces of the lung that are _____ but not _____. An example of normal dead space is the _____ _____. Air that ventilates this normal dead space moves in and out of the lung but does not participate in _____ _____. An example of abnormal dead space occurs in _____ _____, when a blood clot, or _____, blocks blood flow to part of the lung. In this condition, total dead space (i.e., normal plus abnormal dead space) increases/decreases (pick one), which means that a greater/smaller (pick one) than normal fraction of _____ ventilation participates in alveolar ventilation. By definition, dead space ventilation equals _____ ventilation minus _____ ventilation.

44. When blood is "shunted," it moves directly from the _____ circulation to the _____ circulation, without being exposed to a functioning _____ _____ surface in the lung. The result is that _____ blood pours directly into the _____ circulation. This type of defect is sometimes called a right-to-left/left-to-right (pick one) shunt, because venous blood normally enters the _____ side of the heart and arterial blood normally exits the _____ side of the heart. During lung disease, shunting can occur when areas of the lung are _____ but not _____. Severe pneumonia with consolidation can cause shunting because _____ are filled with _____, which entirely blocks _____ from reaching the _____ surface. Alveolar/interstitial (pick one) edema can also cause shunting for the

same reason. _____, which refers to the collapse of airspaces, also can cause shunting, because there is no _____ in the collapsed airspaces.

45. Assuming that all else stays constant, the following will cause arterial PCO_2 to increase: rise/fall (pick one) in minute ventilation, rise/fall in alveolar ventilation, rise/fall in dead space ventilation, rise/fall in CO_2 production.

46. The term "minute ventilation requirement" refers to . . . (complete the sentence). If minute ventilation requirement rises but minute ventilation stays constant, what happens to arterial PCO_2? If minute ventilation requirement rises and minute ventilation rises more than proportionately, what happens to arterial PCO_2.

47. The following will usually increase the minute ventilation requirement: rise/fall (choose one) in CO_2 production, increase/decrease in dead space, worsening/improvement in lung disease.

48. It is possible to conceptualize hypercapnia as being caused by an imbalance between respiratory _____ and neuromuscular _____. This conceptualization is sometimes called the _____-_____ model of hypercapnia. According to this model, a rise in PCO_2 can be caused by either a decrease in _____ or an increase in _____.

49. Name three major components of respiratory load. The term _____, which is sometimes used to describe the "stiffness" of the lung or chest wall, can be thought of as the opposite, or reciprocal, of _____. One component of load, the _____ _____ requirement, tends to increase when there is a rise in either _____ production or _____ _____.

50. Decreases in neuromuscular strength are caused by a lesion in one or more "links" in the neuromuscular chain. List the links, starting with the respiratory center in the brain.

51. Lung disease usually increases respiratory load. But it also may decrease neuromuscular strength. In patients with lung disease, a decrease in strength is most commonly due to a defect at which "link" in the neuromuscular chain?

52. List three common causes of respiratory muscle weakness. These factors can increase susceptibility to muscle _____ when respiratory load is increased/decreased.

53. Lung diseases characterized by increased airflow resistance are termed _____, whereas those characterized by increased elastance (stiffness) are termed _____. Are these two categories mutually exclusive? Name two classic examples of obstructive lung disease. Name one classic example of restrictive lung disease. Many other problems can increase lung stiffness, and hence restriction. Try to give two common examples.

54. Chronic obstructive pulmonary disease (COPD) can have two distinct presentations, which may overlap in any particular patient. Name these two forms of COPD. Which of these usually does not produce respiratory acidosis? Which is associated with extensive destruction of alveolar tissue? With abnormal mucous production?

55. Respiratory alkalosis almost always involves some pathologic factor that acts, directly or indirectly, on the _____ _____ to increase ventilatory _____. The result is that alveolar ventilation exceeds the level required by _____ production.

56. Acute pulmonary diseases often present with hypocapnia (i.e., respiratory alkalosis). What two factors most commonly mediate the hyperventilation in hypocapnic patients?

57. Acute pulmonary disease, when mild, usually presents with respiratory alkalosis. In severe pulmonary disease, respiratory acidosis is increasingly likely to supervene. When respiratory acidosis supervenes, a common contributor to the rise in PCO_2 is _____ _____ _____. Muscle _____, which can be corrected with muscle rest (e.g., using mechanical ventilation) may contribute to muscle failure. Muscle fatigue is a specific type of muscle _____. Muscle fatigue always/sometimes (pick one) is a factor in respiratory muscle failure.

58. The clinical causes of respiratory alkalosis are either pulmonary or nonpulmonary. List four nonpulmonary causes.

59. Acute/chronic (choose one) respiratory acidosis is likely to indicate a medical emergency. In contrast, patients with _____ respiratory acidosis may remain _____ for years. These chronic patients live in a tenuous/secure (choose one) position. An acute medical stress can cause an acute worsening of their hypercapnia. Try to name three examples of such stresses.

60. Consider a patient with acute pulmonary disease (say, pneumonia) who presents with respiratory alkalosis. Some time later, although the patient remains hypoxemic and appears distressed, a blood gas shows that PCO_2 has normalized, to exactly 40 mm Hg. Is this a good sign? What is the likely cause of the normalization in PCO_2? The next change in PCO_2 is most likely to be a rise/fall (pick one).

61. One of the most common causes of respiratory alkalosis is not pathologic at all, but is a normal response to a normal condition. This condition is _____. The mediator of hyperventilation appears to involve elevated plasma levels of _____, which acts to stimulate the respiratory center. The plasma bicarbonate level in such an individual is normally high/low/normal (pick one). Why? If this individual presented with a plasma $[HCO_3^-]$ of 16 mmol/l, should you be concerned and, if so, why?

Answer Key

1. Metabolic acidosis = hypobicarbonatemic acidosis. Metabolic alkalosis = hyperbicarbonatemic alkalosis. Acidemia = low blood pH. Respiratory acidosis = hypercapnic acidosis. Alkalemia = high blood pH. Respiratory alkalosis = hypocapnic alkalosis.

2. No.

3. Yes, if mixed with an alkalosis of equal or greater magnitude.

4. Primary.

5. Complex. Two, primary. Metabolic acidosis, metabolic alkalosis, respiratory acidosis, respiratory alkalosis.

6. Same-direction.

7. Respiratory.

8. Respiratory alkalosis. Normal range.

9. Steady-state. 12 hours.

10. $[HCO_3^-]$. 2–4. 2–5.

11. Ca^{2+}.

12. Gut, metabolism, kidney, intoxicants.

13. Diarrhea. Protons. Bicarbonate.

14. Hypokalemia (with whole-body K^+ depletion), ECF volume depletion.

15. Anabolism, catabolism, intermediary. Plasma $[HCO_3^-]$.

16. Production, anions. Bicarbonate.

17. Septic, cardiogenic.

18. Oxygen.

19. Bicarbonate. Kidney.

20. Check your structures against those on pages 8 and 143–144.

21. Diabetic ketoacidosis. Insulin. Alcoholic ketoacidosis.

22. Methanol, ethylene glycol. Check page 146 for structures.

23. Aldehyde, carboxylic acid. Protons, lower.

24. Alcohol dehydrogenase, aldehyde dehydrogenase.

25. Metabolic acidosis, respiratory alkalosis. Low. Low.

26. Renal failure, renal tubular acidosis. Tubule. Glomerulus, GFR, creatinine, BUN. Anions.

27. Ammonium. Dropout. No.

28. Type 1: distal defect, sometimes below 10, above 5.5, relatively rare in children and adults, normal, hypokalemia or normokalemia. Type 2: reabsorptive defect, typically 15–20, biphasic, relatively common in children, normal, hypokalemia or normokalemia. Type 4: aldosterone defect, typically 15–20, below 5.5, relatively common in adults, slightly elevated, hyperkalemia.

29. The metabolic acidosis and acidemia that accompany RTA stimulate tubular acidification, so a high urine pH indicates an acidification defect.

30. Type 2, because plasma $[HCO_3^-]$, which stabilizes just below the abnormally low reabsorptive threshold, rises, quickly causing urinary bicarbonate spillage.

31. Diarrhea, septic shock, cardiogenic shock, diabetic, alcoholic, salicylates, methanol, ethylene glycol, renal failure, renal tubular acidosis.

32. Loss of gastric fluid (vomiting, nasogastric drainage), diuretics, posthypercapnic. Volume-resistant metabolic alkalosis. 5.

33. Volume-responsive. Primary hyperaldosteronism, Bartter's syndrome.

34. Spilled, urine.

35. Hypokalemia, aldosterone excess, effective circulating volume depletion (or simply "volume depletion"). HAV. Volume depletion.

36. Rise. Excretion, excess.

37. Urine. Aldosterone, volume depletion.

38. Generation: contraction alkalosis. Maintenance: volume depletion.

39. Thiazide, loop.

40. Yes. By definition, non-compensatory hypercapnia is respiratory acidosis.

41. Yes, by definition.

42. Retaining. Blowing off. Yes. Changing (i.e., rising or falling).

43. Ventilated, perfused. Conducting airways. Gas exchange (or: alveolar ventilation). Pulmonary embolism, thrombus. Increases, smaller, minute (or: total). Minute, alveolar.

44. Venous, arterial (or: systemic), gas exchange. Venous (or: unoxygenated), arterial. Right-to-left, right, left. Perfused, ventilated. Alveoli (or: air spaces), pus, air, alveolar. Alveolar. Atelectasis, ventilation.

45. Fall, fall, rise, rise.

46. . . . the minute ventilation required to keep arterial PCO_2 normal. It rises. It falls.

47. Rise, increase, worsening.

48. load, strength. Load-strength. Strength, load.

49. Airflow resistance, lung or chest wall stiffness, minute ventilation requirement. Elastance, compliance. Minute ventilation, CO_2, dead space.

50. Respiratory center, spinal cord, phrenic (and other peripheral) nerves, neuromuscular junction, respiratory muscles (plus: intact chest cage and patent upper airway).

51. Respiratory muscles (due to muscle failure).

52. Malnutrition, electrolyte imbalance (especially low PO_4 and K^+), sepsis (others also). Failure, increased.

53. Obstructive, restrictive. No, a lung disease may have both an obstructive and restrictive component (as well as an increase in the minute ventilation requirement). COPD, asthma. Pulmonary fibrosis. Pulmonary edema, atelectasis (and others).

54. Emphysema, chronic bronchitis. Emphysema. Emphysema. Chronic bronchitis.

55. Respiratory center, drive. CO_2.

56. Stimulation of lung sense receptors (both chemoreceptors and mechanoreceptors), hypoxemia.

57. Respiratory muscle failure. Fatigue. Weakness. Sometimes.

58. Answers include: sepsis, liver disease, salicylate intoxication, psychogenic hyperventilation, cyanotic heart disease, pregnancy, others.

59. Acute. Chronic, stable. Tenuous. Superimposed lung infection, sepsis, onset of congestive heart failure with pulmonary edema, others.

60. No. Evolving respiratory muscle failure or overwhelming disease. Rise.

61. Pregnancy. Progesterone. Yes. Low. Renal compensation. Yes. This bicarbonate value is too low to represent compensation for the mild hypocapnia of pregnancy. There is likely a superimposed metabolic acidosis or hypocapnia of another cause.

Section 4
Diagnosis

This section presents the essentials of acid-base diagnosis. It can be used in two ways.

For <u>students</u>, the section is a complete, step-by-step, self-paced course. To take this "course," simply read the chapters in order. The chapters contain many new concepts, so take your time and read carefully. Be sure to work through any practice problems that you encounter. When you are finished, you will understand acid-base diagnosis with a depth and clarity that will truly surprise you.

For <u>residents</u> and other practicing physicians, the section allows rapid review of specific topics. Related material is tightly organized and presented in one place. Topics can be found by either consulting the index or scanning the text for the desired boldfaced heading. In addition, whole chapters, or even the whole section, can be read as part of a self-directed enrichment program.

The section has five chapters:

    The Foundation of Diagnosis
    Venous Electrolytes
    Arterial Blood Gases
    Other Tests
    Making the Diagnosis

Each of the first four chapters thoroughly explores one important aspect of acid-base diagnosis. In these four chapters, we keep a tight focus and say little about how the topic being discussed fits into an overall diagnostic strategy. This focus lets readers devote full attention to mastering the fundamentals without getting distracted by the big picture.

In the section's final chapter, *Making the Diagnosis,* we pull everything together. We present a simple and efficient diagnostic strategy that integrates the ideas presented in the previous four chapters. Among other things, we discuss how to decide if a blood gas is necessary. The last page of the chapter (p. 269) is a chart that summarizes, in clinically useful form, key information presented throughout the section.*

---

* **Hint for the reader.** This section presumes a basic knowledge of acid-base pathophysiology. Readers who lack this knowledge are encouraged to review the Pathophysiology section of this text by reading the following: (1) Chapter 14, (2) the "Compensation" subsection of Chapter 15, and (3) the chapter summaries of Chapters 16–19.

The Foundation of Diagnosis

20

Venous electrolytes, arterial blood gases, and other laboratory tests play an essential role in acid-base diagnosis. In subsequent chapters, we will learn what these tests are and how to get the most from them. But more important than any test is a solid foundation of knowledge about which diseases cause which types of acid-base disorders. For example, you need to know that renal failure can cause metabolic acidosis, that COPD can cause respiratory acidosis, and so on. This knowledge is what we mean by "the foundation of diagnosis."

This knowledge is useful in two ways: clinical suspicion and differential diagnosis.

> *Clinical suspicion.* When the history and physical examination of a patient suggest a particular disease, you will have a high index of suspicion for a possible acid-base disturbance. For example, when you see a patient with sustained vomiting, you will immediately recognize the possibility of metabolic alkalosis, which you can then test for using appropriate laboratory methods.

> *Differential diagnosis.* When you see a laboratory value that suggests a particular acid-base disturbance, you will be able to anticipate the most likely causes. For example, if a blood gas suggests metabolic alkalosis, you will know that vomiting, nasogastric drainage, or diuretic use is probably responsible. You can then focus your history and physical examination on these areas.

To learn which diseases cause which acid-base disorders, a two-pronged approach is useful. First, and most importantly, study pathophysiology. It is the ultimate mnemonic. For example, once you know that renal failure impedes ammonium excretion and therefore slows bicarbonate regeneration, you will never forget that renal failure can cause metabolic acidosis.

Second, make use of a chart that summarizes key information. The chart at the end of this section is ideal (p. 269). Copy it, carry it with you, and review it frequently. This frequent review will help you learn the important points by memory. However, the summary chart will prove truly useful only after you have read the entire Diagnosis section carefully.

What about this chapter? This chapter is designed to facilitate review of pathophysiology. It lists alphabetically all the common (and a few less common) causes of acid-base disorders, and briefly summarizes some of the main mechanisms responsible for altering $[HCO_3^-]$ or PCO_2. Although in some respects oversimplified, the list is nonetheless an important learning aid. Beginning students should review it frequently, until the contents become second nature. Additional details on each entry can be found in the Pathophysiology section.

Note: it is important to realize that many of the conditions listed here do not cause acid-base disturbances in every instance. These conditions are *potential* causes of the disturbances, not inevitable ones.

Alcoholic ketoacidosis

Disorder: Metabolic acidosis.
Mechanism: Starvation ketoacidosis from fasting and vomiting, with ketogenesis augmented by high plasma catecholamine levels, which arise secondary to volume depletion from vomiting.

Asthma

Disorder: Respiratory alkalosis.
Mechanism: Hyperventilation is caused by hypoxemia, stimulation of sense receptors in the lung, and anxiety. In severe cases, ventilation may fail, raising PCO_2 and causing respiratory acidosis.

Carbon monoxide poisoning

Disorder: Metabolic acidosis.
Mechanism: Lactic acidosis secondary to reduced O_2 carriage by hemoglobin.

Chronic bronchitis-COPD

Disorder: Respiratory acidosis.
Mechanism: Decreased alveolar ventilation from obstructed airways, respiratory muscle failure, and possibly decreased central drive.

Diabetic ketoacidosis

Disorder: Metabolic acidosis.
Mechanism: Low insulin and high glucagon levels lead to increased production of acetoacetic and beta-hydroxybutyric acids.

Diarrhea

Disorder: Metabolic acidosis.
Mechanism: Secretion of bicarbonate into the lumen of the lower GI tract re-

sults in an equimolar release of protons into blood. Diarrhea increases the rate of these processes.

Diuretics (thiazide and loop agents only)

Disorder: Metabolic alkalosis.
Mechanisms: Volume depletion, contraction alkalosis, hypokalemia, and other factors.

Ethylene glycol ingestion

Disorder: Metabolic acidosis.
Mechanism: Ethylene glycol metabolized to strong acids, especially glycolic and oxalic.

GI drainage

Disorder: With lower GI drainage, metabolic acidosis. With upper GI drainage, metabolic alkalosis.
Mechanism: Lower GI same as diarrhea (see above). Upper GI same as vomiting (see below).

Liver disease

Disorder: Respiratory alkalosis. Metabolic acidosis may also occur, especially in fulminant disease.
Mechanisms: Hyperventilation partly due to progesterone and other chemical mediators. Metabolic acidosis from reduced lactate metabolism by liver.

Methanol ingestion

Disorder: Metabolic acidosis.
Mechanism: Methanol metabolized to formic acid.

Pneumonia

Disorder: Respiratory alkalosis.
Mechanism: Hyperventilation caused by stimulation of lung sense receptors and hypoxemia. In severe cases, ventilation may fail, raising PCO_2 and causing respiratory acidosis.

Pulmonary edema

Disorder: Respiratory alkalosis.
Mechanism: Edema fluid causes hypoxemia and stimulates pulmonary sense receptors, resulting in hyperventilation. In severe cases, ventilation may fail, raising PCO_2 and causing respiratory acidosis.

Pulmonary embolus

Disorder: Respiratory alkalosis.
Mechanism: Hyperventilation due to stimulation of pulmonary sense receptors and, in some cases, pain and/or hypoxemia. In severe cases, ventilation may fail, raising PCO_2 and causing respiratory acidosis.

Recovery in COPD

Disorder: Metabolic alkalosis.
Mechanism: "Post-hypercapnic" metabolic alkalosis may occur in hypercapnic COPD patients if the hypercapnia remits somewhat, or if the patient is mechanically ventilated and PCO_2 drops from its chronic, compensated level. With PCO_2 reduced, hyperbicarbonatemia, which was compensatory, becomes the primary disturbance and persists if the patient is volume and/or potassium depleted.

Renal failure

Disorder: Metabolic acidosis.
Mechanism: Loss ("dropout") of functioning nephrons lowers ammonium excretion and, hence, bicarbonate regeneration. Bicarbonate that is consumed in buffering endogenously produced acid is not fully replaced.

Renal tubular acidosis

Disorder: Metabolic acidosis.
Mechanism: Types 1 and 4 inhibit bicarbonate regeneration; mild urinary bicarbonate spillage also occurs. Type 2 causes massive urinary bicarbonate spillage.

Salicylate intoxication

Disorder: Mixed respiratory alkalosis and metabolic acidosis. In adults, the alkalosis typically predominates. In young children, the acidosis typically predominates.
Mechanism: Salicylate stimulates the medullary respiratory center, causing hyperventilation, and interferes with metabolic pathways, augmenting production of organic (especially lactic and keto) acids.

Sepsis

Disorder: Respiratory alkalosis.
Mechanism: Cytokines and other mediators of hyperventilation. May progress to shock (see below).

Shock

Usual forms: Septic or cardiogenic shock.
Disorder: Metabolic (lactic) acidosis (plus respiratory alkalosis in septic shock).

Mechanism: Tissue hypoperfusion leading to anaerobic respiration. In cardiogenic shock caused by frank cardiac arrest, ventilatory arrest occurs, leading to superimposed respiratory acidosis. For mechanisms of respiratory alkalosis, see "Sepsis" (above).

Strenuous exercise with volume depletion

Disorder: Metabolic acidosis.
Mechanism: Rapid anaerobic metabolism from exertion, and reduced lactate consumption from decreased hepatic perfusion.

Vomiting

Disorder: Metabolic alkalosis.
Mechanism: Liberation of protons into gastric fluid results in an equimolar release of bicarbonate into blood. Alkalosis is maintained by volume depletion and hypokalemia.

The above list provides the essential foundation needed to master acid-base diagnosis. Because the list is itself a summary of the Pathophysiology section of the text, no summary paragraph needs to be provided for this chapter. In the next three chapters, we introduce the laboratory tests that are used in acid-base diagnosis and discuss how to interpret them.

Venous Electrolytes

21

Introduction

An electrolyte is a substance that exists in solution as an ion. Calcium (Ca^{2+}), sulfate (SO_4^{2-}), and magnesium (Mg^{2+}) are electrolytes. Organic ions such as lactate and acetoacetate are also electrolytes. Hundreds of electrolytes exist in body fluids, and over a dozen can be measured in the hospital laboratory. However, only four are routinely and frequently measured:

Sodium, Na^+
Potassium, K^+
Chloride, Cl^-
Bicarbonate, HCO_3^-

When acutely ill patients enter the hospital, it is so common to measure these four electrolytes that they are sometimes called "admission electrolytes." The blood sample may be either arterial or venous (electrolyte concentrations are about the same in both), but venous blood is used because it is easier and less painful to obtain. Thus, this chapter's title, *Venous Electrolytes,* refers to the concentration of Na^+, K^+, Cl^-, and HCO_3^- in the venous blood plasma. Our goal in this chapter is to learn how to get the most information from these four laboratory values.

Note: The concentration of these four ions can be expressed in either millimoles per liter (mmol/l) or milliequivalents per liter (meq/l). Because all four ions carry a single charge, the molar and equivalent values are the same. For example, the normal range for [K^+] can be written as either 3.5–5.0 mmol/l or 3.5–5.0 meq/l. In the clinical setting, the units are often left unstated. For example, instead of saying that [HCO_3^-] is "24 mmol/l," we might simply say "24."

What electrolytes can tell you

For purposes of acid-base diagnosis, venous electrolyte measurements are important because they provide *three* key pieces of data. In a moment, we'll look at each in detail. But first we'll do a quick preview. The three important data are:

221

1. *Bicarbonate Concentration.* An abnormal plasma $[HCO_3^-]$ always indicates that an acid-base disturbance is present. Metabolic disturbances affect $[HCO_3^-]$ directly, as their primary manifestation. Respiratory disturbances affect $[HCO_3^-]$ indirectly, the result of renal compensation for the abnormal PCO_2. In fact, the only acid-base disorders not associated with a clearly abnormal $[HCO_3^-]$ are acute (i.e., not yet compensated) respiratory disturbances and certain mixed disorders (e.g., mixed metabolic acidosis and metabolic alkalosis with offsetting effects on plasma $[HCO_3^-]$).

2. *Anion Gap.* The anion gap is defined as the difference between $[Na^+]$ and the sum of $[HCO_3^-]$ and $[Cl^-]$. That is: Anion gap $= [Na^+] - ([Cl^-] + [HCO_3^-])$. For example, if $[Na^+] = 140$, $[Cl^-] = 105$, and $[HCO_3^-] = 25$, the anion gap is 10. As we will see, calculating the anion gap can help suggest the cause of metabolic acidosis.

3. *Potassium Concentration.* Certain acid-base disorders cause predictable changes in plasma $[K^+]$. For example, the metabolic acidosis caused by diarrhea is consistently associated with hypokalemia. Knowing what usually happens to $[K^+]$ in different situations can help you determine the cause of a disturbance.*

Let's now study each of these three in detail.

Bicarbonate concentration

In most hospitals, when you send a venous blood sample to the laboratory for an $[HCO_3^-]$ measurement, a funny thing happens: the lab report does *not* say "bicarbonate concentration" or "$[HCO_3^-]$." Instead, it says "Total CO_2" or "carbon dioxide" or maybe just "CO_2" (with no "P" in front of it). The reason is that clinical laboratories typically measure $[HCO_3^-]$ indirectly, via a technique that produces carbon dioxide gas. They add strong acid to the plasma sample, and protons from the acid react with plasma bicarbonate, like this:

$$HCO_3^- + H^+ \rightarrow H_2O + CO_2$$

For each mmol of HCO_3^- in the plasma, a mmol of CO_2 is liberated. The concentration of CO_2 is then determined by electronic sensor. It is this concentration that is reported as "CO_2" or "Total CO_2."

---

* **Hint for the reader.** As you may have noticed, the $[Na^+]$ and $[Cl^-]$ values are directly useful for acid-base diagnosis only because they let us calculate the anion gap.

If this were the whole story, the above approach, although indirect, would precisely quantify $[HCO_3^-]$. Bicarbonate in the plasma sample would be quantitatively converted to CO_2, and the reported Total CO_2 value would exactly equal $[HCO_3^-]$. However, in addition to HCO_3^-, several other substances in plasma also contribute to Total CO_2. Taken together, these substances usually increase Total CO_2 by only about 5% above actual $[HCO_3^-]$. Thus, while Total CO_2 is only an approximation for $[HCO_3^-]$, it is a fairly good one.

What are the other substances that contribute to Total CO_2? The most important is carbon dioxide itself, which exists in dissolved form in all body fluids, including plasma. Each mm Hg of PCO_2 represents 0.03 mmol per liter dissolved CO_2 (p. 44). Since normal venous PCO_2 is about 46 mm Hg, venous $[CO_2]_{dissolved}$ is about $0.03 \times 46 = 1.38$ mmol/l. Therefore, Total CO_2 is about 1.4 mmol/l higher than actual venous $[HCO_3^-]$. Even in severe hypercapnia, the contribution of dissolved CO_2 to Total CO_2 is small. For example, a PCO_2 of 100 mm Hg translates into a $[CO_2]_{dissolved}$ of only $0.03 \times 100 = 3.0$ mmol/l.

Several other substances in plasma can also liberate CO_2. These include carbonic acid, H_2CO_3, and the carbonate anion, CO_3^{2-} (note the CO_2 "hidden" in the formulas), as well as CO_2 bound to certain amino groups in plasma proteins ("carbamino compounds"). However, the combined concentration of these substances is low, and they raise Total CO_2 only slightly. As a practical matter, you can disregard them.

Because the difference between Total CO_2 and actual $[HCO_3^-]$ is small, the two quantities are usually treated as being equal. For this reason, we often speak of venous "bicarbonate concentration" or "$[HCO_3^-]$," without referring to the fact that this value is measured as Total CO_2. The normal range for plasma bicarbonate concentration, measured as Total CO_2, is about 24 to 30 mmol/l.

We can now ask, *What does the bicarbonate concentration tell us?*

Because metabolic disturbances directly affect $[HCO_3^-]$, and respiratory disturbances affect $[HCO_3^-]$ indirectly, via renal compensation, most acid-base disturbances can be detected by scrutinizing $[HCO_3^-]$. A low $[HCO_3^-]$ indicates either metabolic acidosis or compensated respiratory alkalosis. A high $[HCO_3^-]$ indicates either metabolic alkalosis or compensated respiratory acidosis. As the following examples show, the history and physical examination often help distinguish among the different possibilities.*

---

* **Reminder.** Compensation follows the "same-direction rule": the primary and compensatory variables both move in the same direction. For example, a primary fall in $[HCO_3^-]$ (i.e., metabolic acidosis) is compensated by a low PCO_2. If you need to review compensation, take a few minutes to read the "Compensation" discussion starting on page 131.

A child with polyuria, polydipsia, and polyphagia has an $[HCO_3^-]$ of 14. Interpretation: The bicarbonate value itself could represent either a metabolic acidosis or compensated respiratory alkalosis. However, in light of the history, metabolic acidosis due to uncontrolled diabetes is a virtual certainty.

An otherwise healthy patient presents with a 3-day history of vomiting and a bicarbonate of 36. Interpretation: Metabolic alkalosis.

A patient with a history of COPD with stable hypercapnia has an $[HCO_3^-]$ of 39 and no other unusual findings. Interpretation: Respiratory acidosis.

These examples show how a venous $[HCO_3^-]$, in conjunction with key historical or physical findings, may be all you need to make a correct diagnosis. Sometimes, however, more information is required. For example:

A patient with liver failure has an $[HCO_3^-]$ of 17. Comment: Liver disease can cause metabolic acidosis or respiratory alkalosis, and either can lower $[HCO_3^-]$. We need more information to decide between these possibilities.

A COPD patient presents with fever, cyanosis, and an $[HCO_3^-]$ of 41. Comment: Is the $[HCO_3^-]$ explained by renal compensation for chronic hypercapnia? Possibly. But we don't know for sure if this COPD patient is normally hypercapnic. Fever in a COPD patient suggests the possibility of respiratory infection, which might be raising PCO_2 acutely, but we can only guess. More information is needed.

An older, chronically hospitalized patient with occasional diarrhea has an $[HCO_3^-]$ of 15. Comment: Is this metabolic acidosis from diarrhea? Or is it metabolic acidosis from another cause? Or is it compensated respiratory alkalosis from, say, undiagnosed hypoxemia or liver disease? We can't be sure. More information is needed.

We will refer to venous $[HCO_3^-]$ at many other points in this section, and this will help deepen your understanding. But for now we move on.

Anion gap

In this subsection, we first explain the anion gap concept. We then examine how this concept is used clinically.

The anion gap concept

The law of electroneutrality tells us that blood plasma, like all solutions, contains an equal number of positive and negative charges. It follows that if we graphically stack up plasma cations ($+$) and anions ($-$) side by side, the resulting "ionogram" will have two columns of equal height:

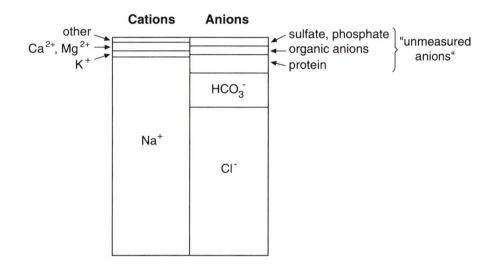

The height of the columns indicates the total ion concentration, measured in equivalents. As illustrated, the major cation is Na^+. The minor cations include K^+, Ca^{2+}, and Mg^{2+}. The major anions are Cl^- and HCO_3^-. The minor anions include the negatively charged groups on plasma proteins (especially albumin), phosphate, sulfate, and organic acid anions such as lactate and acetoacetate. Of the many plasma anions, only Cl^- and HCO_3^- are routinely measured in the hospital laboratory. For this reason, all the other anions are sometimes lumped together and called "unmeasured anions," as shown.

What happens to the ionogram during metabolic acidosis? First, the addition of strong acid to blood releases protons, which are buffered primarily by bicarbonate via the reaction $H^+ + HCO_3^- \rightarrow CO_2 + H_2O$. This reaction causes plasma $[HCO_3^-]$ to fall, shrinking the $[HCO_3^-]$ block of the ionogram. Second, the anions that remain from the strong acid are added to the plasma. For example, if lactic acid is added, the concentration of lactate rises (this increases the total concentration of "unmeasured anions"). If hydrochloric acid, HCl, is added, $[Cl^-]$ rises. Thus, the space left by the shrinking bicarbonate block is filled by the expansion of another region of the anion column. This expansion maintains the height of the anion column and, hence, electroneutrality. These concepts are illustrated in the following ionograms. Be sure you understand why each ionogram looks the way it does.

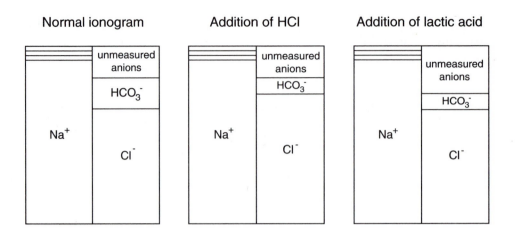

Normal ionogram   Addition of HCl   Addition of lactic acid

Now consider a patient with metabolic acidosis of unknown cause. If you could see the patient's ionogram, you would gain valuable diagnostic information. For example, if the ionogram looked like the one on the right (above), you would suspect the acidosis was of a type that leaves an anion other than chloride (e.g., lactic acidosis, ketoacidosis). If the ionogram looked like the one in the middle, you would suspect a different set of causes.

In reality, clinicians cannot routinely get enough information to construct a complete ionogram. However, it is possible to construct a *simplified* ionogram by assuming (1) that Na^+ is the only cation in plasma and (2) that the anion column is only as tall as the Na^+ column.* These assumptions have the effect of "decapitating" the ionogram at the top of the Na^+ column, like this:

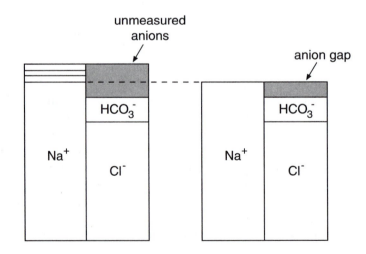

unmeasured anions   anion gap

* **Technical information.** Because sodium is by far the most plentiful cation in plasma, these assumptions are not too unreasonable. Typical concentrations of the four most prevalent plasma cations, in meq/l, are $[Na^+] = 140$, $[K^+] = 4.0$, $[Ca^{2+}] = 4.6$, and $[Mg^{2+}] = 2.2$.

What interests us most in the simplified ionogram is the region labeled "anion gap." This region is filled with unmeasured anions, but only some of the unmeasured anions are included (the rest were decapitated). Although the anion gap of the simplified ionogram is smaller than the unmeasured anion region of the full ionogram, the size of the two regions change in parallel. Thus, when the concentration of unmeasured anions is normal, the anion gap is of normal size. When the concentration of unmeasured anions increases, the anion gap gets bigger. The following "table" illustrates this parallelism:

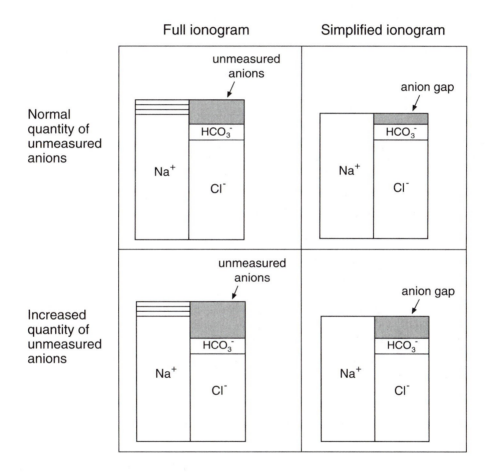

We now arrive at a key point in our discussion. Look at either of the simplified ionograms in this illustration. Notice that the size of the anion gap is equal to the height of the Na^+ column minus the combined heights of the HCO_3^- and Cl^- regions. We can thus describe the size of the anion gap using a simple formula:

$$\text{Anion gap} = [Na^+] - ([Cl^-] + [HCO_3^-])$$

This formula is invaluable. It lets you use readily available laboratory data (i.e., $[Na^+]$, $[Cl^-]$, and $[HCO_3^-]$) to determine if the quantity of unmeasured anions in the plasma is normal, elevated, or decreased. You do not have to draw an ionogram. For example, if $[Na^+]$ = 140 mmol/l, $[Cl^-]$ = 105 mmol/l, and $[HCO_3^-]$ = 25 mmol/l, then the anion gap = 10. If $[Na^+]$ = 140, $[Cl^-]$ = 100, and $[HCO_3^-]$ = 15, then the anion gap = 25. Notice that the units of the anion gap are left unstated; we say simply "25," not "25 meq/l."

The normal range for the anion gap varies somewhat among laboratories. However, the most commonly cited normal range is 8 to 16 (i.e., 12 $\pm$ 4). Thus, in our first example (gap = 10) the patient had a normal plasma concentration of unmeasured anions. In the second example (gap = 25), the concentration of unmeasured anions was elevated, 9 above the top end of the normal range. Although we write "$[HCO_3^-]$" in the gap formula, gap normal ranges are determined using venous Total CO_2 values. Therefore, you should use the Total CO_2 value in your calculation.*

Clinical use of the gap

Let's now see how the anion gap is used clinically. We begin with terminology. During metabolic acidosis, the fall in $[HCO_3^-]$ is always accompanied by a rise in the concentration of either unmeasured anions or chloride (as we have seen, electroneutrality is maintained by this rise). Based on this fact, two general presentations of metabolic acidosis are distinguished. When unmeasured anions rise, the anion gap enlarges and, therefore, the acidosis is considered an "anion gap metabolic acidosis." When $[Cl^-]$ rises, the anion gap does not enlarge and, therefore, the acidosis is considered a "non-anion gap metabolic acidosis." To visualize these two presentations, take a moment to look at the preceding illustration (i.e., the ionogram "table"): the bottom row shows the anion gap pattern and the top row shows the non-anion gap pattern. Note: anion gap metabolic acidosis can also be called "normochloremic metabolic acidosis" because the blood chloride level is normal. Similarly, non-anion gap metabolic acidosis can be called "hyperchloremic metabolic acidosis" because the chloride level is increased.

Different causes of metabolic acidosis tend to be associated with one or the other of these two presentations. When the gap is greater than 16 (the upper

---

* **Terminology.** The actual concentration of unmeasured anions is virtually never discussed; all quantitative references are to the anion gap. Thus, if someone says "The patient's unmeasured anions are at (for example) 25," you can safely assume that the speaker is using "unmeasured anions" loosely, as a synonym for "anion gap," and that the gap is 25. This said, it is possible to estimate unmeasured anion concentration, although this estimation is never done clinically. Here's how. The simplified ionogram assumes that Na^+ is the only cation; in fact, K^+, Mg^{2+}, and Ca^{2+}, as well as a small quantity of cationic proteins, are also present. The combined concentration of these cations is normally about 11 meq/l. Since these are neutralized by an equivalent number of anions, you can estimate unmeasured anion concentration, in meq/l, by adding about 11 to the anion gap.

limit of normal), you should suspect one of the anion gap causes. The higher the gap above 16, the more suspicious you should be. Conversely, when the gap is normal, you should suspect one of the non-gap causes. Let's now look at the causes of gap and non-gap acidosis.

Anion gap (normochloremic) metabolic acidosis

Three disorders account for most cases of anion gap metabolic acidosis: ketoacidosis, lactic acidosis, and renal failure. The next most common cause is toxic ingestions (especially of methanol, ethylene glycol, or salicylates). The following table lists these causes, along with the anions most responsible for enlarging the gap:

Condition	Predominant anions
Ketoacidosis	Acetoacetate, beta-hydroxybutyrate
Lactic acidosis	Lactate
Renal failure	Sulfate, phosphate, urate, hippurate
Methanol	Formate
Ethylene glycol	Glycoxylate, glycolate, oxalate
Salicylate	Only partially characterized. Include ketoacid anions, lactate, and salicylate*

How large is the anion gap in these conditions? There are no absolute rules, but general comments are possible. Salicylates tend to raise the gap only modestly, often not even to 20 and rarely to 30. Renal failure may raise the gap to around 25. Diabetic ketoacidosis can produce gaps to around 35 or 40. Lactic acidosis, methanol, and ethylene glycol can produce gaps greater than 35 and, uncommonly, even greater than 50 (a gap greater than 35 usually suggests one of these three conditions). Note that the numbers just given are the upper extremes. All causes of gap acidosis can present with a range of gap values, including values that are only slightly elevated. For example, a gap of 22 can represent any cause of gap acidosis.

The largest gaps are caused by ketoacidosis, lactic acidosis, and poisoning with methanol or ethylene glycol. Why? In these conditions, the acidosis tends to develop rapidly, with acid production overwhelming the body's capacity to metabolize the anions. Other factors also contribute. In some

---

* **Mnemonic.** An acronym for the common causes of gap acidosis is MEG'S LARD. MEG'S lists the intoxicant causes: Methanol, Ethylene Glycol, Salicylates. LARD lists the non-intoxicant causes: Lactic acidosis, Alcoholic ketoacidosis, Renal failure, Diabetic ketoacidosis.

cases, the anions are not readily metabolized (e.g., formate). In lactic acidosis, urinary anion spillage is prevented because the kidney's capacity to reabsorb lactate is high, and this helps maintain high plasma levels. The reabsorptive capacity for ketoacid anions is lower. Thus, during ketoacidosis, profound ketonuria can occur, which tends to limit the size of the gap. However, in diabetic ketoacidosis, GFR will decrease if the osmotic diuresis causes severe volume depletion. This fall in GFR slows ketonuria, increases retention of ketoanions, and thus tends to maintain the gap at high levels.

Non-anion gap (hyperchloremic) metabolic acidosis

Let's now consider the non-gap acidoses. There are three common causes of non-gap metabolic acidosis: diarrhea, renal tubular acidosis, and renal failure. Note: although renal failure "classically" presents with an elevated anion gap, excretion of unmeasured anions is sometimes adequate, so the gap may be normal.

Where does the additional Cl^- come from in non-gap (i.e., hyperchloremic) acidosis? If hydrochloric acid (HCl) is ingested or infused, hyperchloremic acidosis develops. In this case, the source of the additional plasma Cl^- is apparent. But what about the more common causes of non-gap acidosis? It appears that the chloride comes from the combination of dietary chloride intake and augmented renal chloride reabsorption. That is, the body retains more chloride than usual, raising $[Cl^-]$ in the extracellular fluid. In diarrhea and RTA, renal chloride reabsorption is increased partly because these conditions cause mild volume depletion, which promotes reabsorption of both Cl^- and Na^+. Note that in Type 2 RTA, bicarbonate is lost via urinary spillage, not via the buffering of strong acid. However, plasma $[HCO_3^-]$ falls, and $[Cl^-]$ rises, just the same.

A final note. The anion gap is sometimes called "delta", symbolized by the Greek letter of that name, Δ. Thus, "$\Delta = 21$" means that the anion gap is 21. Although Δ is often used to symbolize a change in a variable, in this context Δ does not refer to the change from normal in the gap. It refers to the size of the gap itself. Thus, if the gap rises from 12 to 22, $\Delta = 22$, not 10.*

---

* **Going further.** Some clinicians include potassium in the anion gap formula, like this: $\Delta = ([Na^+] + [K^+]) - ([Cl^-] + [HCO_3^-])$. Including $[K^+]$ has the effect of "decapitating" the ionogram at a slightly higher level (i.e., the level of $[Na^+] + [K^+]$). This raises the normal range of the gap by the value of $[K^+]$ (about 4), to 16 ± 4, but otherwise has little practical effect.

Potassium concentration

Introduction to [K+]

Plasma [HCO_3^-] and the anion gap are the most important acid-base data obtained from the venous electrolyte assay. In addition, evaluating plasma [K+] can sometimes provide important diagnostic information. Because the evaluation of plasma [K+] is relatively complex, yet is somewhat less important than [HCO_3^-] and the anion gap for acid-base diagnosis, first-time readers should not worry about absorbing all the details presented here. Read for understanding, which will help you learn the main concepts, but don't try to memorize. You can always review the details later.

Let's begin with the obvious. When potassium enters the extracellular fluid (ECF), plasma [K+] rises. When potassium leaves the ECF, plasma [K+] falls. Less obvious is that these K+ movements can take place in two different ways: between the ECF and the outside environment, and between the ECF and the intracellular fluid (ICF). The former are called either "environmental" or "external" movements. The latter are called either "cellular" or "transcellular." We look at these two types of potassium movement individually.

"Environmental" or "external" K+ movements

K+ moves between the ECF and the outside environment at two major interfaces: gut and kidney. These organs can act as environmental interfaces because their lumina are effectively outside the body: the gut lumen is like the hole in a doughnut, and the nephron lumen is, in essence, a branched extension of the ureter, which is itself contiguous with the external environment via the urethra and bladder.

So how do external K+ movements occur? External potassium <u>losses</u> occur when K+ exits the body in stool, gastric fluid, or urine. Because volume depletion raises plasma aldosterone levels, and aldosterone augments urinary K+ excretion, volume depletion itself speeds K+ losses. As a result, vomiting, gastric drainage, and diarrhea cause K+ to be lost via both gut fluids *and* urine, with the urinary losses being secondary to volume depletion from the gut fluid losses. External potassium <u>gains</u> occur when renal failure or Type 4 RTA inhibits the excretion of normal dietary K+ loads, or when patients receive additional K+ in intravenous fluids, oral KCl supplements, or from K+-containing dietary salt substitutes.

"Cellular" or "transcellular" K+ movements

Fluxes (or "shifts") of potassium between cells and ECF can have a profound effect on plasma [K+], largely because intracellular [K+] is much higher than extracellular [K+] (roughly 150 mmol/l versus 4 mmol/l). Although both external and cellular fluxes affect plasma [K+], only external fluxes alter the total amount of K+ in the body. This schematic illustrates the two types of K+ fluxes:

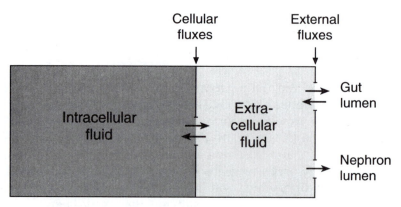

Density of shading indicates [K$^+$]

How a particular disorder affects plasma [K$^+$] depends on the net effect of external and cellular fluxes. For example, if K$^+$ enters the ECF via both external and cellular routes, plasma [K$^+$] will rise. Conversely, if K$^+$ exits the ECF via both routes, [K$^+$] will fall. However, if K$^+$ enters the ECF via one route and exits via the other, plasma [K$^+$] can rise, fall, or remain constant, depending on which route predominates. For example, if moderate kaliuresis (i.e., urinary K$^+$ excretion) is accompanied by massive cellular shifts into the ECF, plasma [K$^+$] will rise.*

The following illustrations show how external losses of potassium can be accompanied by either hypokalemia or hyperkalemia. As you study the illustrations, pay special attention to the size of each arrow, as this indicates the magnitude of the flux:

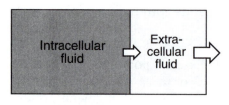

Hypokalemia with whole-body potassium depletion

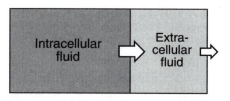

Hyperkalemia with whole-body potassium depletion

What causes cellular K$^+$ shifts? In the setting of acid-base disorders, five factors are especially important:

1. *pH.* Acidemia tends to shift K$^+$ out of cells, thus raising plasma [K$^+$]. Alkalemia tends to shift K$^+$ into cells, thus lowering plasma [K$^+$]. Although the mechanism of pH-induced shifts is unknown, a useful mnemonic is to think of these shifts as being due to an H$^+$−K$^+$ exchange across cell membranes.

---

* **Terminology.** In this case, hyperkalemia develops even though total-body K$^+$ stores decrease. This situation might be termed "paradoxical hyperkalemia."

2. *Bicarbonate level.* When plasma [HCO_3^-] falls, a gradient is created for the exit of bicarbonate from cells. As bicarbonate exits cells, K^+ (the major intracellular cation) follows to maintain electroneutrality. Thus, a fall in extracellular [HCO_3^-] causes K^+ to exit cells, raising plasma [K^+]. Conversely, a rise in extracellular [HCO_3^-] causes bicarbonate to enter cells, and K^+ follows, lowering plasma [K^+]. In general, changes in [HCO_3^-] have a much greater effect on plasma [K^+] than do changes in pH (i.e., factor 1.)

3. *Organic vs. inorganic acids.* The effect of hypobicarbonatemia in raising plasma [K^+] (i.e., factor 2) is much greater for inorganic acids than for organic acids. Thus, hyperchloremic acidoses tend to shift K^+ out of cells (the Cl^- anion is inorganic), whereas, for example, lactic acid has little effect. The basis for this difference is not known.

4. *Insulin.* The $Na^+-K^+-ATPase$ pumps K^+ into cells and thus helps maintain normal intracellular potassium stores. Insulin has a stimulatory effect on this transporter. Thus, if plasma insulin levels fall acutely, the transporter slows and K^+ tends to exit cells, which raises plasma [K^+]. If insulin levels are restored, K^+ returns to cells.

5. *Osmolarity.* If the osmolarity of the blood and ECF rises, water is osmotically pulled out of cells, and potassium moves out with the water. This raises plasma [K^+]. When osmolarity returns to normal, water and K^+ move back into cells, lowering plasma [K^+].

Specific disorders

With this background, we can now examine how specific acid-base disorders affect plasma [K^+]. To begin, take a moment to scan the following table, which provides a summary of typical [K^+] patterns in the common disorders:

Disturbance	Typical [K^+]
Metabolic alkalosis (all causes)	Low
Metabolic acidosis	Depends on the cause, as follows:
Diarrhea	Low
Renal failure	Slightly elevated but often in normal range
Renal tubular acidosis	Types 1 and 2: low or normal Type 4: high
Diabetic ketoacidosis	Usually normal or high, but can be low
Lactic acidosis, alcoholic ketoacidosis, methanol, ethylene glycol, salicylates	No typical value
Respiratory disturbances	Acute: slightly high with acidosis; slightly low with alkalosis Chronic: normal

We now look in detail at each disorder contained in this table. As you read, you may find it useful to refer back to the five factors, listed above, that explain why cellular K^+ shifts occur.

Metabolic alkalosis

Virtually all causes of metabolic alkalosis present with hypokalemia or, at least, a low-normal $[K^+]$. The fall in plasma $[K^+]$ is due to both cellular shifts and external losses. Cellular shifts occur via the pH- and HCO_3^--mediated mechanisms (i.e., factors 1 and 2). External losses occur primarily in the urine, secondary to high plasma [aldosterone] levels. In "volume-responsive" (p. 168) causes of alkalosis, such as diuretics, vomiting, and nasogastric drainage, plasma [aldosterone] rises due to volume depletion. In some of the "volume-resistant" (p. 168) causes, such as primary hyperaldosteronism, the rise in [aldosterone] is primary. During vomiting and gastric drainage, some K^+ is also lost in the gastric fluid.

Metabolic acidosis

Metabolic acidosis lowers pH and $[HCO_3^-]$, both of which act to raise plasma $[K^+]$. However, other factors that influence $[K^+]$ also come into play. To determine the net effect, we must consider each cause of metabolic acidosis individually, as follows:

Diarrhea.   Diarrhea causes hyperchloremic acidosis (i.e., inorganic anions; see factor 3), which results in marked cellular shifts of K^+ into the ECF. Opposing this hyperkalemic effect, external K^+ losses occur via both diarrhea fluid and urine. On balance, the external losses predominate over the cellular shifts, so diarrhea characteristically produces hypokalemia. Note that the combination of cellular shifts plus external losses produces a one-way K^+ flux from ICF to ECF to urine. This flux can substantially reduce body potassium stores.

Renal failure.   The loss of functioning nephrons, which occurs in renal failure, inhibits urinary K^+ excretion. Therefore, renal failure tends to raise plasma $[K^+]$. This elevation may be mild, with $[K^+]$ remaining within the normal range. However, an acute K^+ load (e.g., intravenous potassium, tissue breakdown with cellular K^+ spillage, salt substitutes) can cause frank hyperkalemia, which usually resolves gradually as the injured kidneys slowly excrete the excess K^+.

Renal tubular acidosis.   Distal (Type 1) and proximal (Type 2) RTA both cause urinary spillage of K^+. In general, these urinary losses more than offset the shift of K^+ out of cells (factors 1 and 2). Thus, RTA Types 1 and 2 tend to cause hypokalemia, although $[K^+]$ may sometimes be normal. In contrast, Type 4 RTA causes hyperkalemia (p. 154).

Diabetic ketoacidosis (DKA).   Because the ketoanions are organic (factor 3), the hypobicarbonatemia of DKA does not shift K^+ out of cells. However, large cellular shifts nonetheless occur because of hypoinsulinemia (factor 4) and hyperosmolarity (factor 5), which results from the hyperglycemia. Simultaneously, large amounts of K^+ are excreted in the urine as part of the osmotic diuresis that occurs with DKA. The final $[K^+]$ varies, depending on the interplay of these cellular and external shifts. Usually, the hyperkalemic influences equal or exceed the hypokalemic influences, so most patients are either normokalemic or hyperkalemic. However, a few percent of patients are hypokalemic. The lack of a predictable kalemic pattern means $[K^+]$ is of little help in making the diagnosis of DKA.*

Lactic acidosis.   As an organic acid, lactic acid does not promote cellular K^+ shifts (factor 3). Thus, uncomplicated lactic acidosis tends to present with a relatively normal $[K^+]$ (keep in mind that factor 1 shifts are relatively minor). However, complicating factors are common, and these may independently move $[K^+]$ in either direction. Examples include K^+ release from ischemic cells, decreased renal K^+ excretion secondary to hypotension with renal hypoperfusion, and intestinal K^+ losses from diarrhea. Thus, plasma $[K^+]$ usually is not helpful in diagnosing lactic acidosis. However, marked hyper- or hypokalemia in the setting of already-diagnosed lactic acidosis suggests the presence of other pathologic influences on $[K^+]$.

Alcoholic ketoacidosis.   Patients with alcoholic ketoacidosis can present with a $[K^+]$ that is normal, high, or low. However, hyper- or hypokalemia, when they occur, are usually not severe. For example, of those patients who present with hyperkalemia, $[K^+]$ is on average less elevated than the $[K^+]$ of hyperkalemic DKA patients. One reason for this difference may be the lower plasma [glucose], and hence lower osmolarity, in alcoholic ketoacidosis.

Methanol, ethylene glycol, and salicylate intoxication.   Metabolic acidosis from these intoxicants can present with a $[K^+]$ that is normal, high, or low. However, the limited data available suggest that hyper- or hypokalemia, when they occur, are usually not severe. This said, ethylene glycol can cause acute renal failure (due to deposition of calcium oxalate in the kidney); if it does, more severe hyperkalemia may develop.

Respiratory disturbances

Traditional teaching is that acute respiratory acidosis causes a slight rise in $[K^+]$, and acute respiratory alkalosis causes a slight fall in $[K^+]$. These changes are usually attributed to pH-induced shifts (factor 1). In chronic respiratory disturbances, compensation almost normalizes pH and, as a result, plasma $[K^+]$ returns to its previous level.

---

* **Clinical note.** Because of urinary K^+ losses, all DKA patients (including those with hyperkalemia) have low total-body K^+ stores. When insulin is given, K^+ shifts back into cells, and hypokalemia develops in all patients. This point is discussed further in the Treatment section of the text (p. 292–293).

Diagnostic utility of [K⁺]

How does knowing [K⁺] aid in acid-base diagnosis? To start with, [K⁺] can sometimes increase your confidence in a tentative diagnosis. For example, if you suspect a simple metabolic alkalosis, and you then find a low [K⁺], you will feel more certain your suspicion is correct. Conversely, if [K⁺] does not meet your expectation, you may reconsider the diagnosis. For example, if a patient has metabolic acidosis, and you suspected simple diarrhea as the cause, finding an elevated [K⁺] would lead you to consider a different cause for the acidosis, or to seek an independent explanation for the hyperkalemia.

There is one situation in which plasma [K⁺] can help you differentiate between two primary disorders. If venous [HCO_3^-] is elevated, and the history and physical examination are unrevealing, it will not be immediately apparent whether a metabolic alkalosis or a compensated respiratory acidosis is present. However, in simple metabolic alkalosis, [K⁺] is almost always low. In contrast, in compensated respiratory acidosis, [K⁺] is either slightly high or normal. (We will see later that a blood gas lets you differentiate with certainty among the four primary acid-base disorders, but for now we are considering just venous electrolytes.)

The normal range for plasma [K⁺] is 3.5 to 5.0 mmol/l. As a final review of [K⁺] in acid-base disorders, take a moment to reread the summary table on page 233.

Interpreting venous electrolytes

To help you integrate the ideas discussed in this chapter, we conclude by presenting three complete venous electrolyte reports. Analyze each report as thoroughly as you can before reading the interpretation. Be sure to consider [HCO_3^-], the anion gap, and [K⁺]. To keep things simple, we assume that the venous electrolyte assay is the only lab test available. Concentrations are in mmol/l. Assume that normal ranges are: [HCO_3^-] = 24–30, anion gap = 8–16, [K⁺] = 3.5–5.0.

Lab report 1.   Na⁺   =   143
                 K⁺   =   3.3
                 Cl⁻   =   90
                 HCO_3^- =   40

Interpretation: The high [HCO_3^-] suggests either metabolic alkalosis or compensated respiratory acidosis. The low [K⁺] makes metabolic alkalosis much more likely, since metabolic alkalosis typically presents with hypokalemia, whereas respiratory acidosis tends to present with a normal or slightly high [K⁺]. The anion gap is 13, which is normal, consistent with metabolic alkalosis. A history of vomiting, nasogastric drainage, or diuretic use (the common causes of metabolic alkalosis), would help confirm your diagnosis.

Lab report 2. Na^+ =   140
$\qquad\qquad\quad$ K^+ =   3.1
$\qquad\qquad\quad$ Cl^- =   115
$\qquad\qquad\quad$ HCO_3^- =   15

Interpretation: The low $[HCO_3^-]$ suggests either metabolic acidosis or compensated respiratory alkalosis. Although respiratory alkalosis can lower K^+, it does so only slightly (not to 3.1) and usually only in the acute phase, before compensation fully lowers $[HCO_3^-]$. Therefore, metabolic acidosis is more likely. The normal anion gap (10) effectively rules out the anion gap causes. Of the non-gap causes, diarrhea and Types 1 and 2 RTA can present with marked hypokalemia. If the patient gave a history of recent, severe diarrhea, you could be reasonably confident that the diarrhea caused the acidosis. If there was no history of diarrhea, you would lean toward one of the RTAs.

Lab report 3. Na^+ =   145
$\qquad\qquad\quad$ K^+ =   3.4
$\qquad\qquad\quad$ Cl^- =   81
$\qquad\qquad\quad$ HCO_3^- =   34

$\qquad\qquad\quad$ Note: this one is difficult!

Interpretation: If you solved this one, you deserve much credit. If not, study this explanation carefully so that you will recognize the pattern in the future. The bicarbonate and potassium levels suggest metabolic alkalosis, just like in the first report, above. But the elevated anion gap (30) suggests an anion gap metabolic acidosis. The solution is a mixed disturbance consisting of both these primary disorders. For example: an alcoholic patient experiences several days of severe vomiting (which raises $[HCO_3^-]$ and lowers $[K^+]$) and then develops alcoholic ketoacidosis (from fasting and volume depletion). Were it not for the onset of the acidosis, which consumed some of the excess bicarbonate, plasma $[HCO_3^-]$ would be substantially higher than 34. Conversely, were it not for the metabolic alkalosis, $[HCO_3^-]$ would be very low (perhaps around 5) and the lab report would have looked like a simple anion gap metabolic acidosis. Finally, if both acidosis and alkalosis had been of the same magnitude, $[HCO_3^-]$ would be normal, although the gap would still be elevated.

Summary

Venous electrolytes provide three key pieces of data for acid-base diagnosis: Total CO_2, anion gap, and $[K^+]$. Total CO_2, which closely approximates $[HCO_3^-]$, is low in metabolic acidosis and compensated respiratory alkalosis, and high in metabolic alkalosis and compensated respiratory acidosis. The anion gap, defined as $[Na^+] - ([Cl^-] + [HCO_3^-])$, parallels the concentration of plasma unmeasured anions. When metabolic acidosis is accompanied by an elevated anion gap, the condition is called an "anion gap (or normochloremic) metabolic acidosis." When metabolic acidosis is accompanied by a normal anion gap, it is called a "non-gap (or hyperchloremic) metabolic acidosis." The gap is typically high in ketoacidosis, lactic acidosis, and ingestions of methanol, ethylene glycol, and salicylates. The gap is typically normal in diarrhea and renal tubular acidosis. The gap may be either high or normal in renal failure. Plasma $[K^+]$ is influenced by both cellular and external K^+ movements. In metabolic alkalosis, $[K^+]$ is low. In metabolic acidosis, $[K^+]$ is cause-specific: $[K^+]$ is low in diarrhea, low (or normal) in Types 1 and 2 RTA, high in Type 4 RTA, and high (often only slightly) in renal failure. In lactic acidosis and ketoacidosis, $[K^+]$ is most often normal or high, but it can be low. In acute respiratory acidosis, $[K^+]$ may rise slightly; in acute respiratory alkalosis, $[K^+]$ may fall slightly.

Congratulations. You have just covered a great deal of new material and are now well on your way to mastering acid-base diagnosis. Before reading the next chapter, take a few moments to review anything that is not clear to you. Focus especially on the interpretation of the bicarbonate level (i.e., Total CO_2) and anion gap. The interpretation of the potassium level is slighty more advanced, and if this is your first exposure to the topic you probably should not expect to remember all the details just yet.

Arterial Blood Gases

22

Introduction

The term *arterial blood gas* ("A.B.G." or simply *blood gas*, with "arterial" left unstated) refers to a specific set of tests performed on an arterial blood sample. It provides four key pieces of information: pH, PCO_2, $[HCO_3^-]$, and PO_2. The name *blood gas* is really a partial misnomer since H^+ and bicarbonate are not gases.

The A.B.G. is the only standard test that measures plasma pH or PCO_2 and, for this reason, many consider it the definitive test for making or confirming an acid-base diagnosis. Although PO_2 is important, it is not directly relevant to acid-base. Therefore, this chapter focuses on pH, PCO_2, and $[HCO_3^-]$. These are sometimes described as the "three acid-base variables." The normal arterial ranges are:

$$pH \quad = \quad 7.35\text{–}7.45$$
$$PCO_2 \quad = \quad 35\text{–}45 \text{ mm Hg}$$
$$HCO_3^- \quad = \quad 23\text{–}29 \text{ mmol/l, just slightly below venous } [HCO_3^-]$$

Although the full range of normal values may be encountered in healthy individuals, the "classic" normal values often cited are pH = 7.4, PCO_2 = 40 mm Hg, and $[HCO_3^-]$ = 24 mmol/l. Beginning students often find it a useful mnemonic to note that the numeral "4" is prominent in each.

How are these values measured? In the hospital laboratory, pH and PCO_2 are measured directly, via electrode sensors. Bicarbonate concentration is not measured but is calculated by plugging the values for pH and PCO_2 into a rearranged version of the Henderson-Hasselbalch equation (many blood gas machines perform this calculation automatically). Because arterial and venous bicarbonate levels tend to parallel each other closely, arterial $[HCO_3^-]$ and venous Total CO_2 are usually within 1 or 2 mmol/l of each other.*

---

* **Correcting a misperception.** Because arterial $[HCO_3^-]$ is not directly measured, it is sometimes assumed that the value is inaccurate. In fact, the value is generally quite accurate, and it is a mistake to disregard it or to rely exclusively on venous Total CO_2. Calculated arterial $[HCO_3^-]$ would be inaccurate only if the Henderson-Hasselbalch equation did not apply to blood plasma in vivo, or if the pH or PCO_2 measurements were in error.

The blood sample for an A.B.G. requires special handling. Four points are relevant for the clinician: (1) Blood should be collected in a special low-friction syringe designed to fill under arterial pressure. Pull ("suction") syringes and "vacutainers" are not used because the partial vacuum they create causes dissolved gas to come out of solution, reducing both the PCO_2 and PO_2 of the sample. (2) Most blood-gas syringes contain heparin to prevent clotting. Excess heparin should be expressed from the syringe; too much will dilute the sample, altering concentration values. (3) If bubbles form in the sample (because room air enters through a non-airtight skin puncture), they should be "tapped" to the surface and expressed from the syringe. Otherwise, the atmospheric air in the bubbles can equilibrate with gases dissolved in the sample, artifactually raising PO_2 and lowering PCO_2. (4) If laboratory analysis will be delayed more than a few minutes, the sample should be refrigerated (typically by placing the capped syringe in a cup of ice water). Refrigeration slows the red blood cells' metabolism, which, because it is anaerobic, produces lactic acid and tends to acidify the sample.

This chapter has several subsections. The first provides a "feel" for how the different primary acid-base disorders affect the three acid-base variables. The second subsection presents a step-by-step method for analyzing a blood gas report and determining the major disturbance. The third shows how to determine if an additional, subtle disturbance is superimposed on the major one (i.e., if a subtle "mixed" disturbance is present). The fourth will help you better assess whether a disturbance is simple or mixed. These subsections build on each other. Taken together, they form a short but thorough course on understanding and interpreting blood gas reports.

Getting a "feel" for blood gases

In this subsection we examine graphic blood gas profiles of simple (i.e., not mixed) disturbances. Understanding these profiles is the essential foundation for interpreting blood gas reports. Each profile reflects two distinct processes:

1.   *The disturbance.* This process involves a primary change in either $[HCO_3^-]$ ("metabolic" disturbances) or PCO_2 ("respiratory" disturbances). These primary changes move pH away from its normal set point.

2.   *The compensation.* This process may or may not be present, depending on how much time has elapsed since the disturbance developed. Remember that compensation always follows the "same-direction rule" (p. 132), meaning that the compensatory and pathologic variables change in the same direction. For example, a primary fall in $[HCO_3^-]$ (i.e., metabolic acidosis) is followed by a compensatory fall in PCO_2. Compensation returns pH toward, but not to, its normal set point.

First, let's consider metabolic acidosis. The primary change is a fall in plasma $[HCO_3^-]$. Before respiratory compensation develops, the profile looks like this:

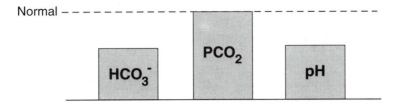

The dotted line indicates (in a qualitative way) normal levels. Note that $[HCO_3^-]$ and pH are both low. When the acidosis is caused by the addition of strong acid, the buffering of protons by bicarbonate liberates a small amount of carbon dioxide. This CO_2 is excreted by the lung and, unless pulmonary function is impaired, there is no rise in arterial PCO_2. Thus, as shown, PCO_2 is normal.

You may occasionally see an entirely uncompensated metabolic acidosis, as shown above. However, because respiratory compensation begins within a few hours and is generally complete within 12–24 hours, most patients will manifest at least partial compensation by the time a blood gas is done. Thus, most profiles will look more like this compensated one:

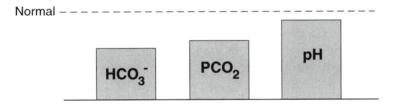

Here we see that the compensation for metabolic acidosis is a fall in PCO_2. This fall is consistent with the "same-direction rule," and it returns the pH toward normal. Note that plasma $[HCO_3^-]$ is still depressed to the same degree that it was before compensation. If you measure a blood gas after respiratory compensation begins but before PCO_2 reaches its new steady-state level, the blood gas will be intermediate between the two profiles just presented.

Next, consider metabolic alkalosis. The pre- and post-compensatory blood gas profiles are:

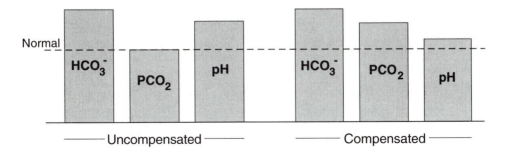

Note that the primary change is a rise in $[HCO_3^-]$. The compensatory change is a rise in PCO_2, which again follows the same-direction rule. Next, consider uncompensated respiratory acidosis:

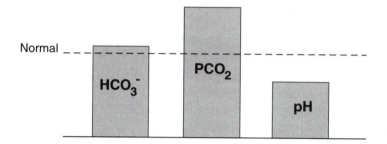

Note the high PCO_2, which is the defining characteristic of the disturbance. Also note that although compensation has not yet set in, $[HCO_3^-]$ is slightly above its normal set point (although it is usually within the normal *range*). This slight, pre-compensatory rise in $[HCO_3^-]$ occurs because the increase in PCO_2 drives the $CO_2 + H_2O \rightleftharpoons HCO_3^- + H^+$ equilibrium to the right, producing a small amount of bicarbonate.

Although renal compensation sets in fairly quickly, it takes 3 to 5 days for plasma $[HCO_3^-]$ to reach its final compensatory level. This delay makes it useful to apply the adjectives "acute" and "chronic" to respiratory disturbances: acute refers to uncompensated disturbances, chronic to compensated ones. Here is a typical profile for chronic respiratory acidosis:

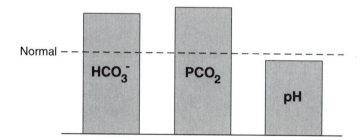

Finally, consider the profiles for respiratory alkalosis, a condition characterized by primary hypocapnia:

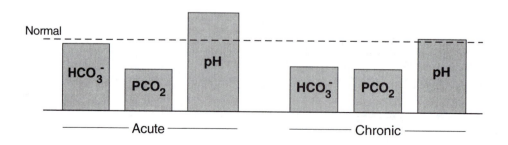

In the acute profile, notice the small, pre-compensatory decline in $[HCO_3^-]$, which is due to a leftward shift in the $CO_2 + H_2O \rightleftharpoons HCO_3^- + H^+$ equilibrium. The acute fall in PCO_2 usually leaves $[HCO_3^-]$ within the normal range. In the chronic profile, notice that pH is almost normal. We said earlier that compensation returns pH towards—but not to—normal. One partial exception occurs during sustained chronic respiratory alkalosis. During the first 2 to 4 days, $[HCO_3^-]$ falls gradually and pH approaches its normal value. This change in $[HCO_3^-]$ is similar to (but the reverse of) what happens in respiratory acidosis. However, unlike in respiratory acidosis, $[HCO_3^-]$ continues to fall gradually for a period of about two weeks. This progressive compensation can normalize pH in chronic respiratory alkalosis.

If you are uncertain about any aspect of these profiles, take a moment to review before continuing.

A step-by-step method for evaluating blood gases

We are now ready to learn a simple method for analyzing arterial blood gas data. The heart of this approach has two steps:

Step 1. *Assess pH.* Is it high or low? Low pH is acidemia. High pH is alkalemia.

Step 2. *Determine the cause of the acidemia or alkalemia.* Acidemia can only be caused by acidosis. Therefore, acidemia implies the presence of acidosis. Similarly, alkalemia can only be caused by alkalosis, so alkalemia implies alkalosis. To determine which type of acidosis or alkalosis is present, see *a.* if acidosis and *b.* if alkalosis:

a. *Acidosis.* An acidosis may be either metabolic or respiratory. If $[HCO_3^-]$ is low, metabolic acidosis is present. If PCO_2 is high, respiratory acidosis is present. If both low $[HCO_3^-]$ *and* high PCO_2 are present, then both metabolic acidosis and respiratory acidosis are present (i.e., a mixed disturbance).

b. *Alkalosis.* An alkalosis may be either metabolic or respiratory. If $[HCO_3^-]$ is high, metabolic alkalosis is present. If PCO_2 is low, respiratory alkalosis is present. If both high $[HCO_3^-]$ *and* low PCO_2 are present, then both metabolic alkalosis and respiratory alkalosis are present (i.e., a mixed disturbance).

The following flow chart portrays these two steps visually. To help you start thinking about numerical A.B.G. data, we have incorporated the normal values for pH, $[HCO_3^-]$, and PCO_2 into the flow chart. Take a moment to study the chart. Make sure you understand the logic behind every step:

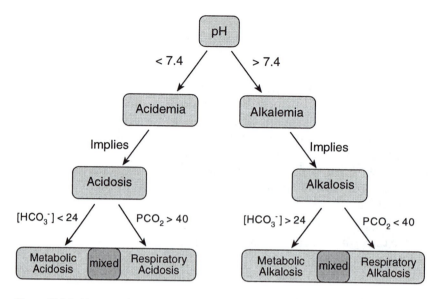

Note: [HCO_3^-] in mmol/l, PCO_2 in mm Hg

For practice, evaluate the following arterial blood gases. Try to analyze all four examples before reading the next paragraph.

Example	pH	[HCO_3^-]	PCO_2
1.	7.30	14	30
2.	7.57	42	47
3.	7.57	18	18
4.	7.60	32	34

Let's analyze example 1. A pH of 7.30 represents acidemia, so you know an acidosis is present. To determine which type of acidosis, look first at [HCO_3^-]. The low [HCO_3^-] indicates metabolic acidosis. In other words, the [HCO_3^-] can account for the low pH. Now look at PCO_2. It is low. A low PCO_2 does not represent an acidosis. It cannot account for the low pH. In fact, if [HCO_3^-] were normal, a low PCO_2 would cause alkalemia. You therefore know that the change in PCO_2 is not causing the acidemia but is the result of respiratory compensation, which follows the same-direction rule. Examples 2 and 3 are also simple disturbances. The approach is the same. Example 4 is a mixed disturbance. Both metabolic alkalosis and respiratory alkalosis are present. In other words, both [HCO_3^-] and PCO_2 can independently account for the pH change. If you are confused about any part of these problems, work them through, step by step, using the flow chart above.*

---

* **Hint for the reader.** If you are unsure why a particular change in [HCO_3^-] or PCO_2 affects pH as it does, you will find it helpful to read the "Respiratory and Metabolic" discussion, which starts on page 124.

You have just completed the most important part of analyzing a blood gas report: finding the major disturbance. You are now ready for the third and final step: determining if a subtle, additional disturbance is present. This last step takes some extra training, which is provided in the next subsection.

The third step: Looking for an additional disturbance

When both [HCO_3^-] and PCO_2 can independently account for the direction of the pH change (as was the case in example 4, just above), a mixed disturbance is obvious. And when a mixed disturbance is obvious, you don't have to keep scrutinizing the blood gas: you have already discovered what you need to know.

However, mixed disturbances usually are not obvious; most are subtle and not immediately apparent. For this reason, when a blood gas indicates a disturbance that appears to be simple and compensated (e.g., metabolic acidosis with low PCO_2), you must check if the *level* of compensation is appropriate. In other words, it is not enough for the compensatory variable to change in the right direction (i.e., that it follows the same-direction rule); it also must change to the quantitatively appropriate degree. If it does not change to the appropriate degree, an additional disturbance, which is affecting the compensatory variable, may be present. For example, during severe metabolic acidosis, you expect PCO_2 to be very low. If PCO_2 is only slightly low, you would wonder if there was a defect in lung function (i.e., a superimposed respiratory acidosis).

How do you assess the degree of the compensation? You do this by comparing the patient's [HCO_3^-] and PCO_2 with previously determined compensatory values. For example, studies have shown that when simple metabolic acidosis lowers [HCO_3^-] to 12 mmol/l, 95% of patients have a PCO_2 between 24 and 28 mm Hg. If a patient's [HCO_3^-] is 12, but PCO_2 is 33 (5 above the maximum expected), you should suspect that a respiratory acidosis is superimposed on the metabolic acidosis.

Where do you find these "previously determined compensatory values" for comparison? You could refer to the original studies. Thus, if you had a patient with respiratory acidosis, you could locate a journal article with a title like "Normal renal compensation in 137 patients with various levels of chronic respiratory acidosis." You would scan the article, looking for subjects whose PCO_2 matched that of your patient. You would then note the compensated [HCO_3^-] values, and see how your patient compared. This approach is obviously slow, labor-intensive, and impractical.

To simplify things, data from many studies have been summarized in various user-friendly ways. Three summary devices have become popular: rules of thumb, confidence bands, and maps. All three summarize the same data, so it doesn't matter which you use. However, it is important to understand (and read about) all of them. We begin with the rules of thumb.

Approach 1: Rules of thumb

Rules of thumb are simple mathematical formulas. To use the "rules," you plug in the value of the pathologic variable (i.e., $[HCO_3^-]$ in a metabolic disturbance, PCO_2 in a respiratory disturbance) and then solve the equation. The solution indicates the expected value of the compensatory variable. By comparing this expected value with the actual value, you can see if compensation is with in the normal range for a simple disturbance. This table lists a few of the more popular rules of thumb:

Rules of thumb for checking if level of compensation is appropriate

Disorder Primary change	Compensatory change	Expected value of compensation
Metabolic acidosis Fall in $[HCO_3^-]$	Fall in PCO_2	$PCO_2 = 1.5 \times [HCO_3^-] + 8 \pm 2$
Metabolic alkalosis Rise in $[HCO_3^-]$	Rise in PCO_2	PCO_2 up by 0.5–1.0 mm Hg for each mmol/l rise in $[HCO_3^-]$
Respiratory acidosis Rise in PCO_2	Rise in $[HCO_3^-]$	Acute: $[HCO_3^-]$ up 1 mmol/l for each 10 mm Hg rise in PCO_2 Chronic: $[HCO_3^-]$ up 4 mmol/l for each 10 mm Hg rise in PCO_2
Respiratory alkalosis Fall in PCO_2	Fall in $[HCO_3^-]$	Acute: $[HCO_3^-]$ down 2 mmol/l for each 10 mm Hg fall in PCO_2 Chronic: $[HCO_3^-]$ down 5 mmol/l for each 10 mm Hg fall in PCO_2

Note: acute changes in $[HCO_3^-]$ during respiratory disturbances are actually due to buffering, not compensation (see text, above).

For practice, use the rules of thumb to determine if the following disturbances are adequately compensated, then check your answers. (In the clinical setting, units are often left unstated. We follow that convention here.)

Patient 1.   A severely bulimic woman. pH = 7.51, $[HCO_3^-]$ = 38, PCO_2 = 49.

Patient 2.   A man with diabetic ketoacidosis. pH = 7.22, $[HCO_3^-]$ = 8, PCO_2 = 20.

Patient 3.   A child has "swallowed" a marble. pH = 7.26, PCO_2 = 60, $[HCO_3^-]$ = 26.

Hint: To find the major disturbance, use the two steps described in the previous subsection: First, assess pH to determine if acidemia or alkalemia is present. Second, look at $[HCO_3^-]$ and PCO_2 to determine which type of acidosis or alkalosis is present. Then, use the rule of thumb that applies to this disturbance.

Solutions: *Patient 1.* Use the metabolic alkalosis rule of thumb. The predicted PCO_2 range is 47–54 mm Hg.* The patient's PCO_2 is

---

* **Hint for the reader.** Why 47–54? The rise in $[HCO_3^-]$ = 38 − 24 = 14; 14 × 0.5 = 7 and 14 × 1 = 14; 40 + 7 = 47 and 40 + 14 = 54.

within this range, suggesting that compensation is appropriate. *Patient 2.* Use the metabolic acidosis rule. Predicted PCO_2 = 18–22 mm Hg. Again, compensation appears to be appropriate. Note: the metabolic acidosis rule given in the table is often called the "Winter's formula," named for one of the researchers who helped formulate it. *Patient 3.* Predicted $[HCO_3^-]$ = 26 mmol/l. The blood gas is consistent with acute (uncompensated) respiratory acidosis.

Approach 2: Confidence bands

Confidence bands are a graphical device for assessing compensation. They are called "confidence" bands because, like the other devices, they present data for the middle 95% of patients, and thus let you work with "95% confidence." They look like this:

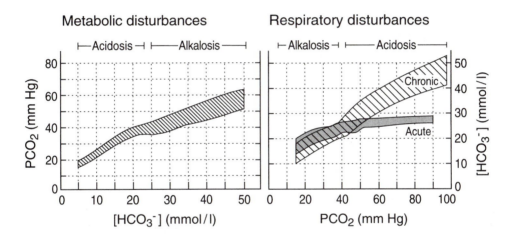

Modified from Valtin H, Gennari FJ: Acid-Base Disorders. Boston: Little, Brown and Company, 1987:68–69. Used by permission of Lippincott-Raven Publishers.

Notice that one box contains the bands for respiratory disturbances (both acute and chronic), and the other contains the band for metabolic disturbances. Because respiratory compensation develops rapidly, only a compensated band is given for metabolic disturbances. To use the bands, choose the box appropriate to the major disorder. Then plot a point using the blood gas values for PCO_2 and $[HCO_3^-]$. If the point falls within the band, compensation is within the normal range. If the point falls above the band, this suggests that the level of the compensatory variable is too high. If the point plots below the band, this suggests that the level of the compensatory variable is too low. Note that in the respiratory disturbance box there is a region of overlap between the acute and chronic bands. If a point plots into this overlap region, it means the blood gas is consistent with either an acute or chronic disturbance. Try these for practice:

Problem: A patient with severe COPD. pH = 7.38, PCO_2 = 70, $[HCO_3^-]$ = 40. What is the disturbance?

Solution: The first two steps tell you that respiratory acidosis is the major disturbance, so you plot the point (PCO_2 vs. $[HCO_3^-]$) in the box for "respiratory disturbances." The point falls in the "chronic" band. This suggests a simple, compensated respiratory acidosis.

Problem: A patient with several days of severe diarrhea. pH = 7.15, $[HCO_3^-]$ = 12, and PCO_2 = 36.

Solution: The first two steps tell you that metabolic acidosis is present, so plot the point in the box for "metabolic disturbances." The point falls above the band for metabolic acidosis. This indicates that PCO_2 is higher than expected and suggests that an additional, respiratory disorder is preventing adequate compensation (i.e., mixed metabolic acidosis and respiratory acidosis).

Approach 3: The acid-base map

An acid-base "map" is really just a set of confidence bands projected onto the same axes (i.e., squashed into the same box). A typical map is shown here:

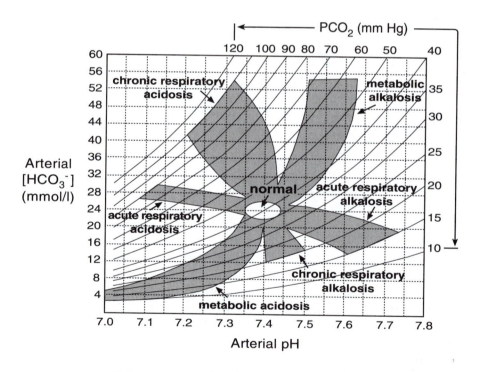

Modified from DuBose TD, Cogan MG, Rector FC. Acid-Base Disorders. In: Brenner BM, ed. The Kidney. 5th ed. Philadelphia: W.B. Saunders, 1996:949.

You use the map in almost the same way you use confidence bands. First, determine the major disturbance using the two steps outlined previously.

Then plot a point using any two of the three acid-base variables (i.e., pH, PCO_2, $[HCO_3^-]$). If the point falls within the band that represents the major disturbance, compensation is in the expected range. Try this example:

> Problem: A patient presents with a history of methanol ingestion. An A.B.G. shows pH = 7.29, $[HCO_3^-]$ = 12, and PCO_2 = 26. What is the disturbance?

> Solution: The first two steps tell you that the disturbance is metabolic acidosis (which you expect because methanol is metabolized to formic acid). Take any two of the three blood gas variables and plot a point. The point falls within the band for metabolic acidosis, suggesting that the disorder is simple and appropriately compensated.

In this example, compensation was normal. If the point had plotted above the band, it would suggest that PCO_2 was high and that the acidosis was incompletely compensated. If the point had plotted below the band, it would suggest that PCO_2 was abnormally low, that is, overcompensated (i.e., a superimposed respiratory alkalosis). If a point plots into a region where the bands intersect, the blood gas is consistent with any of the simple disturbances represented by the overlapping bands.

Finish with a question

So far we have followed a simple, three-step procedure: assess pH, find the major cause of the pH abnormality, and check for a subtle mixed disturbance. This procedure is very effective. But before you consider the results final, you must pause and ask yourself this question: *Is there another possible explanation for these blood gas data?*

This question is what separates the beginner from the expert. It is important for two reasons: (1) simple disturbances sometimes produce A.B.G.s that look mixed and (2) mixed disturbances sometimes produce A.B.G.s that look simple. We will look at these two situations individually.

Simple disturbances sometimes look mixed

A simple disturbance can sometimes produce a blood gas that falsely suggests a mixed disturbance. Let's see how. Consider a patient with a history and physical examination that is consistent with diabetic ketoacidosis. The blood gas shows an $[HCO_3^-]$ of 12 and a PCO_2 of 33. If you use the rules, map, or bands, you will discover that this PCO_2 is high (the expected range is between 24 and 28 mm Hg). Does this high PCO_2 mean that something is wrong with the patient's compensatory response? To answer this question, we need to examine the possible reasons why compensation might not fall into the expected range.

A. Not enough time elapsed

An "insufficient" level of compensation may simply mean that not enough time has elapsed for compensation to become fully manifest. Maximal respiratory compensation usually develops within 12 to 24 hours after the primary disorder is established. Maximal renal compensation requires 2 to 4 days. Thus, during the first day of a metabolic disturbance, and the first 2 or 3 days of a respiratory disturbance, "undercompensation" may in fact be normal. (Note: insufficient time can account only for undercompensation, not overcompensation.)

B. Outlying 5%

"Normal" compensatory values apply to the middle 95% of patients. Thus, 2.5% of patients with an intact compensatory response will have "high" values, and 2.5% will have "low" values. However, most of these outlying values will be just outside the expected range. Any substantial deviation from the norm is almost certainly due to another cause.

C. Defect in compensation

The final possibility is a defect in the compensatory system, which causes true under- or overcompensation.*

How do you use this information? When you see a compensatory value outside the normal range, observe how far it is outside. If it is only marginally outside, it is possible that compensation is actually normal for that particular patient. Next, decide if the abnormal value represents under- or overcompensation. If undercompensation (i.e., too small a change in the compensatory variable), consider how much time has passed since the primary disorder developed. If insufficient time has elapsed, and you have no reason to suspect a defect, then adequate compensation will likely develop (although you can't be sure until you see it). If non-marginal overcompensation exists (i.e., too great a change in the compensatory variable), you know that a mixed disturbance is present.

Mixed disturbances sometimes look simple

On occasion, a mixed disturbance will produce a blood gas that looks like it came from a simple disturbance. We can say that such a mixed disturbance is "masquerading" as a simple one. This point will become clear as you solve the following two problems:

> Problem: A child in status asthmaticus comes to the emergency room. The mother says the attack started several hours ago. A blood gas shows: pH = 7.24, PCO_2 = 65, $[HCO_3^-]$ = 26. What is your diagnosis?

> Solution: You plot these data on an acid-base map. The point falls within the band labeled "acute respiratory acidosis," confirming your clinical suspicion: the child has acute hypercapnia due to asthma.

---

* **Terminology.** A defect in compensation can be referred to in various ways. For example, in a patient with acidemia and metabolic acidosis but an inadequate hyperventilatory response, all of the following phrases can be used: "metabolic acidosis with inadequate compensation," "mixed metabolic acidosis and respiratory acidosis," and "metabolic acidosis with superimposed respiratory acidosis."

Problem: Later that day, a woman with a history of COPD comes to the emergency room. The blood gas is identical to that of the asthmatic child: pH = 7.24, PCO_2 = 65, $[HCO_3^-]$ = 26. What is your diagnosis?

Solution: The map again says "acute respiratory acidosis." However, this time you do not take the map at face value, because you know that COPD can cause chronic hypercapnia. You check the woman's chart and find that her PCO_2 is, in fact, chronically elevated. You question the woman further. She tells you she has had persistent diarrhea for three days. Now you see the whole story: the woman had chronic (compensated) hypercapnia and then developed metabolic acidosis from diarrhea, which lowered the $[HCO_3^-]$ to "normal." The map says "acute" but you know the correct diagnosis is chronic respiratory acidosis with a superimposed metabolic acidosis.

How do you rule out a masquerading mixed disturbance? You do this by considering the results of the blood gas in light of the history, physical examination, and other lab data. Attempt to construct a plausible "mixed explanation" for the apparently simple profile. If you can, then it is possible that the disturbance is mixed. If you cannot, it is likely that the disturbance really is simple.

Summary

The "classic" normal A.B.G. values are pH = 7.4, PCO_2 = 40 mm Hg, and $[HCO_3^-]$ = 24 mmol/l. In collecting an arterial blood sample, use a low-friction syringe, express excess heparin, "tap out" and express air bubbles from the blood sample, and ice the syringe if analysis is not immediate. A.B.G. profiles reflect two distinct processes: the disturbance and the compensation. Compensation may or may not be present, depending on how much time has elapsed since the disturbance developed. The A.B.G. laboratory report can be interpreted in three steps: (1) Look at pH. Determine if acidemia or alkalemia is present. (2) Acidemia implies acidosis and alkalemia implies alkalosis. Determine whether the "-osis" is metabolic or respiratory. Do this by evaluating $[HCO_3^-]$ and PCO_2 to see which can account for the direction of the pH change. Rarely, both $[HCO_3^-]$ and PCO_2 can independently account for the pH change; this indicates an obviously mixed disturbance. (3) If no obviously mixed disturbance is present, check for a subtle mixed disturbance. Compare the patient's level of compensation with established values summarized in bands, rules, or map. Finally, after you complete steps 1–3 and have reached a tentative conclusion, ask yourself if another explanation is possible. Do not be afraid to "contradict" the acid-base map; it is only a tool.

As you know, this chapter was packed with new concepts and information. If you are uncertain about anything you have just read, take some time to review before continuing.

Other Tests

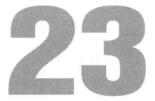

"Other tests," as used here, refers to laboratory tests and calculations other than the arterial blood gas and the common venous electrolytes (Na$^+$, K$^+$, Cl$^-$, HCO$_3{}^-$). In general, these other tests are relatively non-invasive and quick. Some require just a urine dip stick, and few need more than a venous blood sample.

These tests are used in various ways. Most commonly, you will have first looked at the venous electrolytes, and will thus know (or at least suspect) what the major acid-base disturbance is. In these cases, you will use the "other tests" to help determine the cause of this disturbance (i.e., to narrow the differential diagnosis). In other settings, you may see an "other test" result before you know much about the patient. For example, urine dip stick findings may be available almost immediately, and you might thus discover that the urine is positive for ketones or glucose before other laboratory data are available.

For convenience, the tests are arranged in this chapter according to the major disturbances and their subcategories. For example, tests relevant to ketoacidosis are described under the heading *Metabolic acidosis, anion gap*. As just indicated, however, this arrangement does not imply that you must always know the major disturbance in advance.

A note on units. Clinical laboratory values can be reported in two ways: conventional units and International System units (abbreviated "SI," for *Systéme International*). Conventional units are currently more popular in the United States, whereas SI units predominate in Europe. The two systems often overlap. For example, the common venous electrolytes (Na$^+$, K$^+$, Cl$^-$, HCO$_3{}^-$) have the same numerical value whether they are reported in SI units (mmol/l) or conventional units (meq/l). However, for some substances (e.g., glucose) the SI uses particle concentrations (e.g., mmol/l), whereas the conventional system uses mass concentrations (e.g., milligrams per deciliter, "mg/dl"). In this chapter, in cases where the two systems do not overlap, both values are given, with the SI in brackets.*

---

* **Hint for the reader.** Readers accustomed to conventional units often find that molar units yield surprising information; e.g., that normal plasma [glucose], expressed in mmol/l, is just slightly higher than plasma [K$^+$]. Note that normal ranges may vary slightly from hospital to hospital.

Metabolic acidosis, anion gap

In this subsection, we look at tests relevant to the common gap acidoses: renal failure, lactic acidosis, ketoacidosis, and poisoning.

Renal failure. Renal failure should be suspected whenever <u>creatinine and BUN</u> are markedly elevated. In contrast, during lactic- and ketoacidosis, creatinine and BUN are usually normal, but they may be somewhat elevated if circulatory failure or volume depletion reduce renal perfusion ("pre-renal azotemia"). Creatinine and BUN should be scrutinized whenever you suspect renal failure or wish to rule it out. Normal ranges: BUN = 8–25 mg/dl, creatinine = 0.6–1.5 mg/dl [BUN=2.9–8.9 mmol/l, creatinine = 53–133 μmol/l].*

Lactic acidosis. Lactic acidosis can be definitively identified by measuring the <u>plasma lactate</u> level. This assay is generally referred to as "lactate," not "lactic acid," because lactic acid is almost completely dissociated in body fluids. This assay is only reliable when used on plasma: because the kidney's reabsorptive threshold for lactate is high, urinary lactate will often be negative, even with markedly elevated plasma levels. The normal plasma range is 0.5–2.2 mmol/l. Since lactate has a single charge (-1), this normal range can also be expressed as 0.5–2.2 meq/l.

In lactic acidosis, the lactate level is often roughly similar to the *increase* in the anion gap. For example, if lactate is 7 mmol/l and the anion gap is also elevated by about 7, it is likely that the increase in the anion gap is due entirely to lactate. However, if the rise in the anion gap is much greater than the lactate level (e.g., lactate = 5 mmol/l, gap = 28), it is likely that an additional source of unmeasured anions is present. This source is typically a second anion gap metabolic acidosis (i.e., a mixed disturbance is present), such as ketoacidosis or renal failure. Although lactic acidosis usually presents with an elevated anion gap, a modestly elevated lactate level may be "hidden" within the normal range of the anion gap, so lactic acidosis cannot be ruled out just because the anion gap is normal. You should order a plasma lactate level whenever you suspect lactic acidosis or wish to rule it out with assurance.

Ketoacidosis. Ketoacidosis will usually produce a positive <u>ketone test</u> in both plasma and urine. The technical name for the test is the "nitroprusside reaction." Urine will be positive for ketones because, in contrast to lactate, the renal reabsorptive threshold for ketones is relatively low. A positive

---

* Going further. A high [creatinine] may be due to either acute or chronic renal failure. The simplest way to differentiate acute failure from chronic renal dysfunction is to compare the current [creatinine] with past levels recorded in the patient's chart. In older patients, decreased muscle mass often results in reduced creatinine production and, hence, lower normal levels. Thus, in older patients a "normal" [creatinine] may actually indicate reduced renal function. Failure to recognize this fact can lead to overadministration in the elderly of drugs cleared by renal excretion.

ketone test accompanied by hypobicarbonatemia strongly suggests one of the three causes of ketoacidosis: diabetic ketoacidosis (DKA), alcoholic ketoacidosis, or starvation ketoacidosis. Normal individuals are negative for ketones in both plasma and urine. Note: "Acetest" is the commercial name for one of the urine ketone assays.

Glucose levels are key in diagnosing DKA. Presentation plasma glucose levels in DKA are typically 400–800 mg/dl [22–44 mmol/l], but may occasionally be lower. The level almost always exceeds the renal reabsorptive threshold, so urine is positive for glucose. A tentative "bedside" diagnosis of DKA can be made if urine dipsticks (or reagent tablets) are strongly positive for both glucose and ketones. This tentative diagnosis is confirmed by positive findings on the plasma assays. Normal range for glucose: plasma = 70–110 mg/dl [3.9–6.1 mmol/l], urine = 0 mmol/l.*

Poisoning. Whenever you suspect poisoning, toxicology assays that are specific for the suspected toxin should be ordered. There are three intoxicants that commonly cause acid-base disturbances: salicylates, methanol, and ethylene glycol. Salicylates are frequently taken for therapeutic reasons in non-toxic doses, so low plasma levels may be unrelated to an acid-base disturbance. In contrast, even a low level of methanol or ethylene glycol suggests poisoning. Virtually all laboratories have specific assays that can test for the presence of salicylate. In contrast, methanol and ethylene glycol require special equipment that is not available in many hospitals.

Calculating the "osmolar gap" provides another way to help diagnose poisoning. It lets you use information about the osmolarity of blood plasma to help determine if certain toxins are present. It is a valuable supplement to specific toxicology assays, and in hospitals where specific assays are not offered (or are not available rapidly in an emergency) calculating the osmolar gap is indispensable. In the following paragraphs, we will see what the osmolar gap is and how it is used clinically.

The word osmolarity comes from *osmo-*, as in "osmosis," and *molar*, which denotes concentration expressed in moles per liter. *Osmolarity* therefore quantifies the concentration of osmotically active particles. It is approximately equal

---

* **Going further.** There are two clinical situations in which ketoacidosis may present with a plasma ketone test that is only weakly positive or even negative. They are: alcoholic ketoacidosis and combined keto and lactic acidosis ("keto-lactic acidosis"). Keto-lactic acidosis can occur when DKA is complicated by decreased tissue perfusion (with secondary tissue hypoxia) due to either volume depletion or sepsis with hypotension. In both alcoholic and keto-lactic acidosis, mitochondrial NADH levels are elevated, which causes circulating ketoacid anions to exist primarily as beta-hydroxybutyrate (the reduced form, "BHB") as opposed to acetoacetate (the oxidized form). BHB is not a true ketone (p. 143) and is therefore not detected by the assay. Although not usually needed, a special-order assay for BHB is available in some hospitals.

to the total concentration of all particles in solution. (It is not exactly equal because the electrical attraction between ions can slightly reduce their osmotic effect.) For example, if the concentration of all solutes in blood plasma are added together, and the total is 300 mmol/l, then osmolarity will be about 300 milliosmoles per liter (mOsm/l).

Solutes are of two types: charged (i.e., ions) and uncharged (i.e., molecules). Both types are osmotically active, so both must be taken into account when determining osmolarity. Because sodium is the predominant cation in plasma, and plasma (like all solutions) has an equal concentration of positive and negative charges, you can roughly estimate the contribution of ionic solutes to total osmolarity by doubling the sodium concentration. Thus, if $[Na^+] = 140$ mmol/l, ions will account for a total of about 280 mOsm/l.

What about uncharged solutes? Glucose and urea are the major uncharged solutes in normal blood plasma. Therefore, the combined concentration of these two substances (measured in millimoles per liter) gives a good approximation of the contribution of uncharged solutes to osmolarity. The concentration of glucose in mmol/l can be calculated by dividing the mg/dl (i.e., conventional units) value for glucose by 18. The contribution of urea can be calculated by dividing the mg/dl value for BUN ("blood urea nitrogen") by 2.8.* Thus, to estimate the total plasma osmolarity for ions plus uncharged solutes, you can use the following formula:

$$\text{Calculated osmolarity} = 2[Na^+] + [\text{glucose}]/18 + [\text{BUN}]/2.8$$

This sum is called "calculated" osmolarity because osmolarity is determined with a formula and not by actually measuring it with an osmometer. Because the formula takes into account the major osmotically active solutes, calculated osmolarity is normally quite close to the actual measured osmolarity. However, if an abnormal uncharged solute enters the blood, the formula becomes inadequate because it doesn't account for the new solute's osmotic contribution. The result is that measured osmolarity is higher than calculated osmolarity. Such patients are said to have an elevated "osmolar gap," which is defined thus:

---

* **Technical information.** You must convert mg/dl into mmol/l because osmotic activity is a function of the *number* of particles in solution, not the mass of these particles. Why 18 and 2.8? Since glucose weighs 180 grams per mole, and the laboratory gives concentration in mg/(0.1 liter) (*deci-* means one tenth), you divide the reported glucose concentration by 180×0.1, or 18. The procedure is similar for urea [formula: $(NH_2)_2CO$], except that for urea the laboratory assay quantitates the mass only of the two nitrogen atoms (hence, Blood Urea Nitrogen). Since the molecular weight of N_2 is 28, you divide the reported BUN value by 28×0.1, or 2.8. It makes little difference if you use 20 and 3 as divisors instead of 18 and 2.8, and these rounded off numbers may make it easier to work without a calculator. Obviously, when glucose and urea are reported in mmol/l, no conversion is needed.

Osmolar gap = measured osmolarity − calculated osmolarity

For practice: find the osmolar gap if $[Na^+]$ = 140 mmol/l, [glucose] = 90 mg/dl, BUN = 28 mg/dl, and measured osmolarity = 300 mOsm/l.

Healthy individuals may have a small osmolar gap because the formula for calculated osmolarity is only approximate. However, when the gap exceeds 5–10 mOsm/l, an abnormal substance is likely. Because clinical osmometers actually measure the osmolality of plasma water (i.e., osmoles per kg of H_2O), the osmolar gap is sometimes called the osmolal gap. Sometimes, it is called, simply, the osmol gap.

The osmolar gap is used clinically when ingestion of either methanol or ethylene glycol is suspected, especially when specific assays are unavailable or will be delayed. For both methanol and ethylene glycol, blood levels of 50 mg/dl represent major ingestions that can cause permanent harm or even death. At this blood level, methanol (molecular wt. = 32) raises the osmolar gap by 16 and ethylene glycol (molecular wt. = 62) raises the gap by 8. Given these relatively small elevations in the osmolar gap, serious ingestions can sometimes "hide" within the normal range of the osmolar gap. Therefore, while an elevated osmolar gap suggests possible intoxication, a normal osmolar gap does *not* rule it out.

Any non-ionic substance in plasma other than urea or glucose will elevate the osmolar gap. Not all are poisons and not all cause metabolic acidosis. Ethanol (drinking alcohol, molecular wt. = 46) can elevate the gap markedly (each 100 mg/dl elevates the gap by 22). Acetone, the non-ionic "ketone body," can elevate the osmolar gap during ketoacidosis of any cause. Isopropanol (i.e., isopropyl alcohol, rubbing alcohol), which is often ingested as an ethanol "substitute," also raises the osmolar gap. Isopropanol is toxic but it does not usually cause metabolic acidosis. Since isopropanol is metabolized to acetone, a positive ketone test in the absence of metabolic acidosis suggests isopropanol ingestion.

Finally, calcium oxalate crystals observed by microscope in a centrifuged urine sample are a relatively specific marker for ethylene glycol ingestion. These crystals arise when ethylene glycol is metabolized to oxalic acid, which dissociates to oxalate (a divalent anion) and them forms insoluble complexes with Ca^{2+}. The combination of metabolic acidosis, elevated osmolar gap, and urinary oxalate crystals is virtually diagnostic for ethylene glycol. However, a urine negative for the crystals does not rule out ethylene glycol.*

---

* **Important clinical note.** This discussion of poisoning in metabolic acidosis is an introduction. Advanced readers who are actively involved in diagnosing intoxicated patients should also read appendix topic H, which discusses a number of clinically important technical points.

Metabolic acidosis, non-anion gap

Let's now consider tests relevant to the three common causes of non-anion gap (hyperchloremic) metabolic acidosis: diarrhea, renal failure, and renal tubular acidosis.

Diarrhea. Diarrhea can usually be diagnosed by history or by the presence of soiled bedding or underclothing. No "other test" applies specifically to it.

Renal failure. Renal failure can present with either an elevated anion gap or a normal gap (p. 229). However, it always presents with a markedly elevated creatinine and BUN, as discussed above (p. 254).

Renal tubular acidosis (RTA). RTA should be considered any time hyperchloremic metabolic acidosis cannot be attributed to diarrhea or renal failure. The three types of RTA can usually be differentiated by plasma [K+], creatinine, and urine pH. Let's see how.

To begin, take a moment to read through the table on page 150. Given the information in the table, we can say the following: A high plasma [K+] immediately suggests Type 4. The additional finding of a slightly elevated creatine reinforces this impression, and a low urine pH (<5.5) virtually confirms it. Second, a low or normal plasma [K+] immediately suggests Types 1 or 2, and a normal creatinine reinforces this impression. The additional finding of a low urine pH (<5.5) points to Type 2. In contrast, a high urine pH (>5.5) suggests Type 1. However, a high urine pH is also consistent with Type 2 early in its biphasic course.*

Metabolic alkalosis

Metabolic alkalosis falls into two broad categories: volume-responsive and volume-resistant (p. 168). All the common causes of metabolic alkalosis—including vomiting, nasogastric drainage, diuretic use, and post-hypercapnia—are volume-responsive. Together, the volume-responsive entities account for about 95% of metabolic alkalosis cases. Volume-resistant causes comprise a number of rare entities such as primary hyperaldosteronism and Bartter's syndrome. We begin our discussion with volume-responsive alkalosis.

---

* **Going further.** If you suspect an RTA but want to be sure you are not missing an inapparent diarrhea or a hyperchloremic (i.e., non-gap) presentation of renal failure, consider the following. Diarrhea alone usually presents with low [K+]. In contrast, the most common adult RTA (Type 4) presents with high [K+]. Although Types 1 and 2 RTA often present with low [K+], they can be distinguished from diarrhea by urine assay. Type 1 has a urine pH above 5.5 whereas diarrhea usually has a low urine pH. Type 2 is rare in adults (except in patients with myeloma or those taking Diamox) and usually occurs as part of the Fanconi syndrome, which is easily identified by urine assay (p. 154). Because renal failure is sometimes hyperchloremic and hyperkalemic, it might be confused with Type 4 RTA. However, Type 4 usually causes only mild elevations in creatinine, whereas renal failure advanced enough to cause significant acidosis usually presents with sharply elevated creatinine, especially by the time hyperkalemia becomes clinically apparent (p. 155).

Volume-responsive metabolic alkalosis. During volume depletion, which is a key characteristic of volume-responsive alkalosis, filtered chloride is actively reabsorbed by the kidney. Urinary chloride concentration is thus low. In a patient with metabolic alkalosis, a urinary [Cl⁻] of less than 15 mmol/l (it is often below 5 mmol/l) is virtually diagnostic of a volume-responsive cause.

When the history provides a clear-cut explanation for the metabolic alkalosis, checking urinary [Cl⁻] may be unnecessary. For example, in a patient with a plasma bicarbonate of 37 mmol/l and a four-day history of vomiting, volume-responsive alkalosis is a virtual certainty. However, if the history is ambiguous, measuring urinary [Cl⁻] can be invaluable. A few examples: (1) in a patient with no obvious cause for metabolic alkalosis, an elevated urinary [Cl⁻] is likely to be your first indication that a volume-resistant form is present; (2) in a patient with suspected cryptogenic ("hidden cause") metabolic alkalosis, such as surreptitious bulimic vomiting or self-administration of diuretics for weight loss, a low urinary [Cl⁻] tends to support the suspicion; (3) in a patient whose venous electrolytes show an elevated [HCO₃⁻], and the history does not make clear if this elevated [HCO₃⁻] represents metabolic alkalosis or a compensation for respiratory acidosis, a low urine [Cl⁻] strongly suggests metabolic alkalosis whereas a normal urine [Cl⁻] suggests respiratory acidosis.

What about urinary sodium? Like chloride, filtered sodium is actively reabsorbed by the kidney during volume depletion. Thus, a low urinary [Na⁺] also suggests volume depletion and a volume-responsive cause. However, during the early stages of metabolic alkalosis, some bicarbonate is spilled in the urine, and sodium is spilled with it to maintain electroneutrality (p. 165). This Na⁺ spillage can result in a normal urinary [Na⁺] even as volume-responsive alkalosis is evolving. In fact, if vomiting occurs after metabolic alkalosis is already established, urinary [HCO₃⁻] and [Na⁺] may rise transiently following each new episode of gastric fluid loss. In contrast, urinary chloride is generally low in all stages of metabolic alkalosis. Therefore, while a low urine [Na⁺] suggests volume depletion and a volume-responsive cause about as well as urine [Cl⁻], a normal or high urine [Na⁺] does not rule out volume-responsive causes as well as a normal or high urine [Cl⁻] does. Nonetheless, when a urine [Cl⁻] assay is not available (some hospital laboratories do not offer it), [Na⁺] is probably the best substitute. Numerically, a urinary [Na⁺] less than 10–15 mmol/l suggests volume depletion and, thus, volume-responsive metabolic alkalosis.

A caveat. When a patient has recently taken a diuretic, and it is still actively inhibiting salt reabsorption, urinary [Na⁺] and [Cl⁻] will both be elevated, or at least normal, even if volume depletion is severe. Thus, in suspected diuretic abuse, normal or high urinary [Na⁺] or [Cl⁻] do not rule out a volume-responsive cause.*

---

* **Technical note.** Urinary [Cl⁻] may also be greater than 15 mmol/l in volume-responsive metabolic alkalosis associated with severe hypokalemia ([K⁺] < 2.0 mmol/l). Severe hypokalemia interferes with distal nephron Cl⁻ reabsorption, at least acutely.

Volume-resistant metabolic alkalosis. Volume-resistant alkalosis should be suspected whenever metabolic alkalosis presents without a history of volume-responsive causes (i.e., gastric fluid loss, diuretics, or post-hypercapnia). The first diagnostic step is to check urinary chloride. If the alkalosis is volume resistant, $[Cl^-]$ will almost always be greater than 35 mmol/l. Thus, a $[Cl^-]$ greater than 35 mmol/l suggests either a volume-resistant cause or ongoing diuretic abuse. If diuretics are ruled out (e.g., by urinary diuretic screen), a volume-resistant cause is almost certain. Additional diagnostic details are supplied in appendix topic K, which discusses rare causes of acid-base disturbances.

Respiratory disturbances

A number of tests and calculations are useful for diagnosing respiratory disturbances.

Pulse oximetry. Pulse oximetry (or "pulse ox") measures the oxygen saturation of arterial hemoglobin. The normal range is 96–100%. Values below 90% are usually associated with marked tissue hypoxia. Pulse oximetry is especially useful because it is cheap, fast, and non-invasive (the sensor clips on, or is taped to, the finger, ear lobe, forehead, or nose). In fact, in patients with suspected respiratory or cardiac disease, pulse oximetry is increasingly considered a standard screen for hypoxemia. Although pulse oximetry has limitations (its accuracy is affected by intense ambient light near the sensor, nail polish on the sensor finger, sensor motion or malposition, and skin pigmentation) it has proven very useful clinically; some actually call it the "fifth vital sign."

However, it must be understood that oximetry has no direct use in acid-base diagnosis because it tells you nothing about PCO_2, which can be measured only by blood gas. For example, a patient with a pulmonary embolus may have an oxygen saturation ("O_2 sat") of 96% but a PCO_2 of 20 mm Hg. Conversely, a patient with ventilatory suppression who is getting supplemental oxygen may have an oxygen saturation of 100% but a PCO_2 of 100 mm Hg. In both these cases, if you assumed that a normal oxygen saturation ruled out respiratory disease, you would miss a life-threatening diagnosis. Thus, while oximetry can help screen for hypoxemia, it can never screen for changes in PCO_2.*

Alveolar-arterial oxygen difference. In health, the PO_2 of alveolar air is slightly higher than the PO_2 of arterial blood. The difference is quantified as the

---

* **Going further.** A relatively new technology, end-tidal CO_2 monitoring ($P_{ET}CO_2$), analyzes the PCO_2 of expired air as a way to estimate arterial PCO_2. This form of monitoring, which can sometimes obviate the need for a blood gas, has been most widely used on intubated patients in the intensive care setting. For additional comments on the assessment of hypoxemia, see pp. 322–323.

alveolar-arterial oxygen difference. For example, if alveolar PO_2 is 100 mm Hg and arterial PO_2 is 90 mm Hg, the alveolar-arterial oxygen difference is 10 mm Hg. In healthy young people, the alveolar-arterial difference is usually less than 10 mm Hg. The difference tends to increase slightly with age, but it usually remains less than 25 mm Hg in healthy older people. Why does this difference exist? The main reason is that a small fraction of venous blood is normally shunted past the lung, directly into the arterial circulation. The addition of this unoxygenated blood slightly lowers arterial PO_2. Because big "A" symbolizes alveolar, and small "a" symbolizes arterial, the alveolar-arterial difference is sometimes written $P(A-a)O_2$. In routine clinical discussions, it is sometimes called, simply, the "A-a difference" or "A-a gradient."

Lung disease impairs gas exchange and usually causes the A-a difference to rise. Thus, knowing the A-a difference can help you determine if lung disease is present. In fact, this is the main diagnostic use of the A-a difference: to help determine if lung disease is present. If this seems unnecessary—for example, you might be wondering how a blood gas could be abnormal if lung disease was *not* present—remember that hypoxemia and hypercapnia can be caused by a neuromuscular defect (e.g., decreased central drive, phrenic nerve injury, respiratory muscle weakness) even if the lung is normal.

A markedly elevated A-a difference indicates that a gas exchange defect is present in the lung; that is, that some form of lung disease is present. In contrast, while a normal A-a difference is consistent with normal lungs, lung disease, even if severe, sometimes presents with a normal A-a difference as well. Thus, while a markedly elevated A-a helps rule in lung disease, a normal A-a does *not* usually help rule it out.

How do you determine the A-a difference? Although you can directly measure arterial PO_2 by blood gas, you cannot directly measure alveolar PO_2. Thus, alveolar PO_2 ("PAO_2") must be estimated. The following formula, which is called the alveolar gas equation, can be used to calculate PAO_2.

$$PAO_2 = (PB - PH_2O) \times FIO_2 - (\text{arterial } PCO_2 \div R)$$

where

PB   = total barometric pressure (760 mm Hg at sea level)
PH_2O = partial pressure of water vapor in the lung, about 47 mm Hg
FIO_2 = O_2 fraction of inspired air (0.21 if room air, i.e., 21 percent)
R   = respiratory exchange ratio, usually assumed to be 0.8

For practice, calculate alveolar PO_2 (i.e., PAO_2) for a 25 year-old man, hospitalized at sea level, breathing 60% oxygen, whose arterial $PCO_2 = 56$ mm Hg.

$$
\begin{aligned}
PAO_2 &= (760 - 47)(0.60) - (56/0.8) \\
&= 428 - 70 \\
&= 358 \text{ mm Hg}
\end{aligned}
$$

If the blood gas shows that this patient has an arterial PO_2 (i.e., PaO_2) of 167 mm Hg, what is the A-a difference?

$$P(A\text{-}a)O_2 = PAO_2 - PaO_2$$
$$= 358 \quad - 167$$
$$= 191 \text{ mm Hg}$$

An A-a difference of 191 mm Hg is markedly elevated, indicating that lung disease is present. In contrast, if the A-a difference had been normal, this would not rule out lung disease. The derivation of the alveolar gas equation can be found in pulmonology texts.*

Summary

"Other tests" refer to tests and calculations other than venous electrolytes and arterial blood gases. Typical results follow. <u>Metabolic acidosis</u>. Renal failure: creatinine and BUN very high. Type 4 RTA: creatinine slightly high. Lactic acidosis: plasma lactate high. Diabetic ketoacidosis: plasma and urine glucose high. All ketoacidoses: plasma and urine ketones high (may give false negative in alcoholic ketoacidosis or keto-lactic acidosis). Methanol and ethylene glycol intoxication: osmolar gap often high. All poisonings: specific assays positive. Type 1 RTA and early phase of Type 2 RTA: urine pH high. Ethylene glycol intoxication: urinary oxalate crystals often present. <u>Metabolic alkalosis</u>. In volume-responsive cause: urine $[Cl^-]$ and usually $[Na^+]$ are low, except when diuretics are active. In volume-resistant metabolic alkalosis: urine $[Cl^-]$ and $[Na^+]$ usually high. <u>Respiratory disorders</u>. Pulse oximetry can help screen for hypoxemia, but not for abnormal PCO_2. The A-a difference can help rule in lung disease, but it can't help rule it out.

We have now studied all the main components of acid-base diagnosis (Chapters 20-23). The final chapter of this section will help you integrate these components into an efficient and practical diagnostic strategy.

---

* **Going further.** Three points. First, the normal range for the A-a difference tends to rise when supplemental oxygen is given. By the time FIO_2 reaches about 0.6, the normal difference may approach 50 in young people and 100 in older people. This fact must be kept in mind when interpreting the meaning of an elevated A-a in patients on supplemental oxygen. Second, the formula given in the text for estimating PAO_2 can be used at any altitude, by plugging in the appropriate values for PB and PH_2O. Near sea level (i.e., altitudes lower than about 1000 feet) the formula for PAO_2 can be simplified to: $PAO_2 = 7 \times$ inspired oxygen in % $- (1.25 \times$ arterial $PCO_2)$. In patients breathing room air at sea level, the formula can be simplified further to: $PAO_2 = 150 - (1.25 \times$ arterial $PCO_2)$. Third, in patients with lung disease, the actual level of the A-a difference may vary unpredictably with changes in FIO_2. For this reason, unless FIO_2 is constant, even large changes in the A-a difference should not be attributed to improvement or worsening of the underlying gas exchange defect.

Making the Diagnosis

24

We are now ready to bring together the ideas and methods discussed in the previous four chapters (Chapters 20–23). We do this by presenting a step-by-step approach to acid-base diagnosis. Studying this approach will familiarize you with key concepts and give you a simple way to think about the diagnostic process, including how to decide if a blood gas is necessary. Our approach has four steps.

Step 1. Consider history and physical examination

Consider the history and physical examination to determine if the patient has any conditions that might cause an acid-base disturbance. Mentally run down a list of the patient's conditions, asking, *Are any of these likely to cause acidosis or alkalosis?* As you gain experience, this step will become automatic.

> Examples: If a patient reports several days of diarrhea, you would automatically suspect metabolic acidosis. Vomiting or nasogastric drainage should make you think of volume-responsive metabolic alkalosis. Jaundice, which may suggest liver disease, should make you think of either respiratory alkalosis or lactic acidosis (or both). When you see a patient on a ventilator, you should always consider the possibility that an inappropriate ventilatory setting might be causing respiratory acidosis, respiratory alkalosis, or (especially in a volume- or K^+-depleted patient) post-hypercapnic metabolic alkalosis.

Step 2. Consider venous electrolytes

Carefully evaluate plasma $[HCO_3^-]$, the anion gap, and $[K^+]$. Start with $[HCO_3^-]$ (i.e., Total CO_2). Is it high, low, or normal? If it is normal, does this really mean there is no acid base disturbance? Remember that an acute respiratory disturbance, or certain mixed disturbances (e.g., metabolic acidosis and metabolic alkalosis), can give a normal $[HCO_3^-]$. If $[HCO_3^-]$ is abnormal, is it likely that the change is primary (i.e., a metabolic disturbance) or secondary (i.e., renal compensation for a respiratory disturbance)? Next evaluate the anion gap. A markedly elevated gap points to one of the anion-gap metabolic acidoses. Remember that the gap may occasionally be markedly elevated even in the setting of a normal or high $[HCO_3^-]$, and that this combination usually suggests a mixed disturbance. Then evaluate plasma $[K^+]$ and assess if the kalemic pattern is consistent with the disturbance suggested by the $[HCO_3^-]$ and anion gap.

If the $[HCO_3^-]$, anion gap, and $[K^+]$ can all be explained by a single disorder, then a simple disturbance is likely. If the history and physical examination also point to the same disorder, a simple disorder is even more likely. However, if the electrolyte values form a confusing picture, one that cannot readily be explained by a single disorder or that does not fit with your impressions from the history and physical examination, you should suspect a mixed disturbance.

> Example: If you see a patient with a high $[HCO_3^-]$, you would immediately think of either a metabolic alkalosis or a chronic (i.e., compensated) respiratory acidosis. If the patient also has a low $[K^+]$, your suspicion of metabolic alkalosis would rise, since metabolic alkalosis is generally accompanied by hypokalemia. If the patient had been vomiting, this would reinforce your suspicion. If the anion gap is within the normal range, you could assume that there is no superimposed anion gap metabolic acidosis. However, if $[K^+]$ or the anion gap is markedly elevated, or there is no history of gastric fluid loss or diuretic use, you would need to reconsider the diagnosis.

This step is listed as number 2. Sometimes, however, the electrolyte report will be available before you see the patient. In this situation, you may chose to look first at the lab data and, only afterwards, carry out the step listed as number 1. The order is not important so long as you give careful thought to both clinical findings and laboratory data, and interpret one in light of the other.

Step 3. Consider other tests

Look at relevant data from the tests and calculations described in the chapter on *Other Tests* (Chapter 23). Some of these tests may have been ordered before you encountered the patient. For example, it is becoming standard practice to screen all acutely ill patients for laboratory abnormalities (screening tests may include venous electrolytes, BUN and creatinine, a urine dip stick, and plasma glucose). If additional tests are needed, order them. If any of the tests suggest a previously unsuspected disorder, it may be important to return to the patient so you can ask more questions or repeat specific aspects of the physical examination.

> Examples: Markedly elevated BUN and creatinine indicate renal

failure. Lesser elevations of creatinine in a patient with metabolic acidosis and hyperkalemia may indicate Type 4 RTA. If you suspect intoxication, order a plasma osmolarity measurement and calculate the osmolar gap; specific toxin assays will also be needed. A low urine chloride (or sodium) suggests volume depletion and raises the possibility of volume-responsive metabolic alkalosis. Blood or urine that is positive for ketones and glucose should make you think of diabetic ketoacidosis. If glucose is elevated in a patient not known to be a diabetic, it will probably be useful to ask the patient additional questions about conditions such as polydipsia and polyuria.

In some cases, you will look at these "other" laboratory tests only after considering the clinical findings and venous electrolytes. Often, however, you will order some of these tests along with the electrolytes. For example, many hospitals offer "Chem-7" or similar panels, which comprise plasma assays for the four electrolytes plus BUN, creatinine, and glucose. Sometimes, a urine assay will provide your first laboratory data on a patient. As noted, the order of these "steps" is not important. The essential point is that you consider all sources of information and try to form a coherent picture that explains all of the findings.

Step 4. Decide if a blood gas is needed

A blood gas requires arterial puncture. It can be painful, carries a small risk of arterial occlusion, and is relatively expensive and time consuming. Thus, an important step in the diagnostic process is to decide if a blood gas is needed. Except in emergencies, when a blood gas may be needed immediately, you will generally make this decision *after* you have obtained and scrutinized data from other sources.

This point is worth emphasizing because students learning acid-base diagnosis are often encouraged to look at the blood gas report first (the aim being to identify the primary disturbance) and then decide which "additional" tests (e.g., anion gap, BUN and creatinine, glucose) should be ordered to refine the diagnosis. While this approach is a useful learning exercise, in the clinical setting it is more common, and often more appropriate, to first carry out the less invasive methods of data collection—the H & P, venous electrolytes, and other tests—and to use the results to decide if a blood gas is needed.

There is no single "right" method for deciding when to get a blood gas. This decision tree, and the explanatory paragraphs that follow it, provide one good approach. More importantly, the tree and paragraphs are designed to teach key concepts that are valid no matter which approach you ultimately use. Start by scanning the tree. Then read the paragraphs, referring back to the tree as you go.

Based on history and physical exam, venous electrolytes, and other tests, do you suspect an acid-base disturbance?

- yes → Do you suspect a life-threatening acid-base disturbance?
- no → No blood gas

Do you suspect a life-threatening acid-base disturbance?

- yes → Blood gas mandatory
- no → Is the suspected disturbance metabolic or respiratory?

Is the suspected disturbance metabolic or respiratory?

- metabolic → Do data all "fit together" and suggest a simple disturbance?
- respiratory → Is disturbance acute or chronic?

Do data all "fit together" and suggest a simple disturbance?

- yes → Blood gas may not be necessary
- no → Blood gas usually required

Is disturbance acute or chronic?

- acute → Blood gas usually required
- chronic → Do you suspect an acute exacerbation?

Do you suspect an acute exacerbation?

- yes → Blood gas usually required
- no → Do you have a base-line blood gas?

Do you have a base-line blood gas?

- yes → Blood gas probably not necessary
- no → Blood gas usually required

1. Do the less invasive methods of data collection suggest an acid-base disturbance? If not, a clinically significant disturbance is very unlikely and, in general, there is no reason to get a blood gas.

2. If you suspect an acid-base disturbance, do you think it may be either severe (as defined by a large change in $[HCO_3^-]$ or PCO_2) or rapidly progressive (as defined by a rapid rate of change in $[HCO_3^-]$ or PCO_2)? If so, a blood gas is generally considered mandatory. Why? In an unstable patient, more information, including a well-defined baseline in a patient whose condition appears to be deteriorating, could prove critical. For these patients, the decision tree stops here. The following points refer to disturbances that you believe are neither severe nor rapidly progressive.

3. Is the suspected disturbance respiratory and, if so, is it acute? Evaluation of an acute respiratory disturbance, or of an acute exacerbation of a chronic respiratory disturbance (e.g., a hypercapnic COPD patient who develops an acute respiratory infection), usually requires a blood gas because it provides the only way to assess the key pathologic variable, PCO_2. A clinically important degree of hyper- or hypoventilation may not be detectable on

physical examination, so visually scrutinizing a patient's ventilatory pattern cannot substitute for a blood gas.*

4. Do you suspect a chronic respiratory disturbance? The initial evaluation of a chronic respiratory disturbance requires a blood gas. Definitive, subsequent evaluations also require a blood gas. However, when you already have a base-line blood gas, and you do not suspect that any significant change has occurred, a new blood gas is not always necessary. A venous bicarbonate level, which can be compared with previous post-compensation levels, can sometimes act as a partial "check" on PCO_2 and acid-base status.

5. Is the suspected disturbance metabolic and, if so, do you think it is simple? Although definitive diagnosis always requires a blood gas, there are times when all other lab and clinical findings suggest a mild, simple disturbance. In such cases, many physicians will consider not getting a blood gas. For example, some physicians will not get a blood gas for an elevated venous $[HCO_3^-]$ in an otherwise healthy patient with a history of vomiting.

6. Do you suspect a mixed disturbance? Simple disturbances usually produce consistent pictures, with all the data readily attributable to the suspected cause. A confusing picture, in which the cause of certain abnormal findings is not readily apparent, may represent a mixed disturbance and should generally be evaluated by blood gas.

Remember: the above approach is intended to teach key concepts, not to provide an inflexible formula for blood-gas testing. The final decision and its timing must always be based on the physician's informed judgement of whether a blood gas is likely to provide clinically important new information.

If you do obtain a blood gas, how should you proceed? First, study the results carefully. Use the approach discussed in the chapter on blood gases (Chapter 22). What is the major disturbance? Is the level of compensation appropriate? Is a mixed disturbance likely? Next, consider the blood-gas findings in the context of information obtained from the history and physical examination, venous electrolytes, and other tests. Do these other findings suggest an alternate interpretation for the blood gas? You should expect to find a consistent "picture" formed by data from the various sources.

---

* **Clinical note.** For a patient in obvious respiratory distress, it is perfectly appropriate to think of the blood gas primarily as a way to assess respiratory status (i.e., to focus on the PO_2 and PCO_2), and only secondarily to worry about acid-base status *per se*. Additional comments about the decision to get a blood gas in patients with mild acute respiratory disturbances can be found in Chapter 28, *Treatment of Respiratory Alkalosis,* p. 317.

If the blood gas tells you one thing, and the other data tell you another, either you are missing something or there is a lab error.

Summary

Acid-base diagnosis has four components. First, history and physical examination, to see if likely causes of acid-base disorders are present. Second, venous electrolytes, to assess plasma $[HCO_3^-]$, anion gap, and $[K^+]$. Third, other lab tests, such as creatinine, glucose, pulse oximetry, and urine $[Cl^-]$. Fourth, blood gas, but (except in frank emergencies) only if less invasive laboratory or clinical data suggest a need. As a general rule, a blood gas should be obtained when you suspect a disturbance that is severe, rapidly progressive, acute respiratory, or mixed. Although definitive diagnosis always requires a blood gas, a suspected simple metabolic or chronic respiratory disturbance is a "judgement call" for the physician. The goal of acid-base diagnosis is the same as in other areas of medicine: to formulate a coherent pathophysiologic picture that plausibly explains all the data. Until the evidence is unequivocal, realize that your diagnosis is a tentative hypothesis that requires a flexible mindset and an openness to new data.

Carry-along table

The following table summarizes typical presentations of common acid-base disorders. Details pertaining to every aspect of this table can be found in the text. Unusual presentations and mixed disturbances are not included, but knowing the typical will help you recognize the atypical. The table has separate entries for venous Total CO_2 and arterial $[HCO_3^-]$, even though these values usually parallel each other closely. This arrangement is designed to encourage the beginning diagnostician to make full use of the Total CO_2 value, and to remind him or her that it is sometimes appropriate to assess acid-base status without obtaining a blood gas. It should be stressed that this table is designed for use following a careful reading of this section. Feel free to photocopy the table for carry-along reference.

Typical Laboratory Presentations of Common Acid-Base Disturbances

	Venous Electrolytes			
	Total CO$_2$	**Anion Gap**	**Potassium**	**Other Tests, Comments**
Metabolic Acidosis. [HCO$_3^-$] + 8 ± 2		Arterial blood gas: pH ↓, [HCO$_3^-$] ↓, PCO$_2$ ↓. Rule of thumb: Compensated PCO$_2$ = 1.5 ×		
Diarrhea	↓	nl	↓	
RTA: Type 1			↓ or nl	Urine pH > 5.5
RTA: Type 2			↓ or nl	Urine pH biphasic: first > 5.5 then < 5.5. Fanconi urinary profile typical in children
RTA: Type 4			↑	Creatinine slightly ↑: often about 2× nl
Renal Failure		nl or ↑	nl or ↑	Creatinine and BUN markedly ↑
Ketoacidosis	↓	↑	DKA: usually nl or ↑. Falls rapidly with treatment. alcoholic: variable, but extreme ↑ or ↓ uncommon	Plasma and urine glucose and ketones ↑ in DKA. Ketone test may give false negative in alcoholic ketoacidosis and in mixed keto-lactic acidosis. Osmolar gap may be ↑ due to acetone
Lactic Acidosis			variable	Plasma lactate positive but urine negative
Intoxication with Methanol, Ethylene Glycol, or Salicylates			variable, but extreme ↑ or ↓ uncommon	Osmolar gap often ↑ with methanol and ethylene glycol (use freezing point depression osmometer). Specific assays positive. Ethylene glycol may present with urinary calcium oxalate crystals. Salicylate overdose causes mixed metabolic acidosis and respiratory alkalosis. In young children, the acidosis tends to predominate. In adults, the alkalosis often predominates

Metabolic Alkalosis. Arterial blood gas: pH ↑, [HCO$_3^-$] ↑, PCO$_2$ ↑. Rule of thumb: Compensated PCO$_2$ typically ↑ 0.5–1.0 mm Hg per mmol/l rise in [HCO$_3^-$]

	Total CO$_2$	Anion Gap	Potassium	Other Tests, Comments
Vomiting	↑	nl	↓	Urinary [Cl$^-$] 0–15 mmol/l. Urinary [Na$^+$] also less than 15 mmol/l except in early (bicarbonate-spilling) stage of alkalosis
N.G. Drainage				
Posthypercapnic				
Diuretic (loop, thiazide only)				Exception: If diuretic still active, [Cl$^-$] and [Na$^+$] may be nl or ↑
Volume-Resistant Causes			↓ or low nl	Urinary [Cl$^-$] greater than 35 mmol/l. Volume-resistant causes include primary hyperaldosteronism, Bartter's syndrome

Respiratory Acidosis. Arterial blood gas: pH ↓, PCO$_2$ ↑, [HCO$_3^-$] = slightly ↑ if acute and frankly ↑ if chronic. Rule of thumb: Acute [HCO$_3^-$] ↑ 1 mmol/l per 10 mm Hg rise in PCO$_2$. Compensated [HCO$_3^-$] ↑ 4 mmol/l per 10 mm Hg rise in PCO$_2$

	Total CO$_2$	Anion Gap	Potassium	Other Tests, Comments
Pulmonary Diseases	acute = nl or slightly ↑ chronic = ↑	nl	acute = nl or slightly ↑ chronic = nl	Elevated alveolar-arterial (A-a) oxygen difference suggests intrinsic pulmonary disease, but normal A-a does not rule out. COPD usually presents with either normocapnia or hypercapnia Important note: Acute pulmonary diseases most typically present with hypocapnia. Onset of hypercapnia, or even of normocapnia not attributable to repair of underlying disease, may indicate severe disease or respiratory muscle failure
Non-Pulmonary Causes			but influenced by other factors	Non-pulmonary causes include drug overdose, sleep apnea, brain or nerve lesions, neuromuscular disease, low plasma K$^+$ or phosphate, chest cage defect, upper airway obstruction

Respiratory Alkalosis. Arterial blood gas: pH ↑, PCO$_2$ ↓, [HCO$_3^-$] = slightly ↓ if acute and frankly ↓ if chronic. Rule of thumb: Acute [HCO$_3^-$] ↓ 2 mmol/l per 10 mm Hg fall in PCO$_2$. Compensated [HCO$_3^-$] ↓ 5 mmol/l per 10 mm Hg fall in PCO$_2$

	Total CO$_2$	Anion Gap	Potassium	Other Tests, Comments
Pulmonary Diseases	acute = nl or slightly ↓	nl	acute = nl or slightly ↓ chronic = nl	Examples include asthma, pneumonia, pulmonary edema, embolus, interstitial fibrosis. Always consider hypoxemia. (See comments at Respiratory Acidosis)
Non-Pulmonary Causes	chronic = ↓		but influenced by other factors	Causes include anxiety, sepsis, salicylates (see comment at Metabolic Acidosis), brain lesion, liver disease. Compensated respiratory alkalosis is a normal finding in pregnancy

Self-Assessment Quiz

This quiz tests your knowledge of core concepts and facts. More importantly, the process of taking and correcting the quiz will strengthen your understanding of the essentials. To get the most from this process, answer all questions in writing. Use a separate answer sheet if you wish. Take your time. When you finish, check your answers against the key. It doesn't matter whether you ace this quiz or fail it. The important thing is to grapple with the questions and then, for those that you miss, to study the correct answers carefully.

1. Diagnosis of acid-base disorders requires that you know which diseases cause which disorders. List the following ten items: three diseases or conditions that cause metabolic alkalosis, four pulmonary disorders that can cause respiratory acidosis if severe, and three non-pulmonary (i.e., not caused by lung disease) disorders that cause respiratory alkalosis. For each of these diseases, indicate one major pathophysiologic mechanism that causes the primary change in $[HCO_3^-]$ or PCO_2. (Note: causes of metabolic acidosis are tested below.)

2. A high venous $[HCO_3^-]$ indicates one of these primary disturbances: _____ or _____.

3. A low venous $[HCO_3^-]$ indicates one of these primary disturbances: _____ or _____.

4. Which is higher, venous Total CO_2 or actual venous $[HCO_3^-]$? In a healthy person, about how large is the difference in mmol/l? What substance accounts for most of this difference? During the Total CO_2 assay, bicarbonate is converted to carbon dioxide through the addition of strong _____.

5. Write the formula for the anion gap. If $[Na^+] = 140$, $[Cl^-] = 100$, and $[HCO_3^-] = 25$, what is the gap? Does this number represent the actual concentration of plasma unmeasured anions?

6. What is another name for anion gap metabolic acidosis? What is another name for non-anion gap metabolic acidosis?

7. List four causes of anion gap metabolic acidosis. List three causes of non-gap acidosis.

8. Follow-up question. One cause should have appeared as both gap and non-gap. Which one? This condition has traditionally been identified with a gap that is _____, but it is now recognized that the gap may be _____ in some patients.

9. The anion gap is sometimes referred to as _____, symbolized _____.

Does this term refer to the actual value of the gap or the amount it is increased above normal?

10. The normal range of the anion gap can vary from laboratory to laboratory, depending on the type of equipment used and how it is calibrated. Nonetheless, many laboratories fail to publish a normal range for their own equipment. In the absence of more specific guidance, it is reasonable to assume that the normal range is _____. This range is sometimes written as _____ ± 4.

11. The normal range for plasma $[K^+]$ is typically _____ mmol/l. Inside cells, $[K^+]$ is around _____ mmol/l.

12. Estimate what percentage of the body's potassium stores is found in the extracellular fluid. Choose from <1, 1–2, 3–5, 10, 15. If you need help, keep reading . . .

    Hint: Total body water, about 2/3 of which is inside cells, is about 42 liters. Bone contains several hundred mmol K^+.

13. In one sentence, explain how a patient with whole-body potassium depletion can nonetheless present with hyperkalemia.

14. List three factors that play an important role in reversibly shifting K^+ out of cells. Can you name a situation in which K^+ leaves cells irreversibly? (Note: this situation is not discussed in the text.)

15. For each of the following disorders, indicate if there is a distinctive plasma $[K^+]$. If there is, indicate whether $[K^+]$ it is high or low: Volume-responsive metabolic alkalosis, volume-resistant metabolic alkalosis, diarrhea, chronic renal failure, Type 1 RTA, Type 2 RTA, Type 4 RTA, lactic acidosis, ketoacidosis.

16. There are three common causes of metabolic alkalosis: loss of gastric fluid, diuretics, and post-hypercapnic. In each of these, external potassium losses are augmented by high plasma levels of the hormone _____. This hormone is elevated secondary to _____ _____. The volume-resistant metabolic alkaloses, also, are often associated with a primary rise in this hormone, or of some related steroid that acts as an _____.

17. Compensation always follows the "_____-_____ rule." For example, in a patient with compensated metabolic alkalosis, PCO_2 will always be _____.

18. The adjective *chronic,* when applied to a respiratory acid-base disturbance, means _____.

19. A low plasma pH is called _____. A high plasma pH is called _____. A low pH always implies the presence of an _____. A high pH always implies an _____. The two forms of acidosis are _____ and _____. The two forms of alkalosis are _____ and _____.

20. A patient has a low pH and a low $[HCO_3^-]$. What primary disturbance do you know is present? In this patient, you would expect PCO_2 to be _____. Assuming that PCO_2 follows this expectation, is it still possible that the disturbance is mixed?

21. A patient has a high pH and a low PCO_2. What primary disturbance do you know is present? If the disorder was more than a day or two old, you would expect $[HCO_3^-]$ to be _____.

22. A patient has a low pH, a low $[HCO_3^-]$, and a high PCO_2. Is the disturbance simple or mixed? What is the disturbance or disturbances? Would you expect pH to be slightly low or very low? When evaluating this patient, should you consult with one of the devices for assessing the level of compensation (i.e., rules of thumb, confidence bands, acid-base map)?

23. For each of the following five disorders, select the appropriate member of each column: renal failure, ketoacidosis, diabetes mellitus, methanol/ethylene glycol, lactic acidosis.

Plasma test	Sample value	High-normal value
Lactate	Positive	1.5 mg/dl [133 μmol/l]
Ketones	600 mg/dl [35 mmol/l]	5–10 mOsm/l
Glucose	17 mOsm/l	Negative
Osmolar gap	10 mg/dl [900 μmol/l]	110 mg/dl [5.6 mmol/l]
Creatinine	7 mmol/l	2.2 mmol/l

24. Match these disorders with the appropriate column entries: Type 1 RTA, Type 2 RTA, Type 4 RTA.

$[K^+]$	Typical creatinine	Urine pH
High	1.0 mg/dl [88 μmol/l]	Always > 5.5
Low or normal	1.8 mg/dl [158 μmol/l]	Usually < 5.5
		Biphasic: first > 5.5, then < 5.5.

25. If a urine assay is strongly positive for both _____ and _____, it is likely the patient has diabetic ketoacidosis (DKA). If you smell _____ on the patient's breath, the likelihood of ketoacidosis is increased/decreased (choose one). The diagnosis of DKA is confirmed when you find that plasma _____ is low and that _____ and _____ are high.

26. The chemical reaction involved in the ketone test is the _____ reaction. The commercial name for a popular type of urine ketone test is _____ test.

27. Unlike ketones, which appear in the urine during ketoacidosis, _____ does not appear in the urine during lactic acidosis because the renal _____ _____ is relatively high.

28. A patient presents to the emergency room with a Total CO_2 of 15 mmol/l. You are concerned about alcoholic ketoacidosis and order a plasma ketone assay. When it comes back negative you rule out ketoacidosis. Why is this a mistake?

29. A young, apparently healthy woman has the following plasma values: $[HCO_3^-] = 34$, $[K^+] = 3.1$. You ask her if she has been vomiting or taking any medications. She says "No." At this point, it would be reasonable to obtain a sample of this body fluid: _____.

30. Follow-up question. The urine electrolyte assay shows that $[Cl^-]$ is 46 mmol/l. Two major possibilities should come to mind: _____ abuse and _____-_____ _____ _____. How would you rule out the first possibility? Name two examples of the second possibility.

31. A disheveled and confused man presents to the emergency room with an $[HCO_3^-]$ of 14 and an anion gap of 26. You are concerned that the patient may have ingested a toxin, especially _____ or _____ _____. To help assess this possibility, you calculate the _____ _____. To do so, you subtract calculated _____ from _____ osmolarity. To determine the calculated osmolarity value, you sum the following three items: $2 \times$ [_____], [_____]/18, [BUN]/_____. The measured osmolarity value is directly measured by the laboratory from a _____ sample.

32. Follow up question. The osmolar gap in the previous problem is within the normal range. Have you have ruled out the toxins in question? If not, why not?

33. Pulse oximetry measures the _____ _____ of _____ _____. The normal range is _____-_____. Values below _____ usually indicate marked tissue hypoxia. Do you know what PO_2 this O_2 saturation value corresponds to? (This was not mentioned in the main text.) Does a normal O_2 saturation rule out mild hypercapnia? Severe hypercapnia? Mild hypocapnia? Severe hypocapnia? The reason why pulse oximetry is/is not (pick one) useful for ruling out an abnormal PCO_2 is that oximetry measures only _____ saturation, and it has nothing to do with PCO_2.

34. Calculating the "A-a difference" can aid in assessing a patient who has an abnormal blood gas. The A-a difference refers to the difference between the _____ of air in the _____ and the _____ of _____ _____. If the A-a difference is elevated, it suggests that _____ disease is present. In contrast, the A-a difference will not often be elevated if the blood gas abnormalities are caused by a factor outside the lung itself, such as _____ ventilatory drive. This means that the A-a difference will often

be _____ in pneumonia but _____ in a drug overdose. If a hypercapnic patient has a normal A-a gradient, can you assume that lung disease is *not* present? Why or why not? In healthy young people breathing room air (i.e., no supplemental oxygen), the A-a gradient is usually less than _____. This value increases with age, up to a maximum of about _____ in healthy older people.

35. In diagnosing acid-base disorders, there are four main data sources. These data sources were listed as "steps" in Chapter 24, *Making the Diagnosis*. List the sources, arranged roughly from least invasive to most invasive.

36. Follow-up question. Students often learn to diagnose acid-base disorders by first looking at the _____ _____, and interpreting it in light of ancillary data. In reality, it is more common to perform this test only after other laboratory data suggest the presence of an acid-base disturbance.

37. One traditional model of diagnosis portrays the history and physical examination as the only appropriate source of diagnostic hypotheses. Laboratory assays are seen as appropriate only for testing these hypotheses. The model presented in the *Making the Diagnosis* chapter, while emphasizing the essential role of history and physical examination, differs from this traditional model. How?

38. For a respiratory disturbance, a blood gas is generally required if you suspect the disturbance is either _____ or an _____ _____ of a chronic disturbance.

39. For a metabolic disturbance, a blood gas is generally considered mandatory if you suspect the disturbance is either _____ or _____ _____.

40. If a disturbance is not acute, not severe, and not rapidly progressive, you should nonetheless probably get a blood gas if you suspect the disturbance is _____.

41. An otherwise healthy, middle-aged woman develops gastroenteritis and has moderately severe, intermittent vomiting for two days. A venous assay shows $[HCO_3^-] = 34$, $[K^+] = 3.1$, anion gap = 14. What is the likely diagnosis? Would most physicians consider a blood gas mandatory for this patient?

42. Blood gases reflect two processes: the primary _____ and the _____, which may or may not be present. For a patient with a primary metabolic disturbance, respiratory compensation will usually be in place within about _____. In respiratory alkalosis, steady-state $[HCO_3^-]$ will usually be approached within _____-_____ days. In respiratory acidosis, complete compensation usually takes a bit longer, about _____-_____ days.

43. When trying to remember normal values for important acid-base variables, the numeral _____ can be helpful. Here are examples. In the
A.B.G., the following are considered "classic" values: pH = _____,
$[HCO_3^-]$ = _____ mmol/l, PCO_2 = _____ mm Hg. In venous electrolytes, $[HCO_3^-]$ is usually close to _____ mmol/l, $[K^+]$ is around
_____ mmol/l , and the normal range of the anion gap is often equal to
$12\pm$ _____ .

Answer Key

1. See list on pages 215–219.

2. Metabolic alkalosis or compensated respiratory acidosis.

3. Metabolic acidosis or compensated respiratory alkalosis.

4. Total CO_2. 1.4 mmol/l. Dissolved CO_2 gas. Acid.

5. $[Na^+] - ([Cl^-] + [HCO_3^-])$. 15. No, but it provides a way to assess that concentration.

6. Normochloremic metabolic acidosis. Hyperchloremic metabolic acidosis.

7. Ketoacidosis, lactic acidosis, renal failure, toxic ingestions. Diarrhea, renal tubular acidosis, renal failure.

8. Renal failure. Elevated, normal.

9. "Delta," Δ. The actual value.

10. 8–16. 12.

11. 3.5–5.0. 150.

12. 1–2.

13. External K^+ losses are more than offset by cellular shifts of K^+ into the ECF.

14. Hypoinsulinemia; ECF hyperosmolarity; and metabolic acidosis, i.e., primary hypobicarbonatemia, especially when the anion is inorganic (e.g., Cl^-). Cell membrane rupture, e.g., following trauma.

15. Low. Low. Low. Slightly elevated. Low or normal. Low or normal. High. No. No.

16. Aldosterone. Volume depletion. Agonist.

17. Same-direction. High.

18. Compensated.

19. Acidemia. Alkalemia. Acidosis. Alkalosis. Metabolic, respiratory. Metabolic, respiratory.

20. Metabolic acidosis. Low. Yes.

21. Respiratory alkalosis. Low.

22. Mixed. Metabolic acidosis and respiratory acidosis. Very low. No, because you already know that a mixed disturbance is present; the devices are used only when compensation follows the same-direction rule.

23. Renal failure: creatinine, 10 mg/dl, 1.5 mg/dl. Ketoacidosis: ketones, positive, negative. Diabetes mellitus: glucose, 600 mg/dl, 110 mg/dl. Methanol/ethylene glycol: osmolar gap, 17 mOsm/l, 5–10 mOsm/l (also: specific assays). Lactic acidosis: lactate, 7 mmol/l, 2.2 mmol/l.

24. Type 1: low or nl, 1.0, > 5.5. Type 2: low or nl, 1.0, biphasic. Type 4: high, 1.8, < 5.5.

25. Glucose, ketones. Acetone, increased. $[HCO_3^-]$, glucose, ketones.

26. Nitroprusside. Acetest.

27. Lactate, reabsorptive threshold.

28. Alcoholic ketoacidosis and other forms of keto-lactic acidosis can give a weak, or even a negative, ketone assay.

29. Urine.

30. Diuretic, volume-resistant metabolic alkalosis. Urinary diuretic screen. Primary hyperaldosteronism, Bartter's syndrome.

31. Methanol, ethylene glycol. Osmolar gap. Osmolarity, measured. Na^+, Glucose, 2.8. Blood.

32. No. Low but still lethal levels may not raise osmolarity out of the normal range.

33. O_2 saturation, arterial blood. 96–100%. 90%. About 60 mm Hg. No. No. No. No. Is not. Oxygen.

34. PO_2, alveoli, PO_2, arterial blood. Pulmonary. Decreased. High, normal. No. The A-a gradient is suggestive at best, never diagnostic. 10 mm Hg. 25 mm Hg.

35. History and physical examination, Other tests, Venous electrolytes, Arterial blood gas.

36. Blood gas.

37. It sees all of the data sources as valid bases for diagnostic hypotheses.

38.　Acute, acute exacerbation.

39.　Severe, rapidly progressive.

40.　Mixed.

41.　Simple, volume-responsive metabolic alkalosis due to vomiting. No.

42.　Disturbance, compensation. 12 hours. 2–4. 3–5.

43.　4, 7.4, 24, 40, 24, 4.0, 4.

Section 5
Treatment

This section is designed to help you understand key therapeutic concepts. As you will quickly discover, these concepts follow directly and logically from the underlying chemistry, physiology, and pathophysiology. In a world of "empiric" therapies, where the rationale for a particular treatment is not always apparent, seeing these connections is very gratifying.

This section will help you in three concrete ways:

1. *Tailored therapy.* By developing a firm grasp of therapeutic concepts, you will be able to tailor your treatment to best meet the needs of each patient. You will be able to decide if the approach recommended in the therapeutic manual needs to be modified, and in which way.

2. *Iatrogenic complications.* In these chapters, we carefully explore the major complications caused by treatment. By understanding these complications, you will be better equipped to weigh the risks and benefits of a given therapeutic approach. And once you decide on a particular course, you will know which complications to look for and how to reduce the risk that they will occur.

3. *Overview of specific disorders.* The chapters also give a brief overview of the treatment of common disorders. For example, the treatment of diabetic ketoacidosis is broken down into three components, each of which is explained in simple and clear language. For the medical student, these explanations can provide an invaluable introduction to specific therapeutic approaches. For the intern and resident, they can serve as a reminder of how the details fit into the overall therapeutic scheme.

It should be emphasized that this section is *not* intended to replace the specific treatment guidelines presented in therapeutic manuals and other similar sources. Instead, the goal is to provide a foundation of knowledge so that you can use those guidelines more effectively, intelligently, and flexibly.

The section has five chapters. The first four focus on treating the common acid-base disorders. The fifth is on prevention.

Treatment of Metabolic Acidosis 25

This chapter has two subsections. The first explores fundamental treatment concepts that apply to metabolic acidosis in general. The second looks at specific causes of metabolic acidosis and describes key aspects of their treatment.

Fundamental concepts

Consequences of metabolic acidosis

The acidemia of metabolic acidosis suppresses cardiac contractility. However, metabolic acidosis also promotes release of catecholamines, which have an inotropic effect. As long as pH is above about 7.2, these opposing effects tend to cancel, and cardiac contractility remains normal. But when pH falls below about 7.2, myocardial function decreases, in part because the cardiac effects of catecholamines are pH-dependent (i.e., catecholamines have less effect at low pH).* Metabolic acidosis has other cardiovascular effects as well, including arteriolar dilation, increased pulmonary vascular resistance, and heightened susceptibility to malignant ventricular arrhythmias.

Metabolic acidosis can also cause another problem: bone buffering (p. 130). Bone buffering helps mitigate acidosis but consumes bone buffers and mobilizes bone calcium, thereby reducing bone mass and causing disorders such as osteomalacia and rickets. The release of bone calcium raises urinary calcium excretion. This calciuresis, together with an acidosis-induced fall in the excretion of citrate (a substance that helps keep urinary calcium soluble), can cause nephrolithiasis (i.e., pelvicaliceal stones) and nephrocalcinosis (i.e., parenchymal calcifications). Correction of hypobicarbonatemia can prevent or slow the progression of these serious renal conditions. For several decades, it had been thought that chronic metabolic acidosis generally causes substantial, ongoing bone buffering. That assumption has recently been questioned, and the extent of bone buffering in chronic acidosis is currently uncertain.

---

* **Clinical note.** Because beta receptors mediate the cardiac effects of catecholamines, acidemic patients taking beta-blockers can experience myocardial suppression at pH values higher than 7.2.

285

Overall approach to treatment

Treatment of metabolic acidosis has two aspects: (1) treatment of the underlying disorder and (2) raising the plasma bicarbonate level. As a general rule, you always treat the underlying disorder (e.g., give insulin in diabetic ketoacidosis) and only sometimes try to directly raise $[HCO_3^-]$.

Raising $[HCO_3^-]$ can be done by giving either bicarbonate or organic anions such as citrate, lactate, gluconate, or acetate. These organic anions generate bicarbonate when they are metabolized (p. 86–87). The law of electroneutrality makes it impossible to prepare or administer pure bicarbonate or organic anions. Instead, both are given with cations, usually Na^+ or K^+ (e.g., sodium bicarbonate or potassium citrate). These "salts" can be given either orally or intravenously. Bicarbonate is usually preferred over organic anions, both because it is less expensive and because organic anion metabolism can be slowed by hypoxia, poor hepatic perfusion, and other factors.*

In this chapter, for convenience, we generally refer only to treatment with bicarbonate, although organic anions can often be used as well. On occasion, we use the generic term "alkali," which refers to either bicarbonate or organic anions.

Deciding whether to give bicarbonate

In deciding whether to give bicarbonate, three variables must be considered: (1) arterial pH, (2) plasma $[HCO_3^-]$, and (3) how "self-limiting" the acidosis is. In general, the *lower* the pH and $[HCO_3^-]$, and the *less* self-limiting the acidosis, the more important it is to give bicarbonate. We now look at these three variables individually. Later in the chapter, we will see how they apply in specific conditions.

1. pH

Severe acidemia can be life-threatening and is therefore an indication for bicarbonate therapy. However, significant clinical effects of acidemia usually do not appear until pH falls below 7.2, so bicarbonate is frequently withheld until pH is below 7.2. In fact, because of concerns about possible dangers of treatment, bicarbonate is, in some settings, withheld until pH falls much lower (e.g., below 7.0). We will say more about this later in the chapter.

2. Bicarbonate level

When compensatory hyperventilation is active, acidemia may be mild even if $[HCO_3^-]$ is quite low. If treatment decisions were based only on pH, we might never give bicarbonate unless hyperventilation failed. In reality, a

---

* **Clinical note.** However, when large amounts of bicarbonate or organic anions are given orally, organic anions are usually preferred, for two reasons. First, patients tolerate them better. Second, feeding large quantities of bicarbonate has, on rare occasion, led to gastric rupture due to the production of CO_2 from the reaction of bicarbonate with gastric acid.

very low $[HCO_3^-]$ is itself an indication for treatment, irrespective of pH. There are two reasons.

The first reason can be illustrated by comparing two patients who experience a 2 mmol/l fall in plasma $[HCO_3^-]$. In one patient, the initial $[HCO_3^-]$ is 20 mmol/l. In the other, initial $[HCO_3^-]$ is 10 mmol/l. We use the Henderson-Hasselbalch equation to calculate the initial and final plasma pH values for each patient. For simplicity, a PCO_2 of 40 mm Hg is assumed throughout. Here is what happens to pH in the patient with the higher initial $[HCO_3^-]$:

<u>Initial pH</u>
$= pK + \log [HCO_3^-]/PCO_2 \times 0.03$
$= 6.1 + \log 20/(40 \times 0.03)$
$= 6.1 + \log 20/1.2$
$= 7.32$

<u>Final pH</u>
$= pK + \log [HCO_3^-]/PCO_2 \times 0.03$
$= 6.1 + \log 18/(40 \times 0.03)$
$= 6.1 + \log 18/1.2$
$= 7.28$

We see that pH falls by 0.04 units. Here is what happens in the other patient, the one with an initial $[HCO_3^-]$ of 10 mmol/l:

$$\text{Initial pH} = 6.1 + \log 10/1.2 = 7.02$$
$$\text{Final pH} = 6.1 + \log 8/1.2 = 6.92$$

Here, pH falls by 0.10, more than twice as much as in the first patient, even though $[HCO_3^-]$ fell by the same 2 mmol/l. Why did pH fall more? pH is a function of the ratio of $[HCO_3^-]$ to PCO_2. As the initial $[HCO_3^-]$ gets closer to zero, equal decrements in $[HCO_3^-]$ produce increasingly larger drops in the ratio, and in pH. Thus, when the initial $[HCO_3^-]$ is very low, a small additional loss of bicarbonate can cause a large, fatal drop in pH. Giving bicarbonate raises the initial $[HCO_3^-]$, reducing this risk.

The second reason why $[HCO_3^-]$ is important is that it can be risky to rely on respiratory compensation to stabilize pH. Compensation for a severe metabolic acidosis requires heavy muscular work (diaphragm, accessory muscles). In some patients, especially the elderly and debilitated, respiratory muscles are prone to fatigue. If fatigue occurs, ventilation falls, PCO_2 rises, and the patient develops a superimposed respiratory acidosis. By keeping plasma $[HCO_3^-]$ from falling too low, only moderate hyperventilation is needed to maintain an acceptable pH.

3. Self-limiting

Once the cause of the acidosis is removed, the body is usually able to restore plasma $[HCO_3^-]$ to normal. Two mechanisms are involved. First, the kidney regenerates bicarbonate, primarily by increasing ammonium excretion. This process is relatively slow; it takes several days to fully replace lost bicarbonate. Second, in organic acidoses, such as ketoacidosis and lactic acidosis, circulating anions (e.g., acetoacetate, beta-hydroxybutyrate, lactate) can be metabolized to bicarbonate. This process may be extremely rapid and can cause $[HCO_3^-]$ to normalize within hours.

However, these two routes of bicarbonate production are not always present. Renal regeneration of bicarbonate is low in patients with renal failure, because ammonium excretion is impaired, and in patients with severe volume depletion, because renal perfusion is reduced. Metabolism of circulating organic anions requires three things: (1) The acidosis must be of the kind that generates metabolizable anions (lactic or ketoacidosis). (2) A substantial quantity of the anions must remain in the body. Anions lost in the urine obviously cannot be metabolized. In well-hydrated patients, a significant fraction of the anions may spill into the urine. (3) Efficient organic anion metabolism requires that the original defect be corrected. For example, an untreated diabetic cannot metabolize ketoanions because this process requires insulin, and a patient with lactic acidosis who remains hypoxic cannot metabolize circulating anions because lactate metabolism is an oxidative process.

If it appears that renal regeneration and/or metabolism of circulating anions will raise plasma $[HCO_3^-]$ fairly quickly, bicarbonate treatment can generally be withheld, even if pH and $[HCO_3^-]$ are quite low. If not, bicarbonate must usually be given.

Complications of treatment

Giving bicarbonate (or organic anions) can cause seven major complications. As you read about these complications, notice that most can be avoided simply by raising $[HCO_3^-]$ slowly and avoiding overtreatment.

1. *Overshoot metabolic alkalosis.* Overshoot metabolic alkalosis (also called "rebound" or "post-treatment" metabolic alkalosis) refers to the iatrogenic conversion of a metabolic acidosis into metabolic alkalosis due to overadministration of bicarbonate. Such overadministration is most likely during organic acidoses, when the potential contribution of circulating anions to the final $[HCO_3^-]$ is not adequately considered. For example, consider a patient with diabetic ketoacidosis who is treated with insulin, fluids, and enough bicarbonate to repair the hypobicarbonatemia. With insulin and volume replaced, the body becomes able to metabolize circulating anions. The sum of metabolically generated plus physician-administered bicarbonate more than replaces the deficit, and metabolic alkalosis results. By itself, overshoot alkalosis is generally not serious because the kidney can excrete the excess bicarbonate.

2. *Post-correction hyperventilation.* Administered bicarbonate enters the extracellular fluid (ECF). However, the respiratory center, which directs compensatory hyperventilation, is on the other side of the blood-brain barrier, which slows passage of ions. Thus, if ECF $[HCO_3^-]$ is rapidly corrected by bicarbonate infusion, brain $[HCO_3^-]$ and pH rise only gradually, and the respiratory center continues to "perceive" acidosis. Hyperventilation and hypocapnia persist for a time even though ECF $[HCO_3^-]$ has normalized.

By definition, low PCO_2 in the context of normal $[HCO_3^-]$ is respiratory alkalosis. If overshoot metabolic alkalosis (above) also occurs, the combined metabolic and respiratory alkaloses can cause a lethal alkalemia. Giving bicarbonate slowly allows blood-brain equilibration and prevents respiratory alkalosis.

3. *Potassium shifts.* Raising ECF $[HCO_3^-]$ can shift K^+ into cells (p. 232), producing hypokalemia. Hypokalemia is especially likely when pre-treatment $[K^+]$ is low or normal. If bicarbonate is infused rapidly, severe hypokalemia can develop, causing cardiac arrhythmias. Giving bicarbonate slowly reduces this risk. Why? First, K^+ shifts more gradually, which is safer than rapid shifts. Second, when K^+ shifts gradually, the clinician can match K^+ replacement to cellular K^+ shifts. That is, cellular K^+ uptake and exogenous K^+ replacement can take place together and at the same rate, creating an approximate steady-state for plasma $[K^+]$.

4. *Rapid alkalinization.* Rapid alkalinization can directly alter nerve conduction, increasing the risk of cardiac arrhythmia and/or convulsions. These effects are intensified by hypokalemia, which also affects nerve conduction.

5. *Volume overload.* Bicarbonate is usually given with sodium (as $NaHCO_3$ solution), which raises extracellular volume. Most patients will not be harmed by this sodium; they will excrete extra Na^+ and volume in the urine. However, if renal function is poor, or the patient is prone to pulmonary edema (e.g., poor cardiac function), expansion of ECF volume is risky. If hypertonic bicarbonate solutions are used, in an attempt to avoid excess fluid, hypernatremia may result.

6. *Hypocalcemia.* Bicarbonate therapy raises ECF pH, causing protons to dissociate from buffer sites on non-bicarbonate buffers such as plasma proteins. This dissociation exposes additional anionic sites, which can bind calcium ions, thereby lowering the biologically active free $[Ca^{2+}]$ without changing total $[Ca^{2+}]$. Thus, rapid alkalinization in patients with preexisting borderline hypocalcemia (e.g., in chronic renal failure) can cause symptomatic hypocalcemia.

7. *Lactic acid production.* Several studies suggest that bicarbonate therapy for lactic acidosis may actually increase lactic acid production. These studies have led to controversy over the use of bicarbonate in lactic acidosis.

The risk of these complications must be considered when contemplating bicarbonate therapy. As noted, slow and conservative treatment will greatly reduce the risk.

Balancing benefits and risks of treatment

When you are trying to balance the benefits and risks of giving bicarbonate, the key question is: *At what point do you start giving bicarbonate and at what point do you stop?* There is no single answer, and different authorities and therapeutic manuals advocate different numerical levels. Here we discuss one of several reasonable approaches. Our aim is not to advocate this particular approach over others, but to show, by specific example, how conceptual issues influence numerical decisions. Once you understand these issues, you will be better able to understand, and if necessary modify, whichever numerical approach you ultimately use.

When weighing benefits and risks of treatment, it is useful to think of three general categories of metabolic acidosis: acute inorganic acidoses, chronic inorganic acidoses, and organic acidoses (which are virtually always acute).

1. Acute inorganic acidoses

These are acidoses that have relatively rapid onset and produce inorganic anions. The common example is diarrhea.

Issues: Acute onset means renal bicarbonate regeneration may not be fully active for several days. Regeneration may be especially slow if renal perfusion is reduced due to volume depletion from diarrhea fluid loss. Circulating anions cannot be metabolized to bicarbonate, since they are inorganic. These factors suggest that bicarbonate therapy should be started relatively early in the course of the acidosis.

Approach: Give bicarbonate if plasma $[HCO_3^-]$ falls below about 15 mmol/l. Maintain $[HCO_3^-]$ at about 15 mmol/l.

2. Chronic inorganic acidoses

These acidoses develop gradually, are of long duration, and produce inorganic anions. CRF and RTA are the two important examples.

Issues: Renal damage prevents adequate regeneration of bicarbonate. Circulating anions cannot be metabolized. Chronicity may result in bone buffering, causing bone loss, fractures, and renal calcification. Children may be especially susceptible to bone problems. Controversy exists whether aggressive bicarbonate therapy can reduce these problems. Many clinicians believe that it can.

Approach: Maintain plasma $[HCO_3^-]$ between 18 and 20 mmol/l in adults, and between 20 and 24 mmol/l in children. If presenting $[HCO_3^-]$ is very low, raise it slowly to avoid complications.

3. Organic acidoses

Ketoacidosis and lactic acidosis are the common examples.

Issues: These acidoses may develop rapidly, so renal bicarbonate regeneration is initially modest. Circulating anions are metabolizable. Anion metabolism can help raise [HCO_3^-] but can increase the risk of overshoot alkalosis and post-correction hyperventilation. During lactic acidosis, administered bicarbonate may stimulate additional lactic acid production.

Approach: Concerns about lactic acid production and iatrogenic alkalemia have made the treatment of organic acidoses especially controversial. In general, bicarbonate is started late and discontinued early. Some physicians will not even consider starting bicarbonate until [HCO_3^-] falls to around 10 mmol/l and pH drops below 7.1 (in fact, some physicians do not give bicarbonate until much later). Therapy may be discontinued when [HCO_3^-] reaches 10 to 12 mmol/l.

Gauging how much bicarbonate to give

When you want to raise plasma [HCO_3^-] by a specific amount, how much bicarbonate will be required? For example, how much bicarbonate is needed to raise ECF [HCO_3^-] by 1 mmol/l? Since ECF volume is typically about 14 liters, a reasonable guess might be 14 mmol. In fact, much more bicarbonate is needed. Let's see why.

Infused bicarbonate raises extracellular [HCO_3^-]. The increase in ECF [HCO_3^-] creates a gradient for the diffusion of bicarbonate into cells, which in turn raises intracellular [HCO_3^-] and pH, which are also low during metabolic acidosis. In addition, some of the added bicarbonate is consumed in buffering the protons that are released from non-bicarbonate buffers during the pH rise. (Note: as pH rises, the $HA \rightleftharpoons H^+ + A^-$ equilibrium of non-bicarbonate buffers shifts to the right, releasing protons.) Thus, of the total quantity of bicarbonate entering the ECF, only a fraction remains to raise [HCO_3^-].

So how much bicarbonate is needed? In general, the lower the pretreatment [HCO_3^-], the more bicarbonate that is needed to produce a given increase in [HCO_3^-]. In patients with mild or moderate hypobicarbonatemia, about 1/4 to 1/2 of infused bicarbonate remains unneutralized in the ECF. Thus, if 60 mmol bicarbonate is infused, 15–30 mmol will remain, and ECF [HCO_3^-] will rise by about 1–2 mmol/l. In severe hypobicarbonatemia, only 1/8 to 1/4 of infused bicarbonate remains unneutralized in the ECF. Thus, the same 1–2 mmol/l rise in [HCO_3^-] requires about 120 mmol of infused bicarbonate.*

These fractional guides are only approximate; it is extremely difficult to predict accurately how much bicarbonate will be needed. The problem is two-

---

* **Terminology.** You can also describe these differences in terms of the "apparent space of distribution" for bicarbonate. In mild-to-moderate acidosis, this space comprises about 40% of body weight. In severe acidosis, the space comprises about 80%. You can estimate the amount of therapeutic bicarbonate needed as: (Desired mmol/l rise in [HCO_3^-]) × (Body wt. in kg) × (Percent distribution/100). For example, if you want to raise the plasma [HCO_3^-] by 5 mmol/l in a 70 kg patient with an assumed 40% distribution space, you would estimate 5 × 70 × 0.4 = 140 mmol bicarbonate.

fold. First, in many individuals, there is ongoing acid production due to gastrointestinal fluid losses or metabolic derangements. For example, in severe lactic acidosis, more than 200 mmol of bicarbonate per hour may have to be infused just to keep pace with acid production. Second, in individuals with organic acidoses and large anion gaps, it is difficult to predict when, if, and at what rate circulating anions will be metabolically converted to bicarbonate.

Specific disease entities

In this part of the chapter, we focus on approaches to treating the common causes of metabolic acidosis. As noted earlier (p. 283), our goal is to teach key concepts, not to describe every aspect of therapy. In fact, many fine points have deliberately been omitted in order to highlight the main themes. When treating patients, detailed treatment guidelines are needed. These guidelines can be found in therapeutic manuals and, for toxic ingestions, handbooks of poisoning or toxicology.

Diabetic ketoacidosis (DKA)

Not all DKA patients need bicarbonate (some authorities believe that only a few do), but all require volume, insulin, and potassium.*

<u>Volume deficits</u> due to osmotic diuresis can cause hypotension, which may be severe and life threatening. Whole-body water deficits may be greater than 10 liters. In hypotensive patients, volume replacement is urgent and is done rapidly with normal saline (i.e., 0.9% NaCl). In normotensive patients (or after hypotension is corrected), the infusion can be slowed, and many authorities advocate switching to half-normal saline (i.e., 0.45% NaCl) for better intracellular distribution of free water.

<u>Insulin</u> is usually given in three stages. The first stage is intended to rapidly raise plasma insulin to physiologic levels. This stage generally consists of either an intravenous loading dose or an intramuscular injection. The second stage is designed to maintain the insulin level. It consists of either a continuous intravenous drip or periodic intramuscular injections. The third stage is a continuation of the second-stage insulin regimen but with intravenous glucose added (yes, glucose). This stage is usually initiated when plasma glucose falls to between 200 and 300 mg/dl (around 10–15 mmol/l). The glucose helps prevent insulin-induced "overshoot" hypoglycemia and keeps extracellular osmolarity, to which glucose contributes, from falling too rapidly.

<u>Potassium</u> is lost rapidly in the urine during the osmotic diuresis. Therefore, all patients with DKA have total-body K^+ deficits, usually of between 200 and 1000 millimoles. However, because insulin deficits result in a shift of intracellular K^+ into the ECF, most patients are either normokalemic or hy-

---

* **Mnemonic.** All diabetics are VIPs.

perkalemic (p. 235) in spite of the potassium deficits. As soon as insulin is administered, K^+ begins moving back into cells, and severe hypokalemia may develop. Therefore, to prevent hypokalemia, all DKA patients must receive potassium. Because both hypokalemia and hyperkalemia (induced by overly zealous potassium supplementation) can cause cardiac arrhythmias, ECG monitoring is often instituted during the first 12 to 24 hours.

Note. Acetone, one of the ketone bodies, is excreted slowly, much of it in gaseous form by the lung. Because this excretion can take several days, the plasma ketone test may remain positive even though the acidosis has resolved. Thus, to gauge the recovery of a ketoacidosis patient, look for a rise in plasma $[HCO_3^-]$ and a fall in the anion gap. Don't worry about a ketone test that remains positive. Since acetone contributes to osmolarity, the osmolar gap may also remain elevated.

Alcoholic ketoacidosis

Although $[HCO_3^-]$ may fall to 10 mmol/l or even lower, bicarbonate therapy is generally not necessary. In most cases, an infusion of glucose (i.e., dextrose) and saline leads to a rapid conversion of circulating organic anions to bicarbonate. The plasma ketone test is often unreliable. It may initially be only weakly positive or even falsely negative (footnote p. 255) and then transiently become more positive as the patient improves. Why? With improvement, beta-hydroxybutyrate (which is not detected by the assay) is converted to acetoacetate (which is detected). This conversion can make the ketone test more positive even though the total ketone level is falling. As with DKA, improvement can be accurately gauged by a rising $[HCO_3^-]$ and a falling anion gap.*

Starvation ketoacidosis

Acidosis is usually mild and requires no treatment.

Lactic acidosis

Lactic acidosis is so difficult to treat that it is sometimes described as "treatment-resistant." One problem is that lactic acid can be generated as rapidly as 300 mmol per hour. Infusing bicarbonate solutions at anywhere near this rate can produce volume overload or, if hypertonic solutions are used, hypernatremia. Another problem is that giving bicarbonate may actually stimulate lactic acid production (p. 289). However, when the acidosis is acutely life threatening, no alternative currently exists to using bicarbonate. Four general rules can increase the chance of a successful outcome:

---

* **Clinical note.** With dextrose-saline treatment, anion conversion can occur quite rapidly. For example, a venous blood sample taken before anion conversion will show a severe gap acidosis, whereas a blood gas taken a short time later may show a simple respiratory alkalosis. Why? The acidosis self-corrected so rapidly that a transient post-correction hyperventilatory state (p. 288) developed.

1. *Search aggressively for treatable causes:* This search is the key element in therapy. Even with excellent symptomatic treatment, the patient is likely to die if the underlying cause is not found and removed.

2. *Do frequent laboratory work:* Because the rate of lactic acid production can vary greatly, it is difficult to predict how rapidly bicarbonate must be given. The best approach is to frequently measure blood gases and/or venous [HCO_3^-] and to adjust the rate of bicarbonate administration accordingly.

3. *Minimize treatment:* Give as little bicarbonate as possible. Some physicians will not give bicarbonate until pH is less than 7.0 and [HCO_3^-] is less than 8 mmol/l. They discontinue bicarbonate when [HCO_3^-] reaches 10 mmol/l.

4. *Consider hemodialysis:* When much bicarbonate is required, hemodialysis can ameliorate the effects of the large fluid and sodium load.

Methanol intoxication

Methanol is converted in the body to formaldehyde and formic acid. These products cause acidosis and damage the eye, sometimes causing visual disturbances or permanent blindness. The clinical picture of a "blind drunk" immediately suggests the diagnosis. There are four major components to therapy.

1. *Administer bicarbonate.* In methanol-intoxicated patients, the risk of mortality and permanent blindness is related to the degree of hypobicarbonatemia. For this reason, aggressive bicarbonate therapy is often advocated. For example, some physicians give bicarbonate until plasma [HCO_3^-] reaches 20 mmol/l.

2. *Remove residual methanol.* When ingestion is recent and methanol is still in the stomach, residual methanol can be removed using techniques such as drainage with a nasogastric tube, ipecac-induced emesis, or gastric lavage.

3. *Administer ethanol.* Give ethanol (yes, ethanol) either intravenously or by mouth. Alcohol dehydrogenase, a key enzyme in methanol metabolism (p. 147), has a higher affinity for ethanol than for methanol. Thus, ethanol inhibits the metabolism of methanol to toxic products. Because immediate treatment is important, ethanol is typically given whenever methanol ingestion is *suspected.* "Better drunk on ethanol than dead on methanol" is the operative quip. If methanol assays later come back negative, ethanol is discontinued.*

---

* **Going further.** By the time you read this, a new drug called 4-MP (4-methylpyrazole) may be approved for clinical use and may largely replace ethanol. Like ethanol, 4-MP inhibits alcohol dehydrogenase. Unlike ethanol, it does not inebriate and it is convenient to give.

4. *Start dialysis.* Patients with significant methanol ingestions require hemodialysis. Dialysis removes methanol and its toxic products and also corrects the hypobicarbonatemia.

Ethylene glycol intoxication

Therapy is essentially the same as for methanol: bicarbonate, gastric cleansing for recent ingestions, ethanol, and dialysis.

Salicylate intoxication

Following salicylate overdose, respiratory alkalosis develops in most patients. A superimposed metabolic acidosis then develops in some patients. pH can be high, low, or normal, depending on which disturbance predominates (p. 147). Treatment has several components.

1. *Minimize gut absorption.* Gut absorption of recently ingested salicylate can be minimized with activated charcoal. Emesis or gastric lavage may be necessary in some patients.

2. *Minimize tissue absorption.* Because salicylate causes most of its damage within cells, especially brain cells, an important goal is to minimize cellular entry. This goal can be accomplished by keeping arterial pH in the alkalemic range. This is often done by giving the patient bicarbonate. Why is alkalemia desirable? Salicylate (S^-) and salicylic acid (SH) are in equilibrium in the blood:

$$S^- + H^+ \rightleftharpoons SH$$

Salicylate, which is ionic and polar, cannot easily cross lipid cell membranes, whereas salicylic acid, which is uncharged and relatively nonpolar, can. Thus, if the salicylate equilibrium in the ECF is shifted to the left by lowering $[H^+]$ (i.e., raising pH), cellular entry is slowed. Note: in patients with marked pretreatment alkalemia (i.e., when respiratory alkalosis predominates) it may not be possible or desirable to alkalinize the blood further.

3. *Maximize renal excretion.* Renal excretion is maximized by increasing urine production and urine pH. Raising urine pH lowers [SH] in the tubular lumen, which steepens the gradient for SH diffusion from blood. As SH enters the alkaline lumen, it dissociates into S^-, which remains in the lumen ("ion trapping") and is excreted. Urinary alkalinization is usually accomplished with a sodium bicarbonate infusion (the same infusion used to raise arterial pH).

4. *Hemodialysis.* Patients with significant salicylate intoxication require hemodialysis. Dialysis removes salicylate and also corrects the hypobicarbonatemia, if present.

Diarrhea

Diarrhea causes loss of ECF bicarbonate, volume (i.e., water and NaCl), and potassium. These deficits should be monitored and, when appropriate, replaced, either orally or intravenously. A few non-obvious points are worth noting. Regarding bicarbonate, remember that volume depletion can limit the kidney's capacity to (1) regenerate bicarbonate and (2) excrete excess bicarbonate if overly aggressive bicarbonate therapy causes overshoot alkalosis. Regarding potassium, diarrhea causes whole-body K^+ depletion but, since metabolic acidosis causes K^+ to shift out of cells, the extent of K^+ losses may be masked by a near-normal plasma $[K^+]$. Raising $[HCO_3^-]$ can cause K^+ to shift back into cells, precipitating severe hypokalemia, whereas rapidly replacing K^+ before the acidosis is corrected can cause severe hyperkalemia. Therefore, close attention must be paid to the relative rates of bicarbonate and potassium administration. Frequent checks of plasma $[K^+]$ are necessary.

Gastrointestinal drainage

Post-surgical biliary, pancreatic, and small bowel drainage are essentially iatrogenic diarrhea, and most of the considerations relevant to diarrhea apply. With drainage, however, you can quantitatively estimate and replace losses. You make the estimate by measuring drainage volume and electrolyte concentrations, as follows: Potassium losses are calculated as $[K^+] \times$ volume. Bicarbonate losses are measured indirectly, by an anion-gap like calculation, as $([Na^+] + [K^+] - [Cl^-]) \times$ volume. For example, if a patient produces 2 liters of drainage with $[Na^+] = 40$ mmol/l, $[K^+] = 20$ mmol/l, and $[Cl^-] = 35$ mmol/l, the estimated net bicarbonate loss is 50 mmol. Check with the hospital laboratory for details regarding sample preparation. In managing these patients, start fluid and electrolyte replacement when drainage begins. Don't wait for large deficits to develop.

Renal failure

In the past, alkali has been given only to children, in whom acidemia can impair growth, or to those adults who have relatively severe hypobicarbonatemia or other symptoms. However, many physicians now treat even mild acidosis in adults, with the goal of reducing bone loss and muscle wasting and slowing the progression of the renal disease.

Renal tubular acidosis

Therapy depends on the type. In <u>Type 1 RTA</u>, metabolic acidosis is treated with daily maintenance doses of bicarbonate or organic anions. The dosage depends largely on the extent of urinary bicarbonate spillage (which is often present, but mild, in Type 1). It may be helpful to give part of the alkali as citrate. Most of this citrate is metabolized to bicarbonate but the unmetabolized portion, which is excreted by the kidney, forms soluble complexes with urinary calcium, thereby inhibiting stone formation. Hypokalemia may or may not require specific therapy. In some patients, potassium wasting is ameliorated when the acidosis is corrected; in other patients, ongoing K^+ supplementation is needed.

If the presenting acidosis and hypokalemia are severe, emergent bicarbonate and potassium therapy, with ECG monitoring, may be necessary. Sometimes the hypokalemia is so severe that respiratory failure results from muscle (diaphragm) weakness. In such cases, hypercapnia may result and mechanical ventilation may be necessary. It is important to remember that raising $[HCO_3^-]$ can shift K^+ into cells, exacerbating the hypokalemia. Thus, bicarbonate and potassium therapy must be carefully coordinated.

In Type 2 RTA, correction of plasma $[HCO_3^-]$ is important for normal growth in children. Organic anions are generally used, and large maintenance doses may be needed because bicarbonate is spilled into the urine as soon as plasma $[HCO_3^-]$ exceeds the abnormally low renal reabsorptive threshold. This additional bicarbonate spillage augments distal delivery of Na^+ (the Na^+ is dragged along in the tubular fluid by charge attraction). Some of this additional distal Na^+ is reabsorbed and, to maintain luminal electroneutrality, additional K^+ is excreted. Thus, effective alkali therapy induces both bicarbonaturia and kaliuresis, and the latter necessitates K^+ supplementation. K^+ is often supplemented by giving about half of the maintenance alkali as the potassium salt (e.g., potassium citrate).*

Type 4 RTA is generally caused by hypoaldosteronism, with the acidosis largely mediated by hyperkalemia (p. 154). Lowering plasma $[K^+]$ will often correct the acidosis. One or more of the following may be effective: a low-potassium diet, a diuretic (e.g., furosemide), or a cation exchange resin (e.g., Kayexalate). If these approaches are ineffective, mineralocorticoids (e.g., Flourinef) are sometimes given to replace aldosterone. However, mineralocorticoids are often poorly tolerated by patients because they can increase sodium reabsorption, resulting in ECF expansion, volume overload, and hypertension. In patients with cardiac dysfunction, ECF expansion can cause congestive heart failure.

Summary

As a general rule for metabolic acidosis, you always treat the underlying disease and the accompanying volume and potassium imbalances, but only sometimes give "alkali" (bicarbonate, organic anions) to raise plasma $[HCO_3^-]$ directly. In assessing the need for alkali, three variables are considered: pH, $[HCO_3^-]$, and the potential for self-correction, i.e., for timely endogenous restoration of $[HCO_3^-]$ by either renal regeneration or organic anion metabolism. Complications of giving alkali include overshoot meta-

---

* **Going further.** In some cases, patients are also treated with thiazide diuretics, the goal being to lower ECF volume. Lowering volume augments proximal reabsorption of sodium (and hence bicarbonate) and thereby reduces the required maintenance alkali dose.

bolic alkalosis, post-correction hyperventilation, hypokalemia, volume overload, hypocalcemia, and (in lactic acidosis) augmented lactic acid production. The risk of these complications can be reduced by slow and conservative alkali treatment. In ketoacidosis and lactic acidosis, treatment with alkali is especially conservative because of concerns about iatrogenic alkalemia and/or augmented lactic acid production. In diarrhea, treatment with alkali is less conservative. In CRF and RTA, treatment with alkali is relatively aggressive, especially in children. Predicting therapeutic alkali needs is difficult. In general, the lower the starting plasma $[HCO_3^-]$, the greater the quantity of bicarbonate needed to raise $[HCO_3^-]$ by 1 mmol/l. Therapeutic manuals or other reference sources should be consulted for detailed treatment plans.

Treatment of Metabolic Alkalosis

26

Consequences of metabolic alkalosis

Metabolic alkalosis is usually accompanied by hypokalemia (p. 233). The high $[HCO_3^-]$ and pH, and the low $[K^+]$, act individually or together to produce three main types of adverse effects: cardiac arrhythmias, decreased oxygen delivery, and neuromuscular dysfunction. These effects are usually significant only when metabolic alkalosis is severe.

Cardiac arrhythmias

Severe metabolic alkalosis can cause treatment-refractory ventricular and supraventricular arrhythmias. These arrhythmias are most common when pH is above 7.6. The cause appears to be a combination of hypokalemia and alkalemia.

Decreased oxygen delivery

Metabolic alkalosis can adversely affect oxygen delivery in two different ways. First, compensatory hypoventilation raises PCO_2 and thereby helps stabilize pH, but it can also cause hypoxemia. Whether or not hypoxemia occurs depends on the degree of hypoventilation and the state of the patient's lungs. In patients with healthy lungs, hypoxemia will not occur with moderate hypoventilation, but can become apparent, and even profound, as metabolic alkalosis and hence hypoventilation become severe. For example, an increase in $[HCO_3^-]$ to 60 mmol/l can cause arterial PO_2 to fall below 50 mm Hg. In patients with lung disease, lesser levels of hypoventilation can cause hypoxemia.*

Second, alkalemia acutely shifts the hemoglobin saturation curve to the left, reducing oxygen unloading at the tissues. However, within about 24 hours, plasma levels of 2,3-DPG rise, which shifts the curve back toward its original

---

* **Clinical note.** When metabolic alkalosis occurs in a mechanically ventilated patient, the "compensatory" decrease in ventilatory drive may make it difficult to liberate the patient from the ventilator. Repairing the metabolic alkalosis may increase ventilatory drive and facilitate liberation.

position. Thus, oxygen delivery is probably impaired by this second mechanism only during the first day.

Neuromuscular dysfunction

Metabolic alkalosis is associated with various CNS and peripheral neuromuscular disturbances. Patients may experience malaise, lethargy, and weakness. Less common are agitation, confusion, stupor, muscle twitching, tetany, seizures, and coma. The pathophysiology of these disturbances is not fully understood, but one or more of the following factors are probably involved: alkalemia, hypoxia, hypokalemia, decreased plasma free $[Ca^{2+}]$, and reduced cerebral perfusion caused by volume depletion (which commonly accompanies metabolic alkalosis).

When to begin treatment

In deciding if treatment is necessary, it is helpful to distinguish between mild, moderate, and severe metabolic alkalosis.

Mild

Metabolic alkalosis is generally considered mild if plasma $[HCO_3^-]$ is less than 32–34 mmol/l. Plasma $[K^+]$ is typically between 3.5 and 3.9 mmol/l. At these levels of HCO_3^- and K^+, adverse effects are rare and vigilance against further changes is often all that is needed.

Moderate

At a plasma $[HCO_3^-]$ between 32 and 40 mmol/l, signs and symptoms are increasingly likely. Some compensatory hypoventilation is usually present, which may cause hypoxemia in patients with preexisting lung disease. Plasma $[K^+]$ is often between 2.5 and 3.5 mmol/l, a level of hypokalemia typically associated with whole-body K^+ deficits of 200–500 mmol. At these levels of HCO_3^- and K^+, treatment should generally be undertaken without delay.*

Severe

Metabolic alkalosis is generally considered severe if $[HCO_3^-]$ exceeds 40–42 mmol/l. At these levels, patients with preexisting lung disease will likely develop hypoxemia. Patients with normal lungs may also develop hypoxemia if $[HCO_3^-]$ reaches the mid- or high 40s. Plasma $[K^+]$ is typically between 2.0 and 2.5 mmol/l, with whole-body K^+ deficits of 600–1000 mmol. Treatment is mandatory. A pH above 7.6 or the appearance of major alkalemic symptoms (e.g., cardiac arrhythmia, seizures) must be treated as a medical emergency.

---

* **Technical information.** Note that most K^+ deficits are intracellular. For example, at a plasma $[K^+]$ of 2.5 mmol/l, ECF K^+ deficits are only about 28 mmol (i.e., 2 mmol/l decrease in $[K^+] \times 14$ liter ECF).

Treatment of volume-responsive metabolic alkalosis

There are two main forms of metabolic alkalosis: volume-responsive and volume-resistant (p. 168). Gastric fluid loss, diuretics, and post-hypercapnic causes produce metabolic alkalosis that is maintained largely by volume depletion, and which therefore responds to therapeutic volume repletion ("volume-responsive"). In contrast, certain rare causes of metabolic alkalosis, such as primary hyperaldosteronism and Bartter's syndrome, do not respond to volume administration ("volume-resistant"). Volume-responsive causes are much more common, so we consider them first.

Whenever possible, the underlying cause of the alkalosis (i.e., the generating factors) should be removed. For example, nasogastric suction should be discontinued or, if discontinuation is not feasible, gastric acid secretion can be suppressed with H_2 (histamine) blockers such as cimetidine or ranitidine, or with omeprazole, a drug that directly inhibits the gastric $H^+ - K^+$–ATPase (which secretes H^+ in exchange for K^+). If diuretics caused the alkalosis, determine if they can be safely discontinued or, at least, if the dosage can be reduced.

Next, attention should be paid to the factors maintaining the alkalosis. As described elsewhere (p. 158–159), the three major maintenance factors are volume depletion, hypokalemia, and aldosterone excess. These can be corrected as follows:

Volume depletion is usually treated by giving sodium in the form of NaCl solutions ("saline"). NaCl solutions can be given either orally or intravenously. The alkalosis-maintaining effects of volume depletion may be partially mediated by a deficit of chloride in the distal nephron (p. 163). NaCl solutions repair this chloride deficit as well.

Hypokalemia is repaired with K^+ supplementation. If hypokalemia is mild, increasing intake of K^+-rich foods may be sufficient. If hypokalemia is moderate or severe, KCl supplements should be given. Preparations containing organic anions (e.g., potassium citrate or gluconate) should not be used because the anions are metabolically converted to bicarbonate. It is usually preferable to give KCl orally, because intravenous KCl poses a greater risk of hyperkalemia, which may produce cardiac arrhythmias.*

---

* **Going further.** The risk of hyperkalemia is especially great if renal function is impaired. Diabetics and patients on beta-blockers are also at increased risk, because insulin and catecholamines facilitate cellular K^+ uptake, which can mitigate the rise in plasma $[K^+]$. This said, the intravenous route is still sometimes preferred. For example, if hypokalemia is acutely symptomatic (cardiac arrhythmia, severe muscle weakness) or if the patient cannot take food (NPO, vomiting), KCl is usually given intravenously. Also, when large amounts of potassium are needed, some patients may not tolerate oral KCl. When the intravenous route is required, the rate of K^+ inflow must be carefully controlled. Except for slow infusions, the patient should be continuously monitored by ECG (ICU placement is often advised) and watched closely for indications of hyperkalemia.

Aldosterone excess in volume-responsive metabolic alkalosis is secondary to volume depletion. It self-corrects when volume is restored with NaCl.

In other words, treating volume-responsive metabolic alkalosis is a simple three-step process: (1) Remove generating factors when possible, (2) give NaCl solution, and (3) give KCl. With the underlying cause and maintenance factors removed, the kidneys will, over a period of days, excrete excess bicarbonate and return plasma [HCO_3^-] to normal. Repair of the alkalosis can be assessed by serial venous electrolyte measurements, which should show a gradual fall in [HCO_3^-] and a rise in [K^+].*

Considerations in diuretic-induced metabolic alkalosis

Patients with hypertension or edematous conditions (heart failure, hepatic cirrhosis, nephrotic syndrome) are often treated with diuretics. The aim is to create mild, therapeutic volume depletion. In hypertensive patients, volume depletion lowers blood pressure; in edematous patients, it facilitates excretion of excess fluid. Unfortunately, the volume depletion can cause metabolic alkalosis. In these patients, you can't simply give saline because this would undercut the therapeutic volume depletion. Also, in patients with heart failure, saline can precipitate pulmonary edema. The following four techniques are often used, individually or in combination, to lower [HCO_3^-] without raising ECF volume.

1. *Reduce the diuretic dosage.* Metabolic alkalosis may indicate that the patient has been over-diuresed or diuresed too quickly. Reducing the dosage may lower plasma [HCO_3^-] somewhat while still maintaining a satisfactory therapeutic effect. In some patients, especially those receiving diuretics for hypertension, it may be possible to stop the diuretic altogether and replace it with another type of drug.

2. *Give KCl but not saline.* Repairing hypokalemia may partially correct the alkalosis. Because hypokalemia often produces symptoms (muscle weakness, cardiac abnormalities) earlier than alkalemia, raising [K^+] may yield clinical improvement even if no reduction in [HCO_3^-] occurs.

---

* **Going further.** Urine pH and [Cl^-] assays can provide a non-invasive check on therapeutic progress. Urine pH, which is usually less than 5.5 in metabolic alkalosis because of the elevated reabsorptive threshold for bicarbonate, rises to 7.0 or higher as soon as bicarbonate excretion begins. Urine [Cl^-], which is usually less than 15 mmol/l because of volume depletion (p. 259), rises to 50 mmol/l or higher once sufficient volume and chloride are given. In general, bicarbonate excretion and urinary pH rise first; chloride excretion increases later.

3. *Give acetazolamide (Diamox).* Acetazolamide is a mild diuretic that inhibits the enzyme carbonic anhydrase. Since carbonic anhydrase plays a key role in renal bicarbonate reabsorption, acetazolamide can cause bicarbonaturia and thereby lower plasma $[HCO_3^-]$. Depending on the clinical situation, acetazolamide can be added to the usual diuretic, which is continued at either the same or a reduced dosage, or substituted for it. Acetazolamide causes massive urinary K^+ spillage, so KCl must be given prophylactically and plasma $[K^+]$ must be followed even more closely than is necessary with diuretics such as furosemide (Lasix).

4. *Give spironolactone.* Spironolactone is a K^+-sparing diuretic that blocks the effect of aldosterone on the distal nephron. Aldosterone stimulates K^+ excretion and distal H^+ secretion, which is important for distal bicarbonate reabsorption. Blocking these actions reduces hypokalemia and causes some urinary spillage of bicarbonate. As with acetazolamide, spironolactone may be added to, or substituted for, the usual diuretic.

In deciding among these four approaches, the specifics of the clinical situation must be considered carefully. For example, in some patients, the risk of pulmonary edema is so great that you cannot safely reduce the diuretic dosage. Conversely, in a patient who has been over-diuresed, adding acetazolamide might simply exacerbate the volume depletion.

Treatment of volume-resistant metabolic alkalosis

For the volume-resistant causes of metabolic alkalosis, the therapeutic goal is to remove the underlying cause or to interfere with its mechanism. For example, primary hyperaldosteronism is commonly treated either with surgery (e.g., to remove an adrenal adenoma) or spironolactone, which blocks the renal effects of aldosterone. Some of the major causes of volume-resistant metabolic alkalosis are briefly described in appendix topic K. A detailed discussion of therapy for these rare disorders is beyond the scope of this book.

Aggressive treatment of metabolic alkalosis

The usual approach to treating metabolic alkalosis is what might be called "passive": you correct the maintenance factors and let the kidneys naturally excrete the excess bicarbonate over several days. On rare occasions, however, it is necessary to actively lower plasma $[HCO_3^-]$ using relatively aggressive techniques. For example, an active approach might be tried if passive approaches fail, or if alkalemia is severe and life-threatening, or if the patient has renal failure (which inhibits the urinary spillage of excess bicarbonate). Although active approaches should generally be discussed with an experienced specialist, it is worth being familiar with the four most common methods.

1. Acetazolamide (Diamox)

The mechanism by which acetazolamide lowers plasma $[HCO_3^-]$ is described earlier in this chapter.*

2. Dialysis

When patients with metabolic alkalosis are hemodialyzed, excess bicarbonate from the blood diffuses into the dialysis solution (dialysis solution is called "dialysate"), lowering plasma $[HCO_3^-]$. The rate that bicarbonate leaves the blood depends on the bicarbonate concentration gradient between the blood and the dialysate. Thus, the rate of bicarbonate elimination can be increased by lowering $[HCO_3^-]$ in the dialysate. Note: some dialysate contains acetate, not bicarbonate, as the base. Acetate, an organic anion, enters the blood and is metabolized to bicarbonate (p. 86–87), so the effect is roughly the same as occurs with bicarbonate-containing dialysate.

3. Infusion of acid

When strong acid enters the ECF, the protons rapidly react with bicarbonate ($HCO_3^- + H^+ \rightarrow CO_2 + H_2O$), which lowers plasma $[HCO_3^-]$. Specially prepared hydrochloric acid (HCl) solutions with concentrations of 100 or 150 mmol/l are available for this type of infusion. Although relatively dilute, these solutions are still somewhat corrosive and can produce thrombophlebitis in small veins. Therefore, acid solutions must be infused slowly and into a large vein, usually the subclavian or femoral.

4. Infusion of acid precursors

"Acid precursors" are not themselves acids but are metabolized to acids in the body. Ammonium chloride (NH_4Cl) and arginine monohydrochloride are examples. Note that the chloride, which is physiologically inert, is given with the cation for reasons of electroneutrality. Acid precursors are not corrosive and can therefore be administered via peripheral veins. However, they have important drawbacks and are not generally recommended. Ammonium chloride, if infused too quickly, can cause ammonium toxicity, especially in individuals with hepatic dysfunction (since most NH_4^+ metabolism occurs in the liver). Arginine solutions, for unknown reasons, cause K^+

---

* **Clinical note.** Acetazolamide inhibits carbonic anhydrase not only in the kidney but also in red blood cells, where it catalyzes the reaction $H_2O + CO_2 \rightarrow HCO_3^- + H^+$. This reaction occurs in systemic capillaries and facilitates the transport of some CO_2 to the lung in the form of bicarbonate. (At the lung, the reaction is reversed, liberating CO_2 for excretion.) Thus, if a hypercapnic patient is treated with acetazolamide, more CO_2 is carried in dissolved form and plasma PCO_2 rises by a few mm Hg. This rise is usually not clinically significant.

to exit cells, which can lead to life-threatening hyperkalemia. Great care and close [K^+] monitoring are essential.*

When giving HCl or an acid precursor, how much is needed? If we calculated the amount required based on ECF volume (which we will assume to be 14 liters) and wished to lower [HCO_3^-] by 10 mmol/l, we would predict that $10 \times 14 = 140$ meq of acid or acid precursor would be needed. It turns out that this amount is insufficient because the added acid must not only neutralize HCO_3^- in the ECF, but must also (1) neutralize excess HCO_3^- inside cells and (2) titrate non-bicarbonate buffers like hemoglobin and phosphate. A better predictor of the acid requirement is to assume a volume of distribution equal to one-half the body mass in kilograms. For example, for a 70 kg patient, if you wish to lower [HCO_3^-] by 10 mmol/l, you might reasonably estimate the following:

$$(1/2 \times 70) \times 10 = 35 \times 10 = 350 \text{ meq of acid}$$

Summary

Metabolic alkalosis is usually treated when [HCO_3^-] is 32–34 mmol/l or higher. This [HCO_3^-] is often associated with a [K^+] below 3.5 mmol/l and whole-body K^+ deficits greater than 200 mmol. Volume-responsive alkalosis (e.g., vomiting, gastric drainage, post-hypercapnic causes) typically self-corrects after you do three things: (1) remove the underlying cause, when possible, (2) give volume as NaCl solution, and (3) give KCl. With treatment, venous blood [HCO_3^-] falls and [K^+] rises. Diuretic patients usually can't be given volume, but are often treated with one or more of the following: replacement of the diuretic with another class of drug; reduction in the diuretic dosage; administration of KCl, acetazolamide, or spironolactone. Volume-resistant causes (e.g., primary hyperaldosteronism) usually require specific surgical or medical treatment. On rare occasions, it is necessary to use an active approach to lower [HCO_3^-], such as acetazolamide, HCl infusion, or dialysis.

---

* **Food for thought.** In theory, sulfur-containing amino acids, which are also acid precursors (p. 86), might be useful in actively reducing [HCO_3^-], but there is nothing in the clinical literature about this possibility.

Treatment of Respiratory Acidosis* 27

Effects of respiratory acidosis

In patients breathing room air, hypercapnia is always accompanied by hypoxemia. Therefore, it is not always known whether a particular "hypercapnic" effect is due to hypercapnia, hypoxemia, or both. Taken together, hypercapnia-hypoxemia produces three broad types of effects: cerebrovascular, neurologic, and cardiac.

Cerebrovascular

Hypercapnia causes cerebral vasodilation and thus increases cranial blood flow. Therefore, respiratory acidosis, both acute and chronic, can raise intracranial pressure. Headache is common, especially at night, probably because PCO_2 normally rises during sleep. The eyes may be reddened because of increased conjunctival and scleral perfusion. With severe hypercapnia, blurring of the optic disk and papilledema may occur. Focal neurologic signs, such as muscle weakness, paresthesias, and altered reflexes, occasionally develop.

Neurologic effects

Acute hypercapnia can decrease mental acuity and cause anxiety, disorientation, combativeness, asterixis, and muscle fasciculations. A transient psychosis with hallucinations, delusions, delirium, or mania may appear. With severe hypercapnia, stupor or coma may develop. Chronic hypercapnia may have no obvious neurologic effect, although progressive CNS depression, characterized by drowsiness, memory loss, and diminished alertness and attentiveness, can occur.

Cardiac effects

Respiratory acidosis may lower the threshold for various arrhythmias. Arrhythmias may be either atrial or ventricular, with atrial more common and

---

* **Hint for the reader.** This chapter and the next (on the treatment of respiratory alkalosis) assume a familiarity with respiratory pathophysiology and with the concept of load-strength imbalance as a cause of hypercapnia. Readers who are unfamiliar with this material are encouraged to read the first four parts of Chapter 18 (p. 171–184) before proceeding.

ventricular more dangerous. These arrhythmias are often multifactorial in origin, with hypercapnia, acidemia, hypoxemia, underlying cardiac disease, and physiologic stress acting in concert to increase the risk.

Categories of respiratory acidosis

In thinking about the treatment of respiratory acidosis, it is useful to conceptualize patients as belonging to one of three categories: acute, chronic, or acute-on-chronic. We introduced these terms elsewhere in the text, but here we review them systematically.

If a respiratory disorder has a rapid onset, such that hypercapnia develops over a few minutes, hours, or (at most) days, the disorder, and hence the hypercapnia and the respiratory acidosis, is said to be <u>acute</u>. Because PCO_2 rises rapidly, but the compensatory rise in plasma bicarbonate concentration takes several days to develop, patients with acute respiratory acidosis are either uncompensated or only partly compensated. Consequently, they have relatively marked acidemia. This uncompensated, relatively acidemic state is *the* defining feature of acute respiratory acidosis.

In contrast, if the underlying disorder, and hence the hypercapnia, develops more gradually and lasts a long time, the condition, and hence the respiratory acidosis, is said to be <u>chronic</u>. In these cases, the renal compensation is able to keep pace with the rise in PCO_2, such that the ratio of $PCO_2/[HCO_3^-]$ never rises sharply from its normal level. Consequently, acidemia is relatively mild. This compensated, mildly acidemic state is *the* defining feature of chronic respiratory acidosis. Patients with chronic respiratory acidosis are, compared with acute patients, relatively stable. In fact, some patients with chronic respiratory acidosis (e.g., some COPD patients) may remain stable, and hypercapnic, for years.

The disorders that cause acute respiratory acidosis not only arise rapidly, they also tend to resolve rapidly with appropriate treatment. For example, acute episodes of asthma, pneumonia, or pulmonary edema—all of which can cause hypercapnia if severe—tend to resolve (at least partly) within a matter of days or, in some cases, hours or even minutes. Acute respiratory acidosis does not usually go on to become chronic. Why not? The diseases are different entities, with different natural histories and different time courses. In other words, inherently acute disorders cause acute respiratory acidosis, and inherently chronic disorders cause chronic respiratory acidosis. In addition, if an underlying acute disorder is severe enough to cause hypercapnia, and the disorder cannot be limited and repaired quickly, the patient is likely to die. That is, acute disorders are often incompatible with the prolonged survival that characterizes chronic disorders.

The third and last category of respiratory acidosis is called <u>acute-on-chronic</u>. This term refers to patients with chronic respiratory acidosis who have an acute rise in their PCO_2 due to a superimposed acute problem. These patients are compensated, but the compensation is at a level appropriate for their chronic baseline PCO_2, not for the acutely elevated PCO_2. Therefore, for any given PCO_2, their acidemia is more severe than in chronic patients.

Let's look at examples. If a patient with severe asthma develops acute hypercapnia, the blood gas might look like this: PCO_2 = 63 mm Hg, $[HCO_3^-]$ = 25 mmol/l, pH = 7.22. If a patient with COPD has chronic hypercapnia, the blood gas might be: PCO_2 = 63, $[HCO_3^-]$ = 34 mmol/l, pH = 7.35. Notice that pH is much lower in the acute patient, even though PCO_2 is the same. If this COPD patient subsequently develops a superimposed pneumonia, which raises PCO_2 to 75 mm Hg, but not enough time has elapsed for renal compensation to raise $[HCO_3^-]$ further, pH will fall to around 7.29. This patient has acute-on-chronic respiratory acidosis.

How does all this apply to treatment? To the extent that a patient's condition is chronic, compensated, and stable, the respiratory acidosis is not itself dangerous. To the extent that a patient's condition is acute (or contains an element of acuteness, as in acute-on-chronic) and uncompensated, the patient is unstable and has a level of acidemia that is relatively severe. As a general rule, patients with stable, chronic hypercapnia do not need urgent therapy, no matter how high the PCO_2. In contrast, patients with acute (or acute-on-chronic) hypercapnia need urgent attention even if PCO_2 is just slightly elevated.

Note: because PCO_2 rises when ventilation fails, it is common to refer to hypercapnic patients as having "ventilatory failure" (or "hypercapnic respiratory failure"). This term refers not to the hypercapnia itself, but to the underlying decline in ventilatory capacity. Put differently, ventilatory failure *causes* hypercapnia. We will use the term "ventilatory failure" later in this chapter.

The goal of therapy: restore the load-strength balance by treating the underlying conditions

Respiratory acidosis—whether acute, chronic, or acute-on-chronic—is not a disease itself, but is the consequence of disease. This underlying disease (or diseases) should be treated. In general, much can be done when the problem is acute, because the disorders tend to be amenable to therapy. In contrast, in chronic disorders, curative treatment usually does not exist, so efforts tend to be limited to symptomatic amelioration and support.

Hypercapnia can be understood as arising from an imbalance between load and strength (i.e., hypercapnia occurs when respiratory load exceeds neuromuscular strength). Therefore, we can organize our discussion of the underlying conditions and their treatment around the load-strength model. In fact, we can summarize our entire discussion with this one sentence preview: all factors responsible for increased respiratory load or decreased neuromuscular strength should be identified and, if possible, treated. That, in a nutshell, is the whole story. Now let's look at the details. We begin with . . .

Increased respiratory load

We can localize respiratory load to three anatomic regions: <u>upper airway</u>, <u>lung</u>, and <u>perilung</u> (i.e., near or around the lung). In the upper airway, respiratory load can rise due to obstruction, which increases airflow resistance. In the lung, respiratory load can rise because of intrinsic disease, which can increase airflow resistance, lung stiffness, and/or minute ventilation requirement (i.e., the minute ventilation required to keep PCO_2 constant). Near the lung (perilung), respiratory load can increase because of disease or defects that restrict lung expansion, a process analogous to lung stiffness, except that the restriction comes from outside the lung, not inside. To these three anatomic regions, we can add a fourth source of increased load: <u>elevated CO_2 production</u>. High CO_2 production increases the respiratory load by raising the minute ventilation requirement.

The following paragraphs briefly discuss the treatment of these four divisions of increased respiratory load. These paragraphs are not intended to be exhaustive treatment guides. Instead, they are written to give you a sense of the types of approaches that are needed.

Upper airway

Increased airflow resistance can occur from obstruction of the nose, mouth, pharynx, larynx, or trachea. Oral cavity obstruction can often be relieved by removing dentures, food, or other foreign matter. Collapsed pharyngeal passages can be opened by carefully extending the head so as to align the air passages.* A "swallowed tongue," a misnomer for pharyngeal obstruction by the base of the tongue, can be relieved by sliding the mandible (to which the tongue is tethered) forward, or by the placement of a nasopharyngeal or oropharyngeal airway, which are simple devices (usually made of rubber or plastic) that push the tongue out of the way and help maintain a patent upper airway. Deep obstruction can sometimes be removed using a laryngoscope or bronchoscope. Unremovable obstruction can be bypassed by cricothyrotomy or tracheostomy.

Lung

Increased respiratory load from airflow obstruction, as occurs in asthma and COPD, may respond to bronchodilators. Expiratory airflow obstruction that is secondary to emphysematous tissue loss can sometimes be ameliorated by pursed-lip breathing (like blowing up a balloon), which increases intra-airway pressure during expiration and thus inhibits premature airway collapse. Obstruction from excess secretions can be reduced by measures such as suction, hydration, expectorants, postural drainage, chest physical therapy, and humidification of inspired air. Pulmonary edema, which increases restrictive load through the accumulation of extravascular fluid, can be treated with di-

---

* **Clinical note.** In patients with possible spinal injuries, any manipulation of the head or neck must be done with extreme caution, to avoid causing or exacerbating damage to the spinal cord.

uretics and other medications; as a temporizing measure, sitting the patient upright with legs hanging off the bed (which redistributes lung volume to capacitance vessels in the legs) may provide some symptomatic relief. Pulmonary embolism, which increases load by raising the minute ventilation requirement (largely through an increase in alveolar dead space), may respond to anticoagulation; in certain cases, the use of thrombolytic agents, which break up the embolized clot, may be helpful. Pneumonia, which can fill air spaces with purulent debris, thus increasing both lung stiffness and ventilatory requirement, is treated with antibiotics and other measures.

Perilung

Defects near the lung can increase the restrictive component of respiratory load. Examples follow. Broken ribs, pleural effusion, pneumothorax, and extensive thoracic skin burns all reduce lung expansion per given respiratory effort. Ascites hinders diaphragmatic flattening by pressing upward against the diaphragm's inferior surface. Following trauma or surgery to the chest or abdomen, adjacent skeletal muscles may increase resting tone to help immobilize the area ("splinting"), which reduces pain on movement but also restricts ventilation (in addition, central drive may decrease by reflex or voluntary mechanisms, also to reduce movement in the area of injury). In obese individuals or patients with a fatigued diaphragm, a horizontal body position may increase the restrictive load by making the diaphragm work against the weight of the abdominal viscera and fat. Correcting these perilung defects can reduce respiratory load.

Increased CO_2 production

Fever, physical activity, hyperthyroidism, and overfeeding with too many calories all increase CO_2 production by the tissues. The elimination of this excess CO_2 requires a higher minute ventilation and, hence, more work. Reducing these causes of excess CO_2 production will lower the respiratory load. In addition, when patients have an increased respiratory load from any cause (e.g., airflow obstruction from asthma), the respiratory muscles must perform heavy work, which increases the amount of CO_2 they produce, thereby raising total-body CO_2 production. Reducing the respiratory load will thus reduce CO_2 production.

Decreased neuromuscular strength

In seeking possible causes of reduced neuromuscular strength, it may help to visualize the neuromuscular chain (p. 176), thinking about each "link" and asking yourself: Could anything be causing poor function at this locus?

Let's start at the top of the chain (central) and move down (to the periphery). Central ventilatory drive may be reduced due to suppression from narcotics or other medications. These medications can sometimes be discontinued, or their dosages reduced. When overdose or poisoning is involved, specific antagonists can sometimes reverse the ventilatory suppression (e.g., Naloxone for narcotic overdose). Nerve or muscle diseases can sometimes be treated or palliated (e.g., Guillain-Barre syndrome, myasthenia gravis, steroid-induced myopathies). Aminoglycoside antibiotics can cause a myasthenia gravis-like syndrome, and should be considered as a possible cause of decreased neuromuscular output.

Continuing down the chain, we come to the muscles. Muscle weakness has many causes. Among the most common are: electrolyte depletion (e.g., low plasma [K$^+$] and [PO$_4$]); poor nutritional status (which has a specific effect on respiratory muscles); sepsis and acidemia (both of which weaken respiratory muscles); hypoxemia, anemia, and low cardiac output (which reduce oxygen and substrate delivery to muscles); and, in postoperative patients, the residual effects of muscle-paralyzing drugs used in surgical anesthesia. All of these causes of neuromuscular weakness can exacerbate load-associated diaphragmatic failure. They should be sought out and corrected.*

A final note. Hypercapnia sometimes occurs because of an isolated increase in respiratory load or an isolated decrease in neuromuscular strength. For example, severe acute asthma may raise PCO$_2$ purely because load is high (i.e., strength may be normal), and Guillain-Barre syndrome may raise PCO$_2$ purely because strength is low (i.e., load may be normal). However, it is much more common that hypercapnia is *multifactorial* in origin. Therefore—except in cases where an isolated defect is clearly involved—multiple causes of both increased load and reduced strength should be sought. In patients with increased load from lung disease, concomitant reductions in neuromuscular strength are most often due to either central ventilatory suppression (e.g., drugs) or muscle weakness (from one of the causes listed in the previous paragraph). In COPD patients, it is especially common that hypercapnia is not due exclusively to the high load, but is associated with various causes of muscle weakness. Therefore, in COPD patients, it is crucial to systematically search for possible causes of muscle weakness and other defects of neuromuscular strength.

The role of mechanical ventilation

A detailed discussion of mechanical ventilation (MV) is beyond the scope of this book. However, it is important to understand how MV fits into the overall management of patients with ventilatory impairment. The paragraphs that follow are designed to provide this understanding.

---

* **Going further.** Although not a cause of muscle weakness, per se, hyperinflation, as occurs in COPD patients, can reduce diaphragmatic efficiency. Hyperinflation causes the diaphragm to become flatter, less dome shaped. The resulting decrease in inspiratory force is independent of muscle fiber strength and can best be understood by imagining an extreme example: a diaphragm that is completely flat, with the apex (central tendon) lying in the same plane as the attachments to the chest wall. In this extreme, hypothetical position, diaphragmatic contraction will not increase thoracic volume at all, because no descent of the apex can occur. If hyperinflation is relieved, diaphragmatic efficiency increases.

As we have seen, treating respiratory acidosis and, more generally, ventilatory failure, requires that the physician identify and correct factors that increase load and decrease strength. This treatment approach constitutes an attempt to *remove impediments* to normal ventilation. However, there are times when a patient's ventilation is (or will soon become) dangerously inadequate, notwithstanding all efforts to treat the underlying conditions. When this happens, the physician must consider an approach that involves not simply removing impediments to ventilation, but actively intervening to ventilate for the patient, using an external ventilatory apparatus. This approach is called mechanical ventilation, or "MV." Mechanical ventilation may be performed either invasively, via endotracheal tube ("intubation"), or noninvasively, via relatively new technologies that use special air-tight masks applied over the nose or both the nose and mouth. In some patients, invasive MV is required; in others, noninvasive MV can be used and may even be preferable.

What is the role of the physician while the patient is on MV? As we have seen, the treatment of patients with respiratory acidosis requires that the physician identify and correct the causes of the imbalance between respiratory load and neuromuscular strength. The initiation of MV does not change this goal—and it does not substitute for it. What MV does is to keep the patient alive longer than would otherwise be possible, thereby giving the physician more time to correct the underlying problems (or, in some cases, giving the body time to heal itself). Thus, whether or not the patient has been placed on a ventilator, the physician's essential task is the same: to systematically search for, identify, and correct the causes of load-strength imbalance. Insofar as we can take competent ventilator management as a given, this "search and correct" mission is *the* central task of the physician during the time the patient is undergoing MV.

The approach to correcting the load-strength imbalance is essentially the same as in patients who are not on MV. Load is reduced by attacking either the underlying disease (e.g., antibiotics for pneumonia) or those consequences of the disease that increase load (e.g., bronchodilators for airway constriction). Strength is increased by treating defects in the neuromuscular chain, with special attention paid to seeking possible causes of reduced central drive and muscle weakness.

In the patient on MV, muscle fatigue may be an important component of muscle weakness, and this fatigue may improve with a ventilator setting that allows the muscles to rest.* Rest allows repletion of depleted muscle glycogen, repair of cellular damage, and the washout of lactic acid or other metabolites. However, it is a serious mistake to assume that fatigue is the sole

---

* **Going further.** Ensuring respiratory muscle rest requires specialized knowledge and can be much more difficult than one might assume. Patients may actually be doing heavy work while they are ostensibly being "rested" on the ventilator. The most basic rule is to make sure the patient *looks* comfortable and does not appear to be straining, "bucking," or otherwise contracting respiratory muscles. There are many other aspects of ensuring rest, which are beyond the scope of this book.

or even primary cause of muscle weakness. This assumption can lead to a passive management strategy, in which the physician assumes that, if adequate muscle rest is assured, the ventilatory problem will take care of itself. In fact, muscle weakness is often multifactorial, with a variety of nonobvious factors acting to lower the fatigue threshold and slow the restoration of muscle strength. Because these muscle-weakening factors are so important, yet often forgotten, we will again list some of the most common ones: hypophosphatemia, hypokalemia, acidemia, sepsis, malnutrition, hypoxemia, anemia, and low cardiac output. Identifying and treating these factors may be a necessary step in allowing the patient to return to spontaneous ventilation (i.e., to be liberated from the ventilator).

Let's conclude by restating the basic idea. In a patient receiving MV for ventilatory failure, the basic task of the physician is as follows: to ensure safe and adequate ventilation (i.e., good ventilator management), to keep the patient medically stable, to ensure muscle rest when fatigue is a possibility, and to clearly identify and reverse the underlying load-strength problems that got the patient on the ventilator in the first place.

Special considerations in patients with chronic hypercapnia

In patients who have a component of chronic respiratory acidosis (i.e., either chronic or acute-on-chronic patients), it is important to be aware of two special considerations. These pertain to (1) the use of supplemental oxygen and (2) the "target" level for PCO_2 if MV becomes necessary. Let's look at these individually.

Supplemental oxygen

In most hypoxemic patients, supplemental oxygen can safely be given—at least temporarily—at virtually any level above the threshold needed to correct the hypoxemia. For example, if a patient with mild pneumonia needs 2 liters per minute by nasal cannula to achieve adequate arterial hemoglobin saturation (SaO_2), there is no immediate danger to giving 3, 4, 5, or even 10 liters per minute. Eventually (after 24–48 hours), high concentrations of supplemental oxygen (greater than around 50–60%) can lead to life-threatening pulmonary oxygen toxicity. However, because oxygen toxicity is not a concern during the first few hours, patients with severe hypoxemia are usually started on high levels of supplemental oxygen (up to 100%)—that is, levels in excess of their requirements—to ensure rapid arterial saturation.

However, in patients with chronic respiratory acidosis, the situation is somewhat different. In these patients, oxygen therapy that raises arterial PO_2 much above 60–65 mm Hg (corresponding to an SaO_2 of around 90%) can sometimes cause an *additional* rise in arterial PCO_2. This acute rise in PCO_2 alters the compensated ratio of $PCO_2/[HCO_3^-]$ and hence causes pH to fall. In short, in the chronic hypercapnic patient, overly aggressive repair of one blood gas abnormality (hypoxemia) can worsen the other (hypercapnia).

Several factors account for this effect. First, patients with chronic hypercapnia may have a reduced ventilatory response to elevated PCO_2, so the ventilatory stimulus provided by hypoxemia plays a greater role than usual. If this hypoxemic stimulus is completely eliminated by excessive oxygen administration, ventilatory drive, and hence minute ventilation, may fall. Second, the lung has homeostatic mechanisms that reduce blood flow to poorly ventilated airspaces (e.g., hypoxic vasoconstriction). Excessive oxygen therapy may partly override this mechanism. The result is that more blood perfuses poorly ventilated areas, increasing the "shunt fraction" (i.e., the fraction of total blood that is shunted), thus raising PCO_2. Other mechanisms also play a role.

How serious is the risk? Until recently, many physicians believed that excessive oxygen therapy in patients with chronic respiratory acidosis was likely to cause a life-threatening rise in PCO_2, or even complete ventilatory arrest. It now appears that the risks were overstated somewhat. For example, one study of COPD patients found that even using 100% oxygen (a level almost never needed in COPD), PCO_2 rose by only about 20 mm Hg, then stabilized. It also appears that some of the previously observed ventilatory suppression may have been due to simultaneously administered sedatives and narcotics, not to the oxygen therapy. Furthermore, it is now recognized that exaggerated concerns about oxygen therapy led some physicians to undertreat severe hypoxemia, causing hypoxic respiratory collapse and death. Current opinion is that (1) the risk of excessive oxygen therapy is real but modest and (2) notwithstanding any risks, one must always give sufficient supplemental oxygen to alleviate life-threatening hypoxemia. Since the vast majority of patients with chronic hypercapnia have COPD, awareness of these points is most important when treating COPD patients.

How do these concerns translate into action? The basic idea when treating patients with chronic hypercapnia is to carefully titrate oxygen therapy to the patient's needs, avoiding excess. The goal is to prevent tissue hypoxia without causing a major rise in arterial PCO_2. This can usually be achieved by keeping oxygen saturation at or just above 90%, usually equal to a PO_2 around 60 mm Hg. In general, supplemental oxygen is increased to a level where O_2 saturation is adequate. Oxygen is then continued at that level, and the patient is monitored closely by blood gas and oximetry to insure adequate ventilation (assessed by PCO_2) and oxygenation (PO_2, SaO_2). Patients are also closely monitored clinically; for example, a decline in mental status or alertness is an especially useful indication of worsening hypercapnia.

A final comment. For patients with chronic hypercapnia, the bottom line is this: although it is desirable to proceed carefully, you must still give enough O_2 to maintain adequate oxygenation. In fact, a major risk to the severely hypoxemic COPD patient is that the physician, in the name of careful titration, will increase the oxygen flow so gradually that dangerous hypoxemia is prolonged. Thus, while careful titration is desirable, it should never be carried out at the cost of prolonging severe hypoxemia. In severely hypoxemic or otherwise unstable patients, oxygen therapy is initiated in a much more aggressive manner, using a higher level of supplemental oxygen. If severe hypercapnia and acidemia develop, mechanical ventilation may become necessary.

Target PCO_2 in mechanical ventilation

In the mechanically ventilated patient, PCO_2 is determined largely by minute ventilation, which is set by the physician. Thus, the physician must have a "target PCO_2" in mind—that is, a PCO_2 that will become the patient's new steady-state level while on MV. In patients with acute lung disease, the target PCO_2 is most commonly the normal level, approximately 40 mm Hg, although there are times when a higher level is targeted.

In contrast, patients with chronic respiratory acidosis are hyperbicarbonatemic due to renal compensation. Thus, if you reduce PCO_2 to the "normal" value of 40 mm Hg, the patient will be left with hyperbicarbonatemia and normocapnia—that is, metabolic alkalosis with alkalemia. This iatrogenic form of metabolic alkalosis is called "posthypercapnic metabolic alkalosis" (it is discussed in detail on p. 167). To avoid this outcome, many physicians advocate reducing PCO_2 to its prior, stable baseline level. For example, if a COPD patient has a chronic, stable PCO_2 of 60 mm Hg, but a pulmonary infection raises the PCO_2 to 85 mm Hg, you might aim to return PCO_2 to 60 mm Hg if MV becomes necessary.

Summary

Patients with respiratory acidosis can be categorized as acute, chronic, or acute-on-chronic. In general, patients with an acute component (either acute or acute-on-chronic) are unstable, relatively acidemic, and require urgent therapy. In contrast, chronic patients are usually relatively stable and only mildly acidemic. The major goal of therapy, in all patients, is to treat the underlying conditions that caused the hypercapnia. These conditions can be conceptualized as either increased respiratory load or decreased neuromuscular strength, which result in a load-strength imbalance (i.e., load > strength). In many patients, hypercapnia is multifactorial, with several causes of both increased load and decreased strength. In patients with lung disease, concomitant reductions in strength are most often due to either central ventilatory suppression (e.g., drugs) or muscle weakness (e.g., hypophosphatemia, hypokalemia, malnutrition, sepsis, hypoxemia, acidemia, residual muscle paralyzing drugs from surgery). Mechanical ventilation (MV) is used if ventilation becomes dangerously inadequate. In addition to basic MV management (which is not discussed in this text), the physician must search for, identify, and correct the defects of load and strength that caused the patient to need MV in the first place. Two special considerations apply to patients with chronic respiratory acidosis. First, in hypoxemic patients, supplemental oxygen is carefully titrated to the patient's needs, avoiding excess; however, titration should never delay aggressive repair of severe, life-threatening hypoxemia. Second, if MV becomes necessary, the target PCO_2 is usually the patient's prior stable level, not a "normal" PCO_2 of 40 mm Hg.

Treatment of Respiratory Alkalosis 28

Effects of respiratory alkalosis

Acute respiratory alkalosis has three main types of effects: cerebrovascular, neurologic, and cardiac.

Cerebrovascular. Acute hypocapnia causes cerebral vasoconstriction. Therefore, hypocapnia lowers intracranial blood pressure and flow. For example, an acute fall in arterial PCO_2 to 20 mm Hg can reduce cerebral blood flow by 40 percent. This relative ischemia can impair higher mental functioning and cause light-headedness and fainting.*

Neurologic effects. Acute hypocapnia causes peri-oral numbness, paresthesias of fingers and toes (usually a tingling sensation), and carpopedal spasms. These effects are probably due primarily to alkalemia. Occasionally (probably due to the combination of cerebral ischemia and alkalemia), generalized tetany, seizures, or coma may occur.

Cardiac effects. Acute respiratory alkalosis may lower the threshold for both atrial and ventricular arrhythmias. These arrhythmias are uncommon in patients with healthy hearts, but may be more frequent in patients with coronary artery disease. In general, neither the neurologic effects (above) nor cardiac arrhythmias develop unless pH is 7.55 or higher; therefore, arrhythmias are not considered a risk in chronic (compensated) respiratory alkalosis.

Chronic respiratory alkalosis (as may occur, for example, in chronic liver disease) has few sequelae. The slow onset allows renal compensation to develop in tandem with the hypocapnia, so pH is not greatly elevated. Also, for unknown reasons, symptomatic cerebral ischemia occurs only in acute hypocapnia; it may be that changes in cerebral arterial tone are partly mediated by pH, which returns toward normal as renal compensation develops.

---

*Clinical note. This vasoconstrictive effect is sometimes used therapeutically in patients with cerebral edema: when swelling threatens to cause lethal brain herniation through the foramen magnum, mechanical hyperventilation can reduce cerebral blood flow and, hence, blood volume and intracranial pressure. This therapeutic effect lasts only a day or two, after which blood flow returns toward normal.

Approach to the patient

Except when respiratory alkalosis is acute and severe, hypocapnia is not itself dangerous, and no attempt is usually made to directly raise PCO_2. For this reason, the major clinical importance of respiratory alkalosis is that it can indicate the presence of a previously unrecognized disease, which is causing the patient to hyperventilate. In other words, respiratory alkalosis can act as a clinical marker of underlying disease. Because this underlying disease may be acutely life-threatening, it is crucial to search for and identify the cause of respiratory alkalosis without delay.

Accordingly, most of this chapter is designed to help you think clearly about what might be causing respiratory alkalosis. However, before we look at possible causes (i.e., the differential diagnosis) of respiratory alkalosis, we need to make two brief points.

First, as just noted, if you detect respiratory alkalosis, it is essential to identify the cause. However, the converse is not necessarily true. That is, if you diagnose a condition that can potentially cause respiratory alkalosis, it is not always necessary to determine with certainty (i.e., by blood gas) whether the respiratory alkalosis is actually present. For example, if you diagnose mild asthma in a clinically stable patient, you may reasonably expect that a mild respiratory alkalosis is present—but there is often no need to verify the existence of this alkalosis by getting a blood gas. Definitively diagnosing the respiratory alkalosis is often unnecessary because the hypocapnia itself needs no treatment. (However, there may be other reasons to get a blood gas in a patient with suspected respiratory alkalosis, such as ruling out hypoxemia, ruling out other acid-base disturbances, or getting a PCO_2 baseline in a patient who might deteriorate.)

Second, it is important to remember that hyperventilation with hypocapnia may result from either respiratory alkalosis or metabolic acidosis with respiratory compensation. Therefore, when hyperventilation is detected, do not automatically assume that respiratory alkalosis is the primary disorder; metabolic acidosis should also be considered as a possibility.*

The differential diagnosis of respiratory alkalosis

The pathophysiologic mechanisms that increase central ventilatory drive, and thus cause respiratory alkalosis, can be divided into four broad groups:

---

*Clinical note. The only reliable way to distinguish between respiratory alkalosis and metabolic acidosis is by blood gas. It is sometimes taught that the physical examination can be helpful as well. Specifically, it is said that patients with respiratory compensation for metabolic acidosis hyperventilate with deep, regular breaths (Kussmaul ventilation), whereas patients with primary lung disease tend to hyperventilate with rapid, shallow breaths. Although this distinction does have a physiologic basis, many additional variables can affect the ventilatory pattern. Therefore, the physical examination should not be relied on to differentiate primary from compensatory hyperventilation.

(1) arterial hypoxemia or tissue hypoxia, (2) stimulation of pulmonary sense receptors by a disease process in the lung, (3) factors that directly affect the medullary respiratory center, and (4) psychologic factors such as anxiety, fear, and pain. When a patient presents with a low PCO_2 on blood gas, or hyperventilation on physical examination, a list of common underlying causes can be generated by thinking about these four groups. Let's look at each group individually, starting with . . .

Hypoxemia or tissue hypoxia

Hypoxemia is the most acutely dangerous, and one of the most common, cause of hyperventilation. Any time a patient presents with hyperventilation, hypoxemia must be considered as a cause and investigated. If hypoxemia is detected, supplemental oxygen should be given and the specific cause of the hypoxemia should be identified and treated. Note: individuals who have just traveled to higher altitudes occasionally develop mild hypoxemia and physiologic hyperventilation; this condition usually needs no treatment.

A number of conditions can cause tissue hypoxia without causing frank arterial hypoxemia. These conditions can sometimes cause hyperventilation. Examples include severe systemic hypoperfusion from low cardiac output, severe anemia, severe hypotension, and carbon monoxide poisoning. All of these conditions reduce the amount of oxygen that is delivered to, or unloaded at, the tissues. Some readers may find it useful to think of these conditions as "hypoxemia equivalents." These conditions should be considered when frank hypoxemia is not present.

Stimulation of lung sense receptors

Any lung disease, whether or not it causes hypoxemia, can increase ventilatory drive by stimulating stretch and/or chemoreceptors in the lung. Examples include asthma, pneumonia, ARDS, cardiogenic pulmonary edema, and pulmonary embolism. Many of these disorders will quickly be apparent from the history and physical examination. However, pulmonary embolism (PE) should be specifically considered because it often presents with non-specific findings; for example, PE may present with mild hyperventilation and subtle dyspnea as the only findings.

Factors that directly affect the respiratory center

Factors that directly impinge on the medullary respiratory center can simulate hyperventilation. These factors should be considered in the hyperventilating patient, especially when hypoxemia or lung disease do not provide an obvious explanation. One of the most important entities in this category is sepsis (the hyperventilation is mediated largely by cytokines). Sepsis must be considered quickly because the patient's condition may evolve rapidly to lethal septic shock. Other conditions that directly affect the respiratory center, causing hyperventilation, include: liver disease (un-deaminated waste products may account for the hyperventilation), aspirin overdose (salicylate drives ventilation), CNS infection (cytokines), CNS neoplasm (cellular breakdown products), and head trauma (physical trauma of the respiratory center mediates the hyperventilation). In pregnancy, mild hyperventilation is a normal finding due to elevated plasma progesterone levels.

Psychologic factors: pain, anxiety, and fear

Pain, anxiety, and fear can cause hyperventilation through cortical and possibly subcortical neural pathways. Patients who hyperventilate based on these factors fall into two broad groups: those who have an underlying physical cause for the psychologic factor, and those who do not ("psychogenic hyperventilation"). We look at these two groups individually.

Pain, anxiety, and fear attributable to physical causes

Any physical problem that causes pain, anxiety, or fear may lead to hyperventilation. These problems may range in severity from acutely life-threatening to self-limited and benign. A few examples of life-threatening sources of pain and anxiety are myocardial infarction, rupture of an aortic aneurysm, pulmonary embolism, and "acute surgical abdomen" (e.g., appendicitis). It is important to note that these life-threatening events, while sometimes presenting with intense localized pain, may also present with only vague discomfort, anxiety, or a sense of trepidation. Examples of non-life-threatening problems that can lead to hyperventilation are post-surgical "incisional" pain, pain from minor trauma of an extremity, and fear or anxiety about a self-limited disease.

Psychogenic hyperventilation

When hyperventilation is caused by psychologic factors that are not directly attributable to physical disease, the disorder is referred to as psychogenic hyperventilation. (Psychogenic hyperventilation is sometimes referred to by other names, including anxiety hyperventilation, primary hyperventilation, and hyperventilation syndrome.) Psychogenic hyperventilation is sometimes due to underlying anxiety or panic attack, and may be precipitated by an emotionally charged life event. Although the clinical presentation is often suggestive, the diagnosis of psychogenic hyperventilation should not made until life-threatening organic causes are considered and ruled out. That is, psychogenic hyperventilation must be a diagnosis of exclusion.

Patients with psychogenic hyperventilation experience intense, terrifying feelings of breathlessness. The terror can compound the underlying anxiety, creating a vicious circle. Light-headedness is common and frank syncope may occur, probably due to hypocapnia-induced cerebral vasoconstriction. Paresthesias and tetany may develop. Other findings may include tachycardia, palpitations, and substernal tightness or pressure. Like the feelings of breathlessness, these other findings can be frightening to the patient and must be differentiated by the physician from life-threatening emergencies such as pulmonary embolism or myocardial ischemia.

Because the "prior probability" (i.e., the statistical likelihood) of an acute pulmonary or cardiac event is lower in young, healthy people, the diagnosis of psychogenic hyperventilation is easier to make in this population. In these patients, if the presentation is suggestive of psychogenic hyperventilation, and the history and physical examination do not hint at the presence of cardiac or pulmonary disease, many physicians will not get a blood gas.* In older patients, or patients with underlying disease, the prior probability of a pulmonary or cardiac event is higher, which makes the diagnosis of psychogenic hyperventilation more problematic. In these higher-risk patients, most physicians will assume that hyperventilation is either caused by or associated with acute organic disease, unless a work up proves otherwise.

How is psychogenic hyperventilation treated? In all patients, ruling out serious disease, and then reassuring the patient about the benign nature of the hyperventilation, is essential. The reassurance helps relieve secondary anxiety and can thus contribute to normalization of ventilation. Many physicians try to get patients to relax and voluntarily slow their rate of ventilation. Some physicians will actually count off inspirations and expirations (e.g., three counts in, three counts out). Benzodiazepines (e.g., lorazepam, diazepam) are sometimes given, primarily for their anxiolytic effect, but also because they have a direct, mild suppressive effect on ventilation.

Having the patient "rebreath" into a paper (not plastic) bag has traditionally been a component of therapy, and many physicians still use the approach. The rationale is that rebreathing CO_2 rich air raises alveolar and arterial PCO_2. (Expired air contains 3% CO_2, whereas atmospheric air contains less than 0.1%.) The rise in arterial PCO_2 helps relieve symptoms of hypocapnia, and it is thought, but not proved, that it may also help reduce ventilatory drive. Adequate oxygen is maintained through leaks around the mouth of the bag.

When paper-bag rebreathing is used in an otherwise healthy patient with true psychogenic hyperventilation, it is safe and may provide some benefit. However, if used in a patient with unrecognized organic disease, it can be dangerous, because the PO_2 of air in the bag does fall somewhat. For example, in a patient with unrecognized lung disease or myocardial ischemia, paper-bag rebreathing can exacerbate hypoxemia or myocardial hypoxia. For this reason, many physicians recommend that no patient be "paper bagged" without using pulse oximetry to assess oxygenation before, and perhaps during, the rebreathing procedure.

---

*__Clinical note.__ Some non-invasive tests that can help exclude serious disease in these low-risk patients include pulse oximetry, blood pressure measurement, and an ECG rhythm strip. In an otherwise healthy patient with psychogenic hyperventilation, the usual findings are: an oxygen saturation of 99–100% (this is the saturation range usually produced when a person with normal lungs hyperventilates), a normal blood pressure, and an ECG showing a sinus rhythm. An oxygen saturation lower than about 99%, or an abnormal blood pressure, or a non-sinus rhythm, may suggest underlying disease.

In patients with repeat episodes of psychogenic hyperventilation, underlying anxiety or panic disorder is common, and consultation with a specialist (e.g., psychiatrist or psychiatric social worker) should be considered. In these patients, psychotherapy and/or chronic drug therapy with selective serotonin reuptake inhibitors (SSRI's) may help prevent future episodes.

A final point: ruling out hypoxemia

Because hyperventilation is often caused by hypoxemia, it is important to understand how to rule out hypoxemia. The key point to understand is this: in a hyperventilating patient, a blood gas (i.e., PO_2) is the only reliable way to rule out hypoxemia. Measuring O_2 saturation ("O_2 sat") is not sufficient. Why not? There are two main reasons.

First, the oxyhemoglobin curve is relatively flat above a PO_2 of 60 mm Hg, which corresponds to an O_2 sat of about 90%. This means that a PO_2 range of 60–100 mm Hg corresponds with an O_2 sat range of roughly 90–100%. Therefore, as PO_2 falls from 100 mm Hg to 60 mm Hg, O_2 sat changes only gradually and in very small increments. For example, a fall in PO_2 from 95 to 65 may cause O_2 sat to fall from 97% to 92%. Given the inherent inaccuracies of pulse oximetry ($\pm$ a few %), it is easy to see that relying on pulse oximetry could cause you to miss evolving hypoxemia in the PO_2 range above 60 mm Hg.

Second, hyperventilation can mask hypoxemia by raising PO_2. This point requires some explanation. Hyperventilation raises alveolar PO_2 while it lowers alveolar PCO_2. These alveolar changes are reflected in the blood: arterial PO_2 rises at the same time that arterial PCO_2 falls. Thus, hyperventilating patients have a PO_2 that is higher than it would be if they were not hyperventilating.

Let's extend this second point. In patients breathing room air, each 1 mm Hg fall in PCO_2 is associated with a rise in PO_2 of roughly 1 mm Hg (i.e., a 1:1 ratio). We can use this 1:1 relationship to calculate a "ventilation-adjusted PO_2." Consider a patient with a PCO_2 = 15 and a PO_2 = 90. PCO_2 is 25 mm Hg below normal (i.e., $40 - 15 = 25$), so we know that the hyperventilation has raised PO_2 by about 25 mm Hg. This means that adjusted PO_2 is $90 - 25 = 65$ mm Hg. This patient has a significant pulmonary oxygenation defect, but it is masked by the hyperventilation, which raises PO_2 to normal. Furthermore, because the non-adjusted PO_2 of 90 mm Hg "translates" into an O_2 sat above 95%, oxygen saturation is normal as well. Note that the adjusted PO_2 value tells us roughly what PO_2 would be if the patient were to stop hyperventilating.

In the example just given, the oxygenation defect was completely masked by hyperventilation. Such a patient might be said to have "occult hypoxemia." It is also possible for hyperventilation to mask hypoxemia only partly. When this happens, the measured PO_2 is low, but it is still higher than it would be if the patient were ventilating normally. For example, if $PCO_2 = 15$ and $PO_2 = 60$, adjusted PO_2 is $60 - 25 = 35$. In this patient, O_2 sat would be about 90%, which appears much less ominous than an adjusted PO_2 of 35 mm Hg. Only a blood gas lets you identify masked hypoxemia and, by calculating an adjusted PO_2, quantitatively assess the severity of the oxygenation defect.*

Summary

The major clinical importance of respiratory alkalosis is diagnostic, in that it can suggest the presence of potentially serious underlying disease. Hyperventilation with hypocapnia may be due to either respiratory alkalosis or to metabolic acidosis with respiratory compensation, and both these primary acid-base disturbances must be considered in a hyperventilating patient. Respiratory alkalosis is caused by four broad groups of pathophysiologic factors: (1) *Hypoxemia or tissue hypoxia.* Hypoxemia is common and dangerous. In a hyperventilating patient, it should be considered, investigated and, if present, treated. Remember that hypoxemia can be ruled out only by blood gas, not by oximetry alone. Conditions that cause tissue hypoxia without arterial hypoxemia should also be considered (e.g., severe anemia). (2) *Stimulation of lung sense receptors by pulmonary disease.* Almost any lung disease can cause hyperventilation, even if PO_2 is normal. In a patient with few clinical findings, pulmonary embolism must be considered. (3) *Factors directly affecting the respiratory center.* Sepsis or salicylate intoxication must be considered quickly because they may be acutely life-threatening. In pregnancy, mild respiratory alkalosis due to elevated progesterone levels is a normal finding. (4) *Psychologic causes such as pain, fear, and anxiety.* These may be associated with life-threatening disorders or minor problems. Psychogenic hyperventilation, which may be caused by underlying anxiety, is a diagnosis of exclusion, which should be made only after ruling out serious underlying disease.

---

*Going further. The 1:1 ratio cited in the text is an easy-to-remember approximation. The actual ratio is closer to 1:1.25. That is, a 1 mm Hg fall in PCO_2 is associated with a 1.25 mm Hg rise in PO_2. The 1:1.25 ratio is derived from the alveolar gas equation, assuming a respiratory exchange ratio of 0.8 (i.e., $1/0.8 = 1.25$). In addition to the two reasons given in the text, there is a third reason why the blood gas provides a better assessment of hypoxemia than oximetry. The alkalemia associated with respiratory alkalosis shifts the oxyhemoglobin curve "to the left," hindering oxygen unloading at the tissues. This impaired unloading worsens the tissue hypoxia that results from any given level of arterial hypoxemia. This fall in oxygen unloading would not be suspected unless you had a blood gas to assess pH. (Conversely, acidemia, which is associated with respiratory acidosis, shifts the curve to the right, which facilitates oxygen unloading at the tissues.) For a basic explanation of pulse oximetry, the alveolar gas equation, and the alveolar-arterial oxygen difference, see the discussion of "Respiratory disturbances" in Chapter 23, starting on page 260.

Prevention of Acid-Base Disorders 29

This chapter is short, but the awareness it aims to impart is crucial. The basic idea can be summarized in two statements: (1) acid-base disturbances often occur for predictable reasons and can therefore be prevented, and (2) as in all areas of medicine, it is better to prevent than treat. The following paragraphs focus on some common and largely preventable disturbances.

Metabolic acidosis

With early therapy and education, you can often lessen the incidence and severity of metabolic acidosis. For example, treat chronic renal dysfunction, such as failure and renal tubular acidosis, early, before the acidosis becomes severe. Ketone-prone diabetics should receive careful instruction about their disease. In addition to the usual thorough instructions about managing glucose levels, patients should be taught that hyperventilation is part of the body's response to uncontrolled ketosis, and is an indication to immediately seek medical help. In patients taking acetazolamide (Diamox) for glaucoma, check venous electrolytes regularly for indications of hypobicarbonatemia from drug-induced proximal RTA (also check for hypokalemia).

Metabolic alkalosis

Two of the most common causes of metabolic alkalosis lend themselves to prevention: diuretics and nasogastric drainage. Diuretics produce metabolic alkalosis largely by inducing hypokalemia and hypovolemia. Although hypovolemia is difficult to prevent without undercutting the diuretic's efficacy, potassium losses can almost always be anticipated and replaced during therapy. Potassium replacement will often prevent alkalosis or, at least, lessen its severity if it does develop. Placing diuretic patients on a low-sodium diet can also help prevent hypokalemia and metabolic alkalosis (because the reabsorption of Na^+ from the distal nephron facilitates K^+ and H^+ secretion [p. 161]). With nasogastric drainage, losses of both volume and potassium should be anticipated and replaced early, starting when the suction is turned on. If metabolic alkalosis starts to develop, histamine H_2 blockers or omeprazole (p. 301) may be used to reduce proton secretion.

Respiratory acidosis

In patients with chronic hypercapnia, acute increases in PCO_2 can sometimes be prevented or minimized by quickly treating lung infections with antibiotics and carefully titrating supplemental oxygen to the patient's needs, avoiding excess. In patients with limited ventilatory reserves (e.g., due to pulmonary or neuromuscular disease), or those who are currently on mechanical ventilation, care should be taken to avoid overfeeding, which can increase CO_2 production and precipitate or exacerbate hypercapnia. In patients with severe lung disease, who may present with respiratory alkalosis but have a high work of breathing, respiratory muscles can fail, slowing ventilation and precipitating hypercapnia. In such patients, it may be possible to prevent ventilation failure and respiratory acidosis by aggressively treating the underlying disorder, thereby reducing respiratory load. If the patient progresses to the point where it appears that ventilatory failure is imminent, it may be desirable to start mechanical ventilation "preemptively," while the patient is still hypocapnic.

Respiratory alkalosis

Hypoxemia is one of the most important causes of respiratory alkalosis. Recognize it early and administer oxygen. Patients who experience repeated episodes of psychogenic hyperventilation may have an underlying anxiety disorder, perhaps panic disorder. Psychiatric consultation and/or psychotherapy should be considered. Some psychiatrists currently advocate prophylaxis with selective serotonin reuptake inhibitors (SSRIs) as a way to help prevent future attacks. If underlying disease has been clearly ruled out (p. 320–321), some physicians instruct patients to keep a small paper bag in their purse or pocket, so they can attempt to abort evolving episodes. The mere presence of the paper bag may impart a feeling of control, reducing the anticipatory anxiety that can contribute to subsequent attacks.

Self-Assessment Quiz

This quiz tests your knowledge of core concepts and facts. More importantly, the process of taking and correcting the quiz will strengthen your understanding of the essentials. To get the most from this process, answer all questions in writing. Use a separate answer sheet if you wish. Take your time. When you finish, check your answers against the key. It doesn't matter whether you ace this quiz or fail it. The important thing is to grapple with the questions and then, for those that you miss, to study the correct answers carefully.

1. Metabolic acidosis usually does not reduce cardiac contractility until pH falls below _____.

2. As a general rule, in patients with metabolic acidosis, you always treat the _____ and sometimes attempt to raise _____ _____.

3. Patients with metabolic acidosis are sometimes treated with bicarbonate. However, _____ _____ can often be used as well. Three examples of this category are _____, _____, and _____.

4. In deciding whether to give bicarbonate to a patient with metabolic acidosis, what three variables must you consider?

5. Name two factors that act to make metabolic acidosis "self-limiting."

6. "Overshoot metabolic alkalosis" is most likely to occur if you give large amounts of bicarbonate to a patient who has a high plasma concentration of _____ _____.

7. Post-correction hyperventilation occurs when plasma $[HCO_3^-]$ rises to normal but the interstitial fluid $[HCO_3^-]$ around the _____ _____ is still low. When this condition develops, a blood gas may change from one showing metabolic acidosis to one showing _____ _____.

8. In patients with diabetic ketoacidosis, plasma $[K^+]$ may be normal or elevated, even though whole-body potassium stores are depleted. The lack of correspondence between body stores and plasma levels occurs because K^+ shifts out of cells, raising plasma $[K^+]$. Name two factors that lead to this shift in DKA. When you give insulin, what happens to these factors? What happens to extracellular potassium? What happens to plasma $[K^+]$? What happens to whole-body potassium stores?

9. Patients with diabetic ketoacidosis may or may not need bicarbonate, but they almost always need _____, _____, and _____.

10. Alcoholic ketoacidosis can usually be treated with nothing more than intravenous _____ and _____.

11. Dextrose is another name for _____.

12. Complete the sentence: In patients with lactic acidosis, the most important thing you can do is . . .

13. The clinical picture of a "_____ drunk" immediately suggests methanol intoxication. In a methanol-intoxicated patient, gastric lavage may be used to reduce gut _____, and _____ is used to remove methanol that is already absorbed. To inhibit the conversion of methanol to toxic metabolites, _____ is given. This substance is typically given as soon as you _____ methanol has been ingested. Because the degree of hypobicarbonatemia may be correlated with mortality, aggressive therapy with _____ is often advocated.

14. Patients with simple metabolic alkalosis usually have low plasma levels of the _____ ion. Do they also have whole-body depletion of this ion?

15. The treatment of volume-responsive metabolic alkalosis is often a simple three-step process. Name the steps. Can you carry out all these steps at once, or must you assess the results of each step before proceeding to the next?

16. When giving potassium, whether during metabolic alkalosis or for another purpose, is it generally preferable to do so by mouth or by vein?

17. What is the major danger of giving potassium intravenously?

18. In patients with metabolic alkalosis caused by diuretic therapy, you cannot give saline with impunity. Why not? Can you still give potassium?

19. Follow-up question. In patients with metabolic alkalosis from diuretics, several treatment modalities can be helpful, depending on the clinical situation. One is to give potassium. Another is to consider _____ the diuretic dosage. Another approach involves giving _____, also known as _____, which is a drug that increases urinary bicarbonate spillage. This drug also causes massive urinary spillage of _____. Another approach is to give _____, the _____-sparing diuretic.

20. In patients with severe metabolic alkalosis, or moderate metabolic alkalosis plus lung disease, the respiratory compensation can sometimes induce _____.

21. In patients taking Diamox (acetazolamide), venous levels of these two electrolytes should be checked regularly: _____ and _____. In patients taking _____ or _____ diuretics, these same two electrolytes should be checked periodically. In a patient taking Diamox for glaucoma, plasma $[HCO_3^-]$ may be high/low (choose one). In a patient taking furosemide for edema, $[HCO_3^-]$ may be high/low (choose one).

22. In patients undergoing nasogastric suction, replacement of _____ and _____ should begin early.

23. In patients on diuretics, _____ should be administered before plasma $[K^+]$ falls markedly. Which chemical preparation of this substance should be used?

24. Depending on the time course, respiratory acidosis can be _____, _____, or _____-_____-_____. For a given level of PCO_2, which of the three will have the most severe acidemia? The least severe? The term "acute-on-chronic respiratory acidosis" refers to patients who have _____ respiratory acidosis but experience an _____ rise in _____. Of the three categories discussed here, two usually require urgent medical attention. Name them.

25. Because PCO_2 rises when ventilation fails, it is common to refer to hypercapnic patients as having "_____ failure" (or "_____ respiratory failure"). This term refers not to the hypercapnia itself, but to the underlying decline in _____ capacity. Put differently, ventilatory failure _____ hypercapnia.

26. The treatment of ventilatory failure and respiratory acidosis can be summarized in this one sentence: all factors responsible for increased respiratory _____ or decreased _____ should be _____ and, if possible, treated.

    Hint: this sentence is based on a particular model used to explain hypercapnia. The model posits that hypercapnia is due to an imbalance between two variables.

27. Many of the causes of increased load can be localized to three anatomic regions: _____, _____ _____, and _____-lung. Give an example of a defect in the last category. Increased production of _____ by the tissues is an additional cause of increased respiratory load, because it raises the minute _____ _____.

28. In patients with lung disease, hypercapnia is often multifactorial. Although the physician will naturally pay great attention to the lung disease itself because the lung disease increases the respiratory load, it is also essential to identify factors that may be acting to decrease neuromuscular _____. In patients with lung disease, the two "links" in the neuromuscular chain that are most likely to be defective are the respiratory _____ in the brain and the respiratory muscles, especially the _____.

29. Follow-up question. In patients with lung disease, defects of the respiratory center are most commonly due to suppression of central drive by _____. A common example of such a drug is _____, which is sometimes given to relieve pain (this answer is not in the text). List four com-

mon causes of respiratory muscle weakness in patients with lung disease. Hypercapnia is especially likely to be multifactorial in this lung disease: _____.

30. When a patient's ventilatory capacity has declined to the point where _____ is threatened, the physician must consider _____ _____, which involves using an external apparatus to ventilate for the patient. However, the use of this approach does not change the physician's primary goal: to _____ and _____ underlying causes of _____ respiratory _____ and decreased neuromuscular _____. When muscle failure is thought to be caused partly by muscle _____, the physician must ensure that the ventilator is set to allow the respiratory muscles to rest. Achieving this goal may be simpler/more complex (choose one) than it initially appears, and may require _____ training (this point is discussed only in a footnote [p. 313], not in the main text).

31. In patients with chronic hypercapnia, overly aggressive use of supplemental _____ can lead to an additional _____ in _____. The goal in these patients is to carefully _____ oxygen therapy to the patient's needs, raising oxygen saturation to about _____, which corresponds to a PO_2 of about _____. However, titration of oxygen therapy should not be carried out at the expense of prolonging severe _____, which is a greater danger than _____.

32. Because hypocapnia is usually not _____ and needs no _____, the major clinical importance of respiratory alkalosis is that it can indicate the existence of a previously unrecognized problem, which is causing the patient to _____. This underlying problem may be _____ or even acutely life-threatening.

33. Hyperventilation may indicate either respiratory alkalosis or _____ _____, with respiratory _____. Therefore, when _____ is noted on physical examination, metabolic _____ should be considered as a possibility, along with the various causes of respiratory _____. The only reliable way to distinguish between these two primary acid-base disorders is a _____ _____.

34. The pathophysiologic mechanisms that increase central ventilatory drive, and cause respiratory alkalosis, can be divided into four broad groups: (1) arterial _____ or tissue _____, (2) direct stimulation of _____ _____ _____ by a disease process in the lung, (3) chemical or physical factors that directly affect the medullary _____ _____, and (4) _____ factors such as anxiety, fear, and pain.

35. In a hyperventilating patient, the only way to rule out hypoxemia is by measuring _____ by _____ _____. Measuring _____ _____ is not sufficient. Of the many lung diseases that can produce hyperventilation by directly stimulating pulmonary sense receptors, it is especially im-

portant to consider _____ _____, because this disorder tends to present with subtle or _____-_____ findings. In the hyperventilating patient, _____ should be considered quickly, because this disorder is both common and may progress rapidly to _____ shock. In the outpatient setting, overdose with _____ should also be considered as a cause of hyperventilation (this overdose can actually produce two acid-base disturbances: a respiratory alkalosis and a _____ _____ of the _____-_____ type).

36. Psychologic factors that can cause hyperventilation include _____, _____, and _____. When hyperventilation is caused by one of these factors, it is important to distinguish between patients who have an underlying physical problem and those who do not. Underlying physical problems may be benign (for example, post-surgical pain) or catastrophic and life-threatening, such as myocardial _____, pulmonary _____, rupture of an _____ _____, or one of the causes of an "acute _____," such as a ruptured appendix. When no underlying physical problem exists, the patient is said to have _____ hyperventilation, which may be associated with underlying _____ and may represent a _____ attack. Psychogenic hyperventilation is a diagnosis of _____, which requires that potentially serious causes be considered and _____ _____.

Answer Key

1. About 7.2.

2. Cause, plasma $[HCO_3^-]$.

3. Organic anions. Citrate, lactate, acetate.

4. pH, $[HCO_3^-]$, and how self-limiting the disturbance is.

5. High plasma levels of organic anions, which can be metabolized to bicarbonate, and good renal function, which can regenerate bicarbonate.

6. Organic anions.

7. Respiratory center. Respiratory alkalosis.

8. Hypoinsulinemia, plasma hyperosmolarity. They "disappear" (i.e., insulin levels and osmolarity return toward normal). Much shifts back into cells. It falls. No change.

9. Volume, insulin, potassium.

10. Saline solution, dextrose.

11. Glucose.

12. Find and correct the underlying cause.

13. Blind. Absorption, dialysis. Ethanol. Suspect. Bicarbonate.

14. Potassium. Yes.

15. Remove underlying cause, give NaCl solution, give KCl. You can usually do all at once.

16. Mouth.

17. Hyperkalemia with cardiac arrhythmia.

18. The volume depletion is therapeutic; saline reverses it. Yes.

19. Reducing. Acetazolamide, Diamox. Potassium. Spironolactone, potassium.

20. Hypoxemia.

21. Bicarbonate, potassium. Loop, thiazide. Low. High.

22. Volume, potassium.

23. Potassium. KCl.

24. Acute, chronic, acute-on-chronic. Acute. Chronic. Chronic, acute, PCO_2. Acute, acute-on-chronic.

25. Ventilatory, hypercapnic. Ventilatory. Causes.

26. Load, strength, identified.

27. Lung, upper airway, peri (or near). Examples include: broken ribs, pleural effusion, ascites, massive obesity. CO_2, ventilation requirement.

28. Strength. Center, diaphragm.

29. Drugs. Morphine. Examples include: low plasma [K^+], low plasma [PO_4], malnutrition, sepsis, acidemia, hypoxemia, residual effects of muscle-paralyzing drugs used in surgery. COPD.

30. Survival, mechanical ventilation. Identify, correct, increased, load, strength. Fatigue. More complex, specialized.

31. Oxygen, rise, PCO_2. Titrate, 90%, 60 mm Hg. Hypoxemia, hypercapnia.

32. Dangerous, treatment, hyperventilate. Serious.

33. Metabolic acidosis, compensation. Hyperventilation, acidosis, alkalosis. Blood gas.

34. Hypoxemia, hypoxia, pulmonary sense receptors, respiratory center, psychologic.

35. PO_2, blood gas. Oxygen saturation. Pulmonary embolism, non-specific. Sepsis, septic. Salicylate, metabolic acidosis, anion-gap.

36. Examples include: anxiety, fear, pain, stress. Infarction, embolism, aortic aneurysm, abdomen. Psychogenic, anxiety, panic. Exclusion, ruled out.

Appendix

Continuing Education

Why this Appendix?

The five main sections of this book provide a detailed survey of medical acid-base. They are designed to give readers a clear and sophisticated understanding of essential concepts. This optional Appendix is for those who want to learn more.

The Appendix contains twelve short presentations, or "topics." Each explores one area of special interest, usually a new aspect of a subject already presented in the text. These topics are not intended to be exhaustive but are written to help the reader go "one level deeper." Aspiring specialists in areas such as nephrology, critical care, and emergency medicine will find some of the topics of particular relevance.

The topics can be read in any order, depending on one's interest; there is no need to read Topic A before Topic B. However, all the topics presume that the reader has mastered corresponding material in the text. For example, Topic D, which deals with diagnosis, presupposes a thorough understanding of the Diagnosis section. Finally, for those readers who wish to explore still further, citations are listed in the bibliography.

List of Topics

A. Acid-base chemistry

This topic is designed for readers who want to deepen their understanding of acid-base chemistry. For example, it explores the meaning of K and the mathematical basis of the Henderson-Hasselbalch equation. It also discusses the role of carbon dioxide as an acid.

B. Shunting, recycling, and multiplication of renal ammonium

During ammonium excretion, NH_4^+ is secreted into the proximal tubule. It is natural to assume that this NH_4^+ stays in the lumen and is carried down the entire length of the nephron by the flow of tubular fluid. Although some NH_4^+ does just this, most takes a circuitous route. Our goal here is to map this circuitous route and to describe what benefits might result.

C. Estimating endogenous acid production

Estimating how much strong acid the body produces is specialized work, but the underlying principles have broad clinical relevance. Studying these principles can, for example, help the clinician better understand what happens when a ketoacidosis patient spills ketones in the urine.

D. Simultaneous analysis of the anion gap and plasma [HCO_3^-]

You can gain rich diagnostic information from the venous electrolyte report by studying the relationship between [HCO_3^-] and the anion gap. In this topic, we describe the approach in detail. In addition, we explore the possibility that the anion gap's normal range is not really 8–16.

E. Mixed disturbances in depth

This topic explores the subject of mixed acid-base disturbances. We investigate general concepts, common clinical examples, blood gas profiles, and principles of treatment. To get the most from this discussion, read Topic D first. A27

F. Additional comments on the blood gas report

This presentation is designed to increase the clinician's facility with blood gases. For example, it shows how to check blood gas reports for "internal errors," and presents five clinically useful generalizations about normal compensation. A35

G. Is compensation really compensatory?

The secondary changes in PCO_2 or $[HCO_3^-]$ that occur with simple acid-base disturbance are widely assumed to be beneficial. However, this view may be only partly correct. A39

H. Laboratory diagnosis of intoxicant-induced metabolic acidosis

This topic is designed to help clinicians more effectively use the hospital laboratory to diagnose or rule out toxic ingestion as a cause of metabolic acidosis. It discusses a number of specific assays, and explores the importance and limitations of the osmolar gap. A41

I. More on renal tubular acidosis

This topic is designed for readers who wish to deepen their understanding of RTA. For example, it explains RTA nomenclature in detail and gives a step-by-step diagnostic approach for differentiating the various Types and subtypes. A49

J. Urinary anion gap

The urinary anion gap can help the clinician gauge the adequacy of renal ammonium excretion. This information is useful in differentiating a number of disorders. To get the most from this discussion, read Topic I first. ... A57

K. Rare causes of acid-base disturbances

This topic describes some uncommon causes of metabolic acidosis and alkalosis. The topic also briefly introduces the diagnosis of volume-resistant metabolic alkalosis. A61

L. Local anesthesia in arteriopuncture

Arteriopuncture for blood gas analysis may cause patients significant pain and anxiety. Using a local anesthetic can reduce both. This topic discusses two anesthetic approaches that may be useful. A65

Topic A

Acid-Base Chemistry

This topic is intended for readers who wish to deepen their understanding of acid-base chemistry. It focuses on four areas not explored in detail in the text. We start with . . .

What determines acidic strength?

Acidic strength is determined by the relative stabilities of the associated and dissociated forms of the acid. Structures that are relatively stable (i.e., that have low free energy) in their unprotonated form tend to dissociate; they are strong acids. Structures that are relatively stable in their protonated form tend to exist protonated; they are weak acids.

What determines relative structural stability? A highly stable conjugate base (and hence a strong acid) is caused by one of two things: a complete outer electron shell or the effective dispersion of the negative charge over several atoms. For example, hydrochloric acid, HCl, is a strong acid because the electron left behind by the dissociating proton completes chloride's outer shell (in this case, eight electrons). In sulfuric acid, H_2SO_4, charge dispersion is most important. When the first proton dissociates, the negative charge is well dispersed by the four highly electronegative oxygen atoms bound to the central sulfur. (There is a lesser tendency for the second proton to dissociate because two negative charges must be dispersed.) Similarly, organic acids are good proton donors because the oxygen atoms in the carboxylate anion (COO^-) disperse the charge; they do not, however, do so as effectively as the more plentiful oxygens in sulfuric acid. Thus, organic acids are weaker than sulfuric acid.

Mathematical derivation of pK and Henderson-Hasselbalch

Because most students initially study pK and the Henderson-Hasselbalch equation using a mathematical derivation, we present this derivation here and emphasize its basis in the fundamental concepts discussed in the main text.

The "p" in pK is the same "p" as in pH. It indicates a reverse logarithmic transformation on the value that follows. In pH, we know that H represents $[H^+]$. What is K? Just as $[H^+]$ and pH both describe free proton concentration, so do K and pK both describe acidic strength. However, unlike pK, which is inverse and logarithmic, K is direct and linear. Thus, a strong acid has a high K and a weak acid has a low K. K is called the "dissociation constant," which is defined formally like this:

$$K = [H^+][A^-]/[HA]$$

Notice that the denominator consists of the concentration, at equilibrium, of the undissociated acid in a solution, and the numerator consists of the product of the equilibrium concentrations of the acid's dissociated ions. K thus gives a measure of an acid's tendency to dissociate when dissolved. For example, if we dissolve two moles of HA in one liter of water, and half of the acid (i.e., one mole) dissociates, the dissociation constant will look like this:

$$K = 1 \text{ molar} \times 1 \text{ molar} / 1 \text{ molar}$$

K for this acid is thus equal to $(1 \text{ molar})^2/1$ molar, or simply 1 molar. Note that K, like $[H^+]$, is discussed in units of concentration. In contrast, both pK and pH are dimensionless, because they are the negatives of the exponent of, respectively, K and $[H^+]$.

To see more clearly why K changes with acidic strength, consider a strong acid. When dissolved in solution, the equilibrium [HA] will be relatively low. Conversely, the concentrations of H^+ and A^- will be relatively high. Therefore, K for a strong acid can be schematized like this:

$$K = [H^+][A^-]/[HA] = [high][high]/[low] = high/low = \text{very high}$$

This qualitative equation shows that K for a strong acid will be relatively high. Conversely, K for a weak acid can be represented thus:

$$K = [H^+][A^-]/[HA] = [low][low]/[high] = low/high = \text{very low}$$

To better understand these two schematic equations, you may find it useful to derive K for two acids of different strengths. For each acid, assume a total concentration of 1 mole per liter. For the stronger acid, assume a 90% dissociation (i.e., $[H^+]$ and $[A^-]$ = 0.9 mol/l, [HA] = 0.1 mol/l). For the weaker acid, assume a 10% dissociation (i.e., [HA] = 0.9 mol/l, etc.). Use these data to calculate K.*

The Henderson-Hasselbalch equation is derived by rearranging the expression for K, like this:

$$[H^+] = K[HA]/[A^-]$$

and taking the negative log (the "p") of both sides:

$$pH = pK + \log [A^-]/[HA]$$

---

* **Answers.** To check your answers: the correct values for K differ by approximately a factor of 729.

"Alpha" vs. K

"Alpha" (α) indicates the fraction of dissolved acid that is dissociated. It is defined mathematically like this:

$$\alpha = [A^-]/([HA] + [A^-])$$

Note that the numerator consists of the dissociated form of the acid, whereas the denominator consists of the total amount of dissolved acid (i.e., both the undissociated and dissociated forms). Strong acids tend to have high alpha values and weak acids tend to have low alpha values. In this respect, alpha is similar to K. This similarity might lead one to ask why alpha is not used instead of K to quantify acidic strength.

The answer is that unlike K, which describes the *inherent* stability of the associated versus dissociated forms of the acid, and hence is constant no matter what the concentration of the acid in solution, the value of alpha increases as the concentration of the acid decreases. Alpha thus tells us much about the state of an acid at a particular moment but little about the acid's inherent qualities. In fact, two acids with different inherent strengths, and hence different K (and pK) values, can have the same alpha values, as long as their concentrations are sufficiently different.

To understand this distinction better, imagine an experiment in which we add an acid whose K is 1 molar to a one-liter beaker of water. If we add 2 moles of acid, we find that $[H^+]$, $[A^-]$, and $[HA]$ all equal 1 molar (because K = 1 molar = [1 molar H^+] $\times$ [1 molar A^-]/[1 molar HA]). Using these values, we find that alpha = 1/2, or 50%. If we add 4 more moles of the same acid, so the total amount is 6 moles, we find that $[H^+]$ and $[A^-]$ = 2 molar, and [HA] = 4 molar (because K = 1 molar = [2 molar H^+] $\times$ [2 molar A^-]/[4 molar HA]). Using these values, we find that alpha is 1/3, or 33%. This "experiment" shows that alpha falls as more acid is added to the solution.*

Carbon dioxide and carbonic acid

We conclude with a few comments about CO_2 and H_2CO_3 in the bicarbonate buffer system. In the text (p. 7), we discuss two ways to define "acid": as a proton donor and as a substance that can raise a solution's $[H^+]$. When discussing the acidic role of CO_2 in body fluids, the latter definition is more generally applicable because, in the carbonic-anhydrase catalyzed reaction of CO_2 and H_2O, acidification takes place without CO_2 itself donating a proton. (Recall that in the catalyzed reaction, the predominant reaction route does not involve the formation of H_2CO_3; p. 45.)

---

* **Technical information.** However, K is constant only with respect to concentration. K does vary somewhat with the temperature of the solution.

Until fairly recently, it was thought that both the catalyzed and uncatalyzed reactions had the same reaction route, with carbonic anhydrase facilitating the formation of H_2CO_3. This mechanistic misunderstanding explains how the enzyme got its name: carbonic anhydrase means "the enzyme that removes water from carbonic acid" (carbonic = carbonic acid, an = without, hydr = water). Remember that enzymes catalyze equilibrium reactions in both directions. Thus, while the name describes the dehydration of H_2CO_3, it applies equally to the hydration of CO_2.

Before the correct reaction route was discovered, the bicarbonate buffer's conjugate acid was usually said to be H_2CO_3, with CO_2 viewed as a precursor. Once the correct catalysis route (i.e., the direct carboxylation of carbon dioxide) became known, those who worry about names found themselves in a quandary. Since carbonic acid is not present in the predominant catalyzed route, it is incorrect to discuss it at all. The alternative, to designate carbon dioxide as the conjugate acid, is not strictly correct, since CO_2 does not itself donate protons, as is required by the definition of the term conjugate acid. In this text, we have erred on the side of "true substance and false name" and focused on carbon dioxide as the conjugate acid.

It is sometimes said, mistakenly, that it is H_2CO_3, not CO_2, that has a pK of 6.1 and a concentration of 1.2 mmol/l. The actual pK of H_2CO_3 at 37°C is about 3.5 and, in health, plasma $[H_2CO_3]$ is around 0.003 mmol/l. In the uncatalyzed reaction, H_2CO_3 is in equilibrium with dissolved CO_2 (see equation p. 45), which pulls the equilibrium point for the H_2CO_3 dissociation to the left (i.e., decreasing the proton-donating potential). This leftward equilibrium shift explains why the net effective pK for the uncatalyzed reaction is 6.1, just as it is for the catalyzed reaction, even though the pK for carbonic acid is much lower.

Finally, note that carbonic acid is sometimes called a "volatile acid" because it can liberate CO_2 (one meaning of *volatile* is "tending to become gaseous"), whereas all other acids are called non-volatile (or "fixed") acids. In fact, some writers refer to CO_2 itself as a volatile acid. Because of this volatility, the bicarbonate buffer is sometimes called the "volatile buffer" whereas non-bicarbonate buffers are sometimes called "non-volatile buffers."

Topic B

Shunting, Recycling, and Multiplication of Renal Ammonium

During ammonium excretion, NH_4^+ is secreted into the proximal tubule. It is natural to assume that this NH_4^+ stays in the lumen and is carried down the entire length of the nephron by the flow of tubular fluid. Although some NH_4^+ does just this, most takes a circuitous route. Our goal here is to map this circuitous route, and to describe what benefits might result. Begin by scanning the following schematic. Then, as you read the text that follows, refer back to the schematic for visual reference:

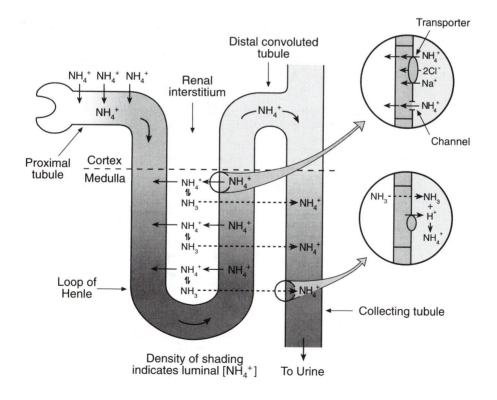

First, notice that proximally secreted NH_4^+ remains in the lumen until it arrives at the ascending limb of Henle's loop. There, much NH_4^+ is reabsorbed and enters the renal interstitium. Reabsorption is thought to occur via two main mechanisms. Most apparently occurs by an $Na^+–K^+–2Cl^-$ cotransporter, with ammonium substituting for K^+. A lesser amount apparently passes through K^+ channels. The presumed substitution of NH_4^+ for K^+ in these mechanisms is chemically plausible; both species are small, monovalent cations. In addition, notice that some NH_4^+ is not reabsorbed, but remains in the lumen.

Second, notice that reabsorbed NH_4^+ reenters the *descending* limb of Henle's loop. This reentry probably occurs by a combination of diffusion and active transport. Once back in the lumen, NH_4^+ again travels downstream, back to the ascending limb, where much is again reabsorbed. A repeating loop is created, as NH_4^+ passes from ascending limb, to descending limb, to ascending limb, etc.

Third, interstitial NH_4^+, like all NH_4^+, participates in the equilibrium reaction $NH_4^+ \rightleftharpoons NH_3 + H^+$. Some of the NH_3, being relatively non-polar, diffuses through the interstitium, across the cells of the collecting tubule, and into the collecting tubule lumen. There, NH_3 combines with protons secreted by the $H^+–ATPase$ (and $H^+–K^+–ATPase$), reforming NH_4^+. Note that these H^+ pumps are the same ones involved in distal bicarbonate reabsorption and titrable acid formation.*

Fourth, the density of gray shading in the lumen indicates luminal $[NH_4^+]$. Notice that the pattern of shading indicates all of the following: $[NH_4^+]$ rises in the descending limb due to the entrance of NH_4^+; $[NH_4^+]$ falls in the ascending limb due to the removal of NH_4^+; $[NH_4^+]$ in the distal convoluted tubule is lower than at the end of the proximal tubule, again due to the reabsorption of NH_4^+ in the ascending limb; $[NH_4^+]$ rises along the length of the collecting tubule, as NH_3 enters and is protonated.

The final passage of NH_3 from the renal interstitium into the collecting tubule depends on a "downhill" diffusion gradient. The steeper the gradient, the more efficient the passage of NH_3. A steep gradient can be created by two conditions: a low $[NH_3]$ in the collecting tubule lumen and/or a high $[NH_3]$ in the interstitium. In fact, both these conditions are present. In the lumen, proton secretion lowers pH, which pushes the $NH_3 + H^+ \rightleftharpoons NH_4^+$ equilibrium to the right, reducing $[NH_3]$. In the interstitium, $[NH_3]$ rises because the repeated passage of NH_4^+ from ascending to descending limb

---

* **Terminology.** The diffusive passage of NH_3 from tubular cell into the nephron lumen is referred to as either non-ionic diffusion, so-called because NH_3 is the non-ionic form of the NH_3-NH_4^+ pair, or as diffusion-trapping, so-called because NH_3 diffuses into the lumen and is "trapped" there when it is converted by protonation into the less permeant ionic form. In fact, although not illustrated, this diffusive mechanism of ammonium transport occurs in the proximal tubule as well, along side of $Na^+–NH_4^+$ exchange.

raises interstitial $[NH_4^+]$. Since NH_3 and NH_4^+ are in equilibrium, interstitial $[NH_3]$ rises as well.

The terms shunting, recycling, and counter-current multiplication are used to emphasize different aspects of the integrated process that we have just described. "Shunting" focuses attention on the fact that ammonium passes directly from the loop of Henle into the collecting tubule, without passing through the distal convoluted tubule (i.e., it is "shunted" across the medulla). "Recycling" emphasizes the fact that ammonium undergoes a repeating cycle of reabsorption and secretion in the loop of Henle. "Counter-current multiplication" emphasizes the fact that $[NH_4^+]$ in the lumen of Henle's loop (as well as $[NH_4^+]$ and $[NH_3]$ in the renal interstitium) rises as a result of transport between the anti-directional streams of the ascending and descending limbs.

At this point, having grasped the mechanistic minutiae, you may reasonably wonder, *What is the point of all this activity?* Put differently: What are the advantages of the above system over a simple system in which proximally secreted NH_4^+ stays in the lumen all the way to the collecting tubule? Three advantages have been proposed:

1. The rate of collecting tubule proton secretion, which affects luminal pH in the collecting tubule, can be regulated. Since a fall in pH lowers luminal $[NH_3]$ and thus increases the interstitium-to-lumen gradient for NH_3 diffusion, augmented proton secretion tends to increase NH_4^+ excretion. Thus, by regulating luminal pH, the kidney may gain a means of regulating ammonium excretion that is independent of the rate of ammonium production by the proximal tubule. Importantly, since distal proton secretion also affects the rate of distal bicarbonate reabsorption and titrable acid formation, the regulation of distal proton secretion may provide a simple, common regulatory mechanism for all three components of net acid excretion. For example, increased collecting tubule proton secretion can simultaneously raise urinary $[NH_4^+]$ and [titrable acid], and lower urinary $[HCO_3^-]$.

2. The rate of ammonium reabsorption by the ascending limb of Henle's loop may be under renal control. Variations in reabsorptive rate would affect interstitial $[NH_3]$ and, in turn, the rate of diffusion into the collecting tubule. For example, increased loop reabsorption would raise interstitial $[NH_3]$, speeding diffusion and raising urinary excretion of NH_4^+. It is thus possible that loop reabsorption and recycling provides yet another means of regulating NH_4^+ excretion that is independent of the rate of proximal NH_4^+ production ("production-independent regulation").

The regulation of ammonium recycling in Henle's loop may be especially important when the kidney retains free water. The removal of water from the collecting tubule, under the influence of ADH, raises the concentration of all solvents that remain in the lumen, including NH_3. High luminal $[NH_3]$ promotes diffusion of NH_3 *out* of the lumen, slowing ammonium excretion. Thus, one might expect ammonium excretion to fall as urine concentration rises. However, it appears that, when urine concentration rises, the kidney may increase loop ammonium reabsorption and hence raise interstitial $[NH_3]$. The increase in interstitial $[NH_3]$ apparently offsets the rise in the luminal $[NH_3]$, thereby allowing interstitium-to-lumen NH_3 diffusion, and hence ammonium excretion, to continue apace. Thus, through its modulation of loop ammonium reabsorption, the kidney retains control of the NH_3 diffusion gradient, and hence ammonium excretion, in spite of changes in urine osmolarity. Put differently, loop reabsorption and recycling makes possible the independent regulation of urine osmolarity and ammonium excretion.

3. The cells of the distal convoluted tubule (DCT) may be somewhat permeable to NH_3 and, to a lesser extent, NH_4^+. Thus, some NH_3 and NH_4^+ can diffuse out of the DCT lumen and enter the blood that is flowing through the peritubular capillaries. This diffusion is especially likely to occur because DCT luminal pH is relatively high (it is substantially higher than pH at the end of the collecting tubule). The high pH keeps the luminal $NH_3 + H^+ \rightleftharpoons NH_4^+$ equilibrium shifted relatively far to the left, raising the concentration of the more permeant species, NH_3. In addition, the rate of blood flow in the renal cortex, where the DCT is located, is high. This high rate of blood flow acts to lower the $[NH_3]$ and $[NH_4^+]$ of peritubular blood by rapidly carrying away, and hence preventing the accumulation of, any NH_3 and NH_4^+ that enters the capillary. The result is a steep lumen-to-blood gradient, which favors the diffusion of NH_4^+ and, especially, NH_3, from the DCT lumen into the capillaries. If loop reabsorption of ammonium did not occur, $[NH_3]$ and $[NH_4^+]$ in the DCT would be relatively high, which might lead to significant diffusion losses to blood, thus decreasing ammonium excretion.

It may be surprising to hear that, even with medullary shunting, which partially bypasses the DCT, about half of all NH_4^+ ultimately enters the blood and is converted to urea. Much of this loss may occur in the proximal tubule, where ammonium is produced. Thus, about half of all NH_4^+ production, and half of all bicarbonate regeneration, is futile. This may sound terribly wasteful, but when you compare the efficiency with that of the internal combustion engine powering your car, which is about 27% (most of the rest is lost to heat), it doesn't seem so bad.*

What's more, when bicarbonate regeneration must increase, the efficiency of NH_4^+ excretion can apparently rise to about 75%. This rise may be partly due to increases in loop NH_4^+ reabsorption and collecting tubule proton secretion.

---

* **Technical information.** Futile NH_4^+ production does not affect the accuracy of the NAE calculation (p. 104) in assessing net bicarbonate regeneration because the nitrogenous end product, which appears in the urine, is urea, not NH_4^+.

Since these mechanisms can increase ammonium excretion only if some NH_4^+ production is normally futile (if all proximally produced ammonium already appeared in the urine, a steeper NH_3 diffusion gradient could not possibly raise NH_4^+ excretion), it may be that the baseline "inefficiency" in ammonium excretion is actually an essential system component, a necessary prerequisite for production-independent regulation of NH_4^+ excretion. Since raising NH_4^+ production requires enzyme induction and/or deinduction, which are slow processes, production-independent regulation may be important when rapid bicarbonate regeneration is necessary. It is even possible that rises in ammonium excretion are generally biphasic: first, excretory efficiency increases; second, ammonium production gradually rises. This possibility is speculative.

Topic C

Estimating Endogenous Acid Production

This topic describes approaches used to quantify endogenous acid production (EAP). The principles that underlie these approaches have broad clinical relevance. Studying them can, for example, help the clinician better understand the significance of phenomena such as the urinary spillage of organic anions during ketoacidosis. In our discussion, we presume a thorough familiarity with Chapter 10, *Endogenous Acid Production*.

Many bodily processes are difficult to observe directly and are therefore studied using a "black box" approach, i.e., by analyzing the body's input and/or output and inferring what occurs inside. The three main methods that have been advocated for estimating EAP are based on this approach. They are: dietary analysis, urinary analysis, and combined dietary-urinary-fecal analysis.

Dietary ash acidity

This approach attempts to infer EAP from diet composition (i.e., from the input to the "black box"). This technique has three steps: (1) a food sample is burned by flame or oven, (2) the ash and evolved gas are collected and dissolved in pure water, and (3) the resulting solution (which is usually acidic) is titrated with strong base to body pH, usually assumed to be 7.4. The amount of strong base needed for the titration is said to represent ash acidity. For example, if 30 mmol of NaOH is needed, the food sample's ash acidity is said to be 30 meq; and it is assumed that this sample would liberate 30 meq acid if oxidized *in vivo*. If the initial pH of the ash solution is above 7.4, the titration is done with strong acid, and the diet is said to be net ash alkaline (often notated as a negative value for ash acidity); such a sample is assumed to produce net bicarbonate *in vivo*. Note that this approach is based on the idea that oxidation of a substrate will produce the same products whether it occurs *in vitro* by burning or *in vivo* by enzymatic catalysis.

A variant of this technique attempts to quantify acidic potential by chemical analysis, instead of burning. It is assumed that all acidity or alkalinity comes from three dietary sources: sulfur (S), organic cations (OC), and organic anions (OA). When fully oxidized, S liberates 2 protons, and organic ions consume or liberate equivalent quantities of protons. Thus, the acid-base effect of a fully oxidized diet should equal $2S + OC - OA$ (note: in this discussion, S is in moles; ions are in equivalents).

Although S can be quantified fairly simply, the many types of OA and OC can make their direct determination difficult. In contrast, the *inorganic* ions can be quantified fairly easily. Thus, an indirect technique, analogous to the plasma anion gap, is used. Because (1) all ions are either organic or inorganic and (2) the law of electroneutrality applies to food, it can be assumed that an excess of inorganic cations over inorganic anions in a food sample exactly quantifies an excess of organic anions over organic cations. In food, the major inorganic ions are Cl^-, phosphate (P^-), Na^+, K^+, Ca^{2+}, and Mg^{2+}. Therefore:

Food organic anion gap $= (Na^+ + K^+ + Ca^{2+} + Mg^{2+}) - (P^- + Cl^-)$

This gap quantifies the excess of OA over OC in food, and hence the net consumption of protons due to excess organic anions in food, assuming complete oxidation of the food. (If OC exceeds OA, which is unusual in non-artificial diets, the OA gap will be negative). Taking S into account, we can say that

Dietary ash acidity $= 2S - (Na^+ + K^+ + Ca^{2+} + Mg^{2+}) + (Cl^- + P^-)$*

How useful is this approach in quantifying EAP? First, the approach does not consider gastrointestinal sources of acid (i.e., GAP), only metabolic (i.e., MAP). Second, the approach assumes that *in vivo* and *in vitro* oxidation are equally complete. In reality, they are not, for several reasons: (1) not all ingested S or OA is absorbed from the gut; some is excreted in stool, (2) some absorbed S (perhaps about 30%) is not converted to sulfate, and this fraction's proton-donating potential is difficult to determine, (3) even in health, a fraction of the ingested neutral substrates is not fully oxidized but is metabolized to organic acids, and (4) humans lack enzymes for the efficient metabolism of certain organic ions (e.g., tartrate). Notwithstanding these shortcomings, it is generally assumed that ash acidity values can be used to compare the *relative* acidogenic potential of different diets, although not to quantify EAP in absolute terms.

Urinary analysis

This approach attempts to infer EAP from urine composition (i.e., one of the outputs of the "black box"). The only direct markers of EAP in urine are OA and sulfate (SO_4^{2-}), which indicate, respectively, endogenous organic acid

---

* **Technical information.** The value of the negative charge on phosphate, a weak acid, varies with ambient pH. Thus, calculating $[P^-]$ in equivalents requires that the food's pH be known. To simplify matters, it is commonly assumed, albeit without much basis, that the average negative charge on phosphate is 1.8, which is what it would be if the food's pH were 7.4, the same as that of blood plasma (vampires take note!). Incorporating this assumption, the formula for ash acidity is often written as follows: $2S - (Na^+ + K^+ + Ca^{2+} + Mg^{2+}) + (Cl^- + 1.8P^-)$, with S and P^- expressed in moles and the other species expressed in equivalents.

production and proton liberation from S metabolism. (Urinary NH_4^+ and titratable acid are not counted because they are considered markers of the renal *response* to EAP.) Thus, this approach quantifies EAP as

$$\text{Urinary } SO_4^{2-} + OA$$

Thus, if urine SO_4^{2-} = 30 meq and urine OA = 15 meq, MAP during the time that the urine was produced is said to be 45 meq. The strength of this approach is that MAP due to metabolic conversion of S to SO_4^{2-} is accurately measured; urinalysis shows the actual products of the proton-liberating reaction (note: only minute quantities of sulfate are excreted in stool). Furthermore, this approach attempts to quantify production of organic acids from the incomplete oxidation of neutral substrates, a process not assessed by ash acidity. However, the approach does not account for the often substantial quantity of net OA in diet, whose metabolism to bicarbonate leaves no urinary markers. GAP is again not considered.

A simple alternative to this approach has been used for patients who are in steady state for bicarbonate (indicated by a stable plasma $[HCO_3^-]$ and no substantial urinary Ca^{2+}, a marker for bone buffering). In this approach, one simply quantitates urinary net acid excretion (NAE) and assumes it is equal to EAP.

Diet-urine-stool analysis

This approach is more complex; it takes into account the input and both major outputs of the "black box." First, to assess complete oxidation of S and incomplete oxidation of neutral substrates, it incorporates both components of the urine-only approach (i.e., urine SO_4^{2-} + OA). Second, to assess the effect of net OA in diet, it incorporates the food organic anion gap. Third, to correct for dietary OA that is not absorbed (and hence cannot be metabolized), it quantifies net fecal OA by determining a *stool* organic anion gap (using the same inorganic ions measured in the food gap) and subtracts this value from the food OA gap. According to this approach,

$$EAP = \text{Urinary } (SO_4^{2-} + OA) - (\text{Food OA gap} - \text{Stool OA gap})$$

Example: If urine SO_4^{2-} = 40 meq, urine OA = 10 meq, food OA gap = 20 meq, and stool OA gap = 10 meq, estimated EAP is 40 meq.

The most confusing part of this calculation involves the offsetting effects of OA in food, stool, and urine. To better understand these offsetting effects, notice that the three OA terms can be rearranged as

$$(\text{OA urine} + \text{OA stool}) - (\text{OA food})$$

which is essentially (OA output) − (OA input). In the example just cited, the total of 20 meq OA excreted in urine and stool is equal to the 20 meq OA ingested in food. Since OA input exactly equals OA output, OA cancels from the equation. That is, it is assumed that OA output does not indicate organic acid production from neutral precursors but simply represents food OA, half of which is absorbed and excreted unmetabolized in the urine and half of which is unabsorbed and thus appears in the stool. Therefore, in this example, EAP is assumed to be quantitatively equal to SO_4^{2-} excretion, or 40 meq. Because the stool gap quantifies not only unabsorbed OA but also stool bicarbonate and OA of bacterial origin (which are markers of gut net bicarbonate secretion), this approach is said to quantify GAP as well as MAP.*

---

* **Caveat.** A full discussion of potential inaccuracies in the described approaches is beyond the scope of this text. Thus, this topic is intended to clarify principles, not advocate specific methods.

Topic D

Simultaneous Analysis of the Anion Gap and Plasma [HCO₃⁻]

This topic, which presumes a firm grasp of the diagnosis section of the text, focuses on the diagnosis of patients who have an elevated anion gap. Our major aim is to learn to fully evaluate the anion gap in the context of the venous bicarbonate level (i.e., Total CO_2). For example, an elevated gap accompanied by a low $[HCO_3^-]$ immediately suggests an anion gap metabolic acidosis. But what if the gap is markedly elevated but $[HCO_3^-]$ is normal or high? We have touched on these questions in the text (e.g., problem no. 3 on p. 237); here we consider them systematically. Specifically, we look at the meaning of an elevated anion gap in the three possible ranges of plasma $[HCO_3^-]$: normal, high, and low. We end our discussion with a few comments on unusual causes of an elevated gap, and on the normal range of the gap.

Normal [HCO₃⁻]

The combination of a markedly elevated anion gap and a normal plasma bicarbonate level is easy to interpret: the patient has a mixed disturbance consisting of an anion gap metabolic acidosis and a second disorder that acts to raise $[HCO_3^-]$. The two disorders that can raise plasma $[HCO_3^-]$ are metabolic alkalosis and compensated respiratory acidosis.

For example, following a drinking-vomiting binge, an alcoholic may present with ketoacidosis and metabolic alkalosis (from vomiting). If bicarbonate consumption and production from these processes are evenly matched, plasma $[HCO_3^-]$ will be normal. However, the anion gap remains elevated because metabolic alkalosis does not eliminate unmeasured anions; in fact, it may reduce ECF volume, slowing renal excretion of ketoanions and thus keeping the anion gap high. Similarly, if a patient with chronic (compensated) hypercapnia (e.g., from COPD) ingests methanol, the anion gap metabolic acidosis may consume the excess bicarbonate, lowering plasma $[HCO_3^-]$ to normal.

These mixed disorders have two components: one lowering and one raising plasma $[HCO_3^-]$. These components do not have to be matched. If the acidosis predominates, $[HCO_3^-]$ will be low; if the bicarbonate-raising process predominates, $[HCO_3^-]$ will be high. Thus, a patient might have an anion gap of, for example, 29 and an $[HCO_3^-]$ of (to give a few possibilities) 24, 16, or 35 mmol/l. In all cases, however, $[HCO_3^-]$ is higher than it would have been if the bicarbonate-raising process were not present.

High $[HCO_3^-]$

Because an elevated anion gap typically presents with a low plasma $[HCO_3^-]$, a markedly elevated gap with a high $[HCO_3^-]$ may seem like a self-contradiction, a clinical oxymoron. However, as described, this combination results when a gap acidosis is accompanied by a bicarbonate-raising process, with the latter process predominating.

When $[HCO_3^-]$ is normal or high, an elevated anion gap may be the only laboratory marker of metabolic acidosis. For example, if metabolic acidosis and alkalosis are evenly matched, pH, PCO_2, and $[HCO_3^-]$ will all be normal. However, if the metabolic acidosis is of the anion gap variety, the anion gap will be elevated. Such a telltale anion gap is sometimes referred to as a "footprint of metabolic acidosis," by analogy to tracks left in snow or mud. Finding such a gap should always cause you to scrutinize the history carefully; it may lead you to get a blood gas as well. (Remember that hyperchloremic metabolic acidosis leaves no "footprint," so your suspicion of a mixed disturbance must be based on other factors.)

Traditionally, it was taught that an elevated anion gap accompanied by a high $[HCO_3^-]$ always indicates a hidden gap acidosis. It is now clear that simple metabolic *alkalosis* can itself elevate the gap, especially when the alkalosis is severe. The four mechanisms responsible, in roughly decreasing order of importance, are: (1) Anionic sites on plasma albumin normally account for over half of all unmeasured anions. Volume depletion, which usually accompanies metabolic alkalosis, concentrates plasma proteins and hence raises the anionic equivalence (i.e., the negative charge concentration) of plasma. (2) Anionic sites on plasma proteins act as buffers. With alkalemia, these buffers liberate protons, exposing additional anionic sites, again raising the anionic equivalence. (3) Cellular alkalinization stimulates mild lactic acid production; lactate raises the gap slightly. (4) Volume depletion may cause prerenal azotemia, which can slightly elevate plasma sulfate, phosphate, and other unmeasured anions.*

Thus, elevation of both $[HCO_3^-]$ and the gap suggests either (1) simple metabolic alkalosis, or (2) a mixed disturbance composed of a gap acidosis and either (a) metabolic alkalosis or (b) compensated respiratory acidosis. Although data are limited, it appears that simple metabolic alkalosis usually raises the gap only modestly: 4 or 5 meq/l above baseline may be average. Therefore, it is probably reasonable to say that gaps up to around 20 (assuming a baseline gap range of 8–16) can be attributed to either a mixed distur-

---

* **Technical information.** Mechanisms 2 and 3 also arise during acute *respiratory* alkalosis, which can raise the gap slightly, typically 2–3 meq above baseline.

bance or a simple, severe metabolic alkalosis, whereas gaps much exceeding 20 suggest a mixed disturbance.

Low [HCO$_3^-$]

Unlike in patients with a normal or high [HCO$_3^-$], an elevated gap in a hypobicarbonatemic patient is not anomalous; it is just what you expect with a simple gap acidosis. Although it seems that there is little else to say, there is actually much.

In patients with metabolic acidosis, it is traditional to calculate the size of the anion gap and then classify the presentation as either anion gap or hyperchloremic (non-gap). In addition, clinicians sometimes compare the elevation in the gap with the decrement in plasma [HCO$_3^-$]. This comparison is often made by calculating a ratio. For example, if the gap has risen by 10 meq/l and [HCO$_3^-$] has fallen by 10 mmol/l, then the ratio is:

$$\text{Rise in anion gap/Fall in [HCO}_3^-] = 10/10 = 1$$

Or, if the gap rises from 12 to 33 (an increase of 21) and bicarbonate falls from 24 to 10 (a decline of 14), the ratio looks like this:

$$\text{Rise in anion gap/Fall in [HCO}_3^-] = 21/14 = 1.5$$

As a shorthand, we can call this the "rise/fall" ratio, symbolized R/F. Thus, in this example, R/F = 1.5. As we will see in a moment, calculating the R/F ratio provides an additional, useful way to conceptualize patients with metabolic acidosis.*

It might seem that, in a patient with simple gap acidosis, R/F should always be 1. We usually think of the offending acid as entering the extracellular

---

* **Terminology.** This ratio is sometimes called the "delta/delta" (symbolized Δ/Δ), because delta is the Greek letter used to indicate a change in a variable. Thus, for the example just given, you would write Δ/Δ = 1.5 or say "delta delta is 1.5." However, the Δ/Δ terminology can lead to confusion. First, the symbol Δ, when used alone, indicates the actual value of the anion gap, but when used in the Δ/Δ, it refers to the change in the gap. Beginners sometimes miss this fact and put the absolute value of the gap in the numerator of the Δ/Δ. Second, the terminology does not indicate which Δ refers to the gap and which refers to bicarbonate, and the ratio is therefore sometimes mistakenly inverted, with the Δ gap placed in the denominator. Third, the symbol Δ indicates the magnitude of a change but it does not indicate direction. However, when calculating the Δ/Δ, the numerator Δ must refer to a positive change (increased gap) and the denominator Δ must refer to a negative change (decreased [HCO$_3^-$]). Beginners sometimes make the mistake of calculating Δ/Δ for hyperbicarbonatemic patients who have an elevated gap, using the increase in bicarbonate to calculate the denominator's Δ. All these problems can be avoided by using the "rise/fall" terminology, which automatically reminds you how to correctly calculate the ratio ("automatically," because everyone knows that, in gap acidosis, the gap rises and bicarbonate falls). Note that, when calculating the ratio, you must assume pre-acidosis values for both the gap and [HCO$_3^-$]. Unless baseline values are available, it is reasonable to use the midpoints of the lab's normal ranges.

fluid (ECF), where it deposits the anion and consumes an equivalent amount of bicarbonate. This buffering sequence does, in fact, lead to an R/F of 1. However, other processes that affect R/F also come into play. For instance, some H^+ are buffered by non-bicarbonate buffers (e.g., phosphate, plasma proteins) and some are buffered inside cells. These processes mitigate the fall in plasma $[HCO_3^-]$ and thus raise R/F. At the same time, some plasma unmeasured anions enter cells, mitigating the rise in the anion gap and therefore lowering R/F. Just as important, the kidney may regenerate new bicarbonate and excrete unmeasured anions in the urine. These renal processes, depending on their relative rates, can cause R/F to increase, decrease, or stay the same. Thus, R/F is determined by a constellation of factors that vary over time and from patient to patient. Nonetheless, the various factors often partially *cancel*, frequently resulting in an R/F close to 1. Therefore, as a rough approximation, it is often useful to think of the "normal" R/F ratio in simple gap acidosis as being around 1.

For patients with simple metabolic acidosis, the R/F ratio puts "gap acidosis" and "hyperchloremic acidosis" on a continuum, and tells you where on the continuum each patient falls. If R/F is less than 1, the acidosis is not purely anion gap *or* hyperchloremic, but a bit of both. For example, an R/F of 0.6 means that 60% of lost plasma bicarbonate has been replaced by unmeasured anions; the rest has been replaced by chloride. If R/F is exactly 1, then the acidosis is purely anion gap in nature, with lost plasma bicarbonate replaced, one for one, by unmeasured anions. If R/F is greater than 1, then the gap more than accounts for the fall in $[HCO_3^-]$. For example, an R/F of 1.8 means the patient has 80% more gap than might be expected based on the $[HCO_3^-]$. That is, all of the lost plasma bicarbonate, plus some plasma chloride, has been replaced by unmeasured anions. Such a patient has, in effect, more gap than acidosis.

Let's now use R/F to deepen our understanding of the five most common forms of metabolic acidosis: ketoacidosis, lactic acidosis, renal failure, diarrhea, and renal tubular acidosis.

1. Ketoacidosis

Ketoacidosis typically presents with a markedly elevated gap. The mean R/F is about 1, and the majority of patients fall within a few tenths of a point of this value. However, R/F may range from 0 (i.e., a pure hyperchloremic pattern) to around 2. Because the renal reabsorptive threshold for ketoanions is relatively low, virtually all ketoacidosis patients excrete a significant quantity of unmeasured anions in the urine. Thus, an R/F of 1 does not indicate complete retention of unmeasured anions, but only that the loss of anions has been balanced by other processes (especially by intracellular buffering, which mitigates the fall in plasma $[HCO_3^-]$).

An R/F much below 1 (e.g., R/F = 0.3) suggests that urinary ketoanion excretion may have been unusually rapid. A low R/F is especially likely when volume status and renal function are good, because these conditions pro-mote rapid anion spillage. Conversely, an R/F much above 1 (e.g., R/F = 1.8) suggests that normal urinary ketoanion excretion may have been slowed by renal impairment, which can be either functional (e.g., volume depletion secondary to osmotic diuresis) or due to intrinsic renal disease (e.g., diabetic nephropathy). Elevated BUN and creatinine levels will help clarify this possibility.

R/F can help predict how fast plasma [HCO_3^-] will normalize once insulin and volume are administered. A low R/F suggests that a large fraction of the ketoanions has been excreted and will thus be unavailable for metabolism to bicarbonate. A high R/F suggests the opposite. Because renal bicarbonate re-generation is relatively slow, a low R/F might reasonably reduce a clinician's threshold for giving bicarbonate (a low R/F would also be expected to min-imize the risk of overshoot alkalosis). In general, R/F will correlate with the size of the anion gap. Thus, a low R/F will usually be accompanied by a small gap and a high R/F will be accompanied by a large gap.*

2. Lactic acidosis

The renal reabsorptive threshold for lactate is relatively high. Thus, unlike in ketoacidosis, urinary organic anion excretion is minimal, and this keeps the gap, and R/F, relatively high. Although data are sparse, it is sometimes said that typical R/F values for lactic acidosis are around 1.7. Because anion spillage is low in all patients, an especially high R/F does not necessarily suggest impaired renal function.

3. Chronic renal failure (CRF)

Although "classically" described as producing an elevated anion gap, CRF sometimes presents with a gap that is only slightly elevated (resulting in a low R/F) or even normal. CRF involves two partially independent defects: (a) in the filtration and/or secretory functions responsible for eliminating ex-cess unmeasured anions, and (b) in ammonium excretion and associated bi-carbonate regeneration. If these defects appear together, the anion gap rises as [HCO_3^-] falls. However, if ammonium excretion deteriorates first, the gap may be normal or only slightly increased, even in severe acidosis. Re-

---

* **Clinical note.** During treatment of diabetic ketoacidosis, it is common to find that the anion gap normalizes before plasma [HCO_3^-] does; that is, the gap acidosis "converts" to a hyperchloremic pattern. There are two reasons why this conversion takes place. (1) Because some ketoanions have been lost in the urine, metabolism of circulating anions cannot replace all lost bicarbonate. This quantity of lost ketoanions thus represents a "post-metabolism bicarbonate deficit." If the rate of renal bicarbonate regeneration is not sufficient to replace this deficit by the time ketoanion metabolism is complete, then the gap will normalize while plasma [HCO_3^-] is still low. (2) Ketoacidosis patients are frequently given saline solutions, which are bicarbonate-free and essentially "hyper-chloremic"; these solutions dilute the unmeasured anions in body fluids.

cent data suggest that a pure hyperchloremic pattern may be relatively common, even in end-stage disease.

4. Diarrhea

Although diarrhea directly causes hyperchloremic acidosis, it sometimes presents with an elevated gap. This elevation can occur by one or more of the following mechanisms. First, anorexia, which may accompany diarrhea, can lead to mild starvation ketoacidosis. Second, volume depletion due to intestinal fluid losses can be so severe that lactic acidosis develops secondary to decreased tissue perfusion. Strictly speaking, these two mechanisms represent mixed metabolic acidoses (i.e., hyperchloremic from the diarrhea plus a gap organic acidosis), although, if mild, they are not likely to be recognized as such. Third, fluid loss with volume depletion can raise the anionic equivalence of plasma and also reduce GFR, which can slightly reduce unmeasured anion excretion (just as described above for metabolic alkalosis). Thus, in a patient with metabolic acidosis from diarrhea, an elevated anion gap may indicate the presence of one or more of the following: semi-starvation, volume depletion with or without hypovolemic shock, and renal impairment, either functional or intrinsic.

5. Renal tubular acidosis

Renal tubular acidosis presents with hyperchloremia, unless an unrelated defect is acting to raise the gap.

Summary

For three of the five most common causes of metabolic acidosis (i.e., ketoacidosis, CRF, diarrhea), no absolute distinction can be made between the anion gap and hyperchloremic presentations. Instead, a range of presentations exist for these conditions, with the anion gap and R/F deviating from their "expected" values based on volume status, renal function, the progression of therapy, and other factors. Thinking carefully about R/F and the size of the gap can give the clinician additional insight into a patient's condition. In addition, unusual R/F values can suggest a mixed disturbance, as we shall now see . . .

The R/F in mixed disturbances

We have seen that an elevated anion gap accompanied by a normal or high plasma $[HCO_3^-]$ often suggests a gap acidosis plus a process that raises $[HCO_3^-]$. Similarly, when $[HCO_3^-]$ is low but R/F is unusually high, a mixed disturbance involving a bicarbonate-raising process is likely. Thus, hypobicarbonatemic patients with unusually high R/F values are part of a continuum that also includes gap patients with normal or high $[HCO_3^-]$ values. The only difference is that in hypobicarbonatemic patients, the metabolic acidosis predominates.

For example, if a DKA patient has a high R/F, say 1.7, this may mean that volume depletion and/or intrinsic renal disease are inhibiting anion excretion, or it may mean that a bicarbonate-raising process is present. (Note that a rise in R/F can be caused by either an increase in the gap or a decrease in the fall in [HCO$_3^-$]). If R/F exceeds 2.0 in ketoacidosis, a mixed disturbance is nearly certain. In both DKA and alcoholic ketoacidosis, vomiting is the most common endogenous source of additional bicarbonate. Similarly, if a patient with metabolic alkalosis from gastric drainage develops lactic acidosis, the venous electrolyte assay may show a low [HCO$_3^-$] and an unusually high R/F.

Conversely, an R/F ratio that is *lower* than expected may suggest a gap acidosis plus a process that is acting to lower [HCO$_3^-$], specifically hyperchloremic metabolic acidosis or compensated respiratory alkalosis. For example, lactic acidosis tends to cause relatively high R/F values. Thus, in a patient with lactic acidosis, an R/F of, say, 0.5 may point to a mixed disturbance.

A caveat on applying the R/F concept. Data on typical R/F ranges, especially for conditions other than DKA, are extremely limited. For this reason, some experts believe that detailed R/F analysis, while a useful intellectual exercise, involves an over-extrapolation of data and yields pseudo-"information" that may not reflect what is actually happening in the patient. Given the limited data, it seems prudent to consider conclusions based on R/F analysis as tentative.

Other causes of abnormal anion gaps

In addition to acid-base disturbances, a number of relatively uncommon conditions can raise the anion gap. These include hyperalbuminemia due to either severe dehydration or albumin therapy; administration of exogenous anions, especially large doses of carbenicillin or penicillin; combined hypocalcemia, hypokalemia, and hypomagnesemia; and laboratory errors that result in the overestimation of [Na$^+$] or underestimation of [Cl$^-$] or [HCO$_3^-$]. With the exception of laboratory errors (which can be substantial), these conditions, like simple metabolic alkalosis, commonly raise the gap by only a few meq/l. Thus, a markedly elevated gap generally indicates an anion gap metabolic acidosis.

A different set of uncommon conditions can lower the gap. These conditions can cause abnormally low anion gaps. Rarely, the gap may even be negative. If the conditions occur in a patient with gap acidosis, they can suppress the expected elevation in the gap. These conditions include hypoalbuminemia*; ab-

---

* **Clinical note.** Hypoalbuminemic patients tend to have low baseline gaps. Thus, when calculating R/F in hypoalbuminemic patients, some authorities advocate that the assumed baseline gap value be reduced by 2.5 meq/l for each g/dl decrement in plasma albumin. Because of the low baseline gap, hypoalbuminemic patients (e.g., chronic alcoholics) who develop simple metabolic alkalosis will generally not present with supranormal gaps.

normally high concentrations of plasma cations other than Na^+, especially as seen in lithium overdose and IgG multiple myeloma; and laboratory errors, whether random or "systematic" (i.e., due to a predictable and identifiable cause), that result in the underestimation of $[Na^+]$ or overestimation of $[Cl^-]$ or $[HCO_3^-]$. Examples of systematic laboratory errors include the underestimation of $[Na^+]$ sometimes observed in patients with severe hypernatremia, hyperlipidemia, or hyperproteinemia; or the overestimation of $[Cl^-]$ that can occur with hyperlipidemia or with intoxication with bromide (e.g., overdose of pyridostigmine bromide) or iodine (e.g., absorbed topical Betadine, especially in patients with renal insufficiency).

What is the normal anion gap?

The most widely cited normal range for the anion gap, 8–16, was determined during the 1970s using the "autoanalyzer" machines then in widespread use. Many laboratories now use newer machines. Although the normal plasma level of unmeasured anions has not changed, these new machines (specifically, the popular ASTRA, made by Beckman) tend to produce a lower normal range for the anion gap, which can be as low as about 3–9 (6 ± 3) when calculated as $[Na^+] - ([Cl^-] + [HCO_3^-])$. It appears that the normal range is reduced mostly because the new machines tend to overestimate plasma $[Cl^-]$ (try this yourself; plug two different $[Cl^-]$ values into the gap formula; the higher value will give a lower gap). Some laboratories recalibrate the chloride electrode in a way that lowers reported $[Cl^-]$, which increases the normal range of the gap back toward the traditional 8–16, but other laboratories do not. Because of this variability, laboratories should always report the gap's normal range, as well as which anion gap formula (K-exclusive or K-inclusive; see footnote p. 230) was used in determining the range. Surprisingly, many laboratories do not provide this information. Note that no matter what the gap's normal range, increases in the gap have the same physiologic meaning. For example, a gap of 10 with a normal range of 3–9 and a gap of 17 with a normal range of 8–16 both indicate that the concentration of plasma unmeasured anions is 1 meq/l above the upper limit of normal.

Topic E

Mixed Disturbances in Depth

This topic has four parts: a conceptual introduction; a list of common mixed disturbances, with comments on their pathophysiology; a discussion of blood gas profiles; and information about aspects of treatment. These seemingly disparate subjects have actually been carefully selected to help the reader develop a deeper and more integrated understanding of mixed disturbances. Our discussion presumes a careful reading of the text sections on pathophysiology, diagnosis, and treatment (Chapters 14–29). In addition, readers may also find it useful to first read Appendix Topic D.

Conceptual introduction

As discussed in the main text (p. 127), mixed disturbances consist of a combination of two or more primary disturbances. For purposes of conceptualization and communication, it is convenient to subdivide mixed disturbances into four general groupings. These groups have no absolute significance (other categorization schemes are possible), but reading about these groups can help you better appreciate the range of combinations that are encountered clinically.

The four groups are: (1) combinations of the same type of primary disturbance, most commonly two different metabolic acidoses (e.g., keto- and lactic acidosis); (2) combinations of different types of primary disturbance (e.g., metabolic acidosis and respiratory alkalosis); (3) an acute (uncompensated) respiratory disturbance superimposed on a chronic (compensated) respiratory disturbance (e.g., a hypercapnic COPD patient with a superimposed acute elevation in PCO_2 due to a pulmonary infection)*; and (4) a predominant disorder for which adequate compensation fails to develop. Note that inadequate compensation can be conceptualized as a separate primary disorder in the compensatory system; thus, this last group can be said to represent a subset of group 2, above.

The primary disorders that compose a mixed disturbance may result from the same underlying condition (e.g., respiratory failure may cause both

---

* **Clinical note.** Because metabolic disturbances are rapidly compensated, the "acute-on-chronic" combination occurs only with respiratory disturbances.

respiratory acidosis and lactic acidosis secondary to hypoxemia) or from different underlying conditions (e.g., a patient with RTA develops respiratory acidosis from a traumatic pneumothorax). Sometimes a mixed disturbance involves three ("triple disturbance") or more primary disorders. However, it is uncommon that more than two of these disorders are clinically important, or that the third or fourth disorder can be diagnosed with assurance.

Some clinicians believe that the subject of mixed disturbances has been unduly emphasized. They note the following: (a) that most mixed disturbances involve a predominant disorder, (b) that this predominant disorder is generally the only one that requires specific therapy, and (c) that focusing on the mixed nature of the disturbance can lead to diagnostic hair-splitting, which distracts attention from the clinically important problem. To avoid this trap, get in the habit of asking yourself if focusing on the additional disturbance(s) will make a difference to the patient.

Common mixed disturbances

You are more likely to suspect, and hence detect, a mixed disturbance if you are familiar with the clinical conditions that are most commonly responsible. The following list describes these conditions. The pathophysiology of each component primary disorder is discussed in the Pathophysiology section, Chapters 16–19. Additional comments are offered here only when relevant information is not contained in those chapters.

Alcoholic patients

Following a sustained drinking-vomiting episode, alcoholic patients may present with a mixed metabolic acidosis (keto- or keto-lactic) and metabolic alkalosis (secondary to vomiting).

Asthma

Status asthmaticus can sometimes cause respiratory acidosis. A subset of these patients develop a superimposed lactic acidosis, primarily as a result of hypoxemia. In addition, patients may increase expiratory effort to overcome pathologically high airway resistance, which can raise intrathoracic pressures during expiration. This increased pressure can inhibit cardiac filling, reduce cardiac output, and thereby diminish tissue perfusion.

Cardiac arrest

All cardiac arrest victims experience at least a degree of lactic (metabolic) acidosis secondary to tissue hypoperfusion. A simultaneous respiratory acidosis due to ventilatory standstill is also present; it may persist due to inadequate mechanical or mouth-to-mouth ventilation. In addition, diminished circulation can hinder removal of CO_2 from the tissues, raising intracellular

PCO_2 even when ventilation is adequate. This cellular hypercapnia will not elevate arterial PCO_2 because, if artificial ventilation is adequate, the lung will normalize the PCO_2 of the reduced quantity of blood that passes through it (in some cases, rapid ventilation may even produce arterial hypocapnia; i.e., respiratory alkalosis). However, the PCO_2 of mixed venous blood samples will be elevated.

COPD patients treated with diuretics, theophylline, or steroids

These medications can all cause metabolic alkalosis. In a hypercapnic COPD patient, this alkalosis is superimposed on respiratory acidosis. Diuretics are often used to treat COPD-associated cor pulmonale or peripheral edema. Theophylline is sometimes used to reduce pulmonary air resistance; it can induce nausea and vomiting, especially when plasma levels exceed the pharmacologic range. Glucocorticoids, which have some mineralocorticoid (aldosterone-like) activity, are sometimes used for their anti-inflammatory effect on the lung.

COPD patients with an acute respiratory disturbance

COPD patients with stable, compensated hypercapnia may experience acute changes in PCO_2, yielding an acute (uncompensated) respiratory acidosis or alkalosis superimposed on a chronic (compensated) respiratory acidosis. Acute elevations in PCO_2 are most frequently caused by pulmonary infection. Acute reductions in PCO_2 can occur if the patient decompensates and is mechanically ventilated.

Poisoning

Toxic ingestions sometimes cause metabolic (lactic) acidosis secondary to hypotension or interference with metabolic pathways, and respiratory acidosis, generally due to respiratory suppression.

Pulmonary edema

Pulmonary edema may cause either respiratory alkalosis or acidosis. When the edema is due to left ventricular failure (i.e., cardiogenic pulmonary edema), a superimposed lactic acidosis frequently develops secondary to tissue hypoperfusion.

Salicylate overdose

See text (p. 147).

Septic shock

Septic shock can sometimes produce a mixed lactic acidosis (which is secondary to hypoperfusion) and respiratory alkalosis.

Severe liver disease

Decompensated liver disease can cause a number of mixed disturbances. The most common is combined respiratory alkalosis and metabolic alkalosis, with the latter usually secondary to either diuretics (given to treat ascites) or vomiting (which may accompany liver failure).

Hospitalized patients

A common mixed disturbance in hospitalized patients is metabolic alkalosis and respiratory alkalosis. The metabolic alkalosis can result from diverse factors, including diuretics, vomiting or gastric drainage, glucocorticoids, alkaline antacids, or infusion of HCO_3^- or metabolizable anions (e.g., lactate from Ringer's solution or citrate from massive blood transfusions). The respiratory alkalosis can result from sepsis, liver disease, hypoxemia, stimulation of pulmonary sense receptors by lung disease, CNS disease, pain, anxiety, or other factors.

Triple mixed disorder

Two of the most common triple disturbances are (1) a vomiting alcoholic (metabolic acidosis and alkalosis, see above) who develops a superimposed respiratory alkalosis from sepsis, liver disease, or other factors, and (2) a hypercapnic COPD patient with an acute change in PCO_2 (see above) who develops either metabolic alkalosis from diuretics or vomiting, or lactic acidosis from sepsis, hypotension, or hypoxemia.

Blood gas profiles

In the text, we studied the blood gas profiles of simple disturbances in detail. We now do the same for mixed disturbances. There are seven possible "double disturbances" (i.e., mixed disturbances composed of two primaries). In the following paragraphs, we briefly discuss each.

Metabolic acidosis and metabolic alkalosis

These two primary processes have opposite effects on plasma $[HCO_3^-]$. Whether the final $[HCO_3^-]$ (and hence pH) is low or high depends on which disturbance predominates. Because the compensatory level for PCO_2 is determined by the final $[HCO_3^-]$, just as it would be in a simple disturbance, the blood gas is indistinguishable from that of a less severe case of the predominant disorder alone. For this reason, correct diagnosis depends heavily on the history, physical examination, and venous electrolytes. Since the two disturbances have opposite effects, the final $[HCO_3^-]$ and pH can be close to normal. Rarely, the two processes are exactly equal in magnitude, producing a completely normal $[HCO_3^-]$, pH, and PCO_2.

Metabolic acidosis and respiratory acidosis

Here, one process lowers [HCO_3^-] and the other raises PCO_2; thus, both act to reduce pH, which can be dangerously low even if neither primary disorder is severe. If the metabolic acidosis predominates, the drive to compensatory hyperventilation may reduce PCO_2 to 40 mm Hg or below. Thus, the diagnosis of respiratory acidosis (when it is part of a mixed disturbance) does not require absolute hypercapnia, only a PCO_2 above the predicted compensatory level. Conversely, if the respiratory acidosis predominates, renal compensation may produce a normal or even supranormal [HCO_3^-]; again, the defining characteristic is an insufficient compensatory response.

Metabolic alkalosis and respiratory alkalosis

Both disorders raise pH, which can be dangerously high without either [HCO_3^-] or PCO_2 being greatly deranged. If the metabolic disturbance predominates, the drive to compensatory hypoventilation can give an apparently normal, or even supranormal, PCO_2. If the respiratory disorder predominates, renal compensation can result in an apparently normal or even subnormal [HCO_3^-]. In either case, assessing the adequacy of compensation may be the only way to determine if the non-dominant disorder is present. If the two disorders are co-dominant, both the respiratory and metabolic components will be obviously alkalotic.

Metabolic acidosis and respiratory alkalosis

These disorders have opposing effects on pH. If the acidosis predominates, the final pH is low; if the alkalosis predominates, pH is high; if the two disorders are co-dominant, the pH will be normal. This mixed disturbance is sometimes mistaken for an especially well-compensated simple metabolic acidosis or respiratory alkalosis, but quantitative assessment of the compensatory response reveals the actual situation.

Metabolic alkalosis and respiratory acidosis

This mixed disturbance can be mistaken for a well-compensated simple metabolic alkalosis or respiratory acidosis. The pH may be normal, or slightly above or below normal, depending on which disorder is dominant. A metabolic alkalosis superimposed on an acute (uncompensated) respiratory acidosis can masquerade as a simple chronic respiratory acidosis, because the elevated [HCO_3^-] may be mistaken for compensation.

"Acute-on-chronic" respiratory disturbances

This pattern occurs when a patient with a chronic respiratory acidosis or alkalosis experiences a substantial, acute rise or fall in PCO_2. (Four "acute-on-chronic" combinations are therefore possible.) In chronic hypercapnic patients, an acute rise in PCO_2 can give a blood gas profile identical to a simple respiratory acidosis in the early stages of renal compensation.

"Same-type" mixed disturbances

This pattern refers to disturbances consisting of two varieties of the same primary disorder, such as mixed keto- and lactic acidosis. The blood gases for these mixed disorders look no different from a single, simple disturbance of the same type.

Triple disturbances

The blood gas profile of disturbances with three (or more) primaries can be extremely difficult to sort out. Often, a double disturbance is diagnosed, and the third primary is "unmasked" when one of the others is treated.

Treatment of mixed disturbances

Although a vast number of mixed disturbances are possible, most treatment decisions can be made by considering a few simple guidelines.

1. Accurate diagnosis

When evaluating any acid-base disturbance, always consider the possibility of a mixed disturbance, and do so early because it may affect your assessment of urgency. For example, if venous Total CO_2 is 17 mmol/l and you suspect a simple metabolic acidosis, you may not view the situation as urgent. However, if you suspect superimposed hypercapnia, you will recognize the possibility of lethal acidemia.

2. Treat individual disturbances

The next step is dictated by common sense: treat each of the component disorders. The approaches are the same as they would be if the disturbances were simple. First, the underlying cause must be identified and, if possible, corrected. Second, if necessary, abnormal $[HCO_3^-]$ and PCO_2 can be treated.

3. "Additive pH change" metabolic-respiratory disturbances

When both primary disorders move pH in the same direction (e.g., metabolic acidosis and respiratory acidosis), acidemia or alkalemia may be life threatening. If so, the primary goal of therapy is emergent correction of pH. This correction is accomplished most quickly by treating both metabolic and respiratory components. Correction of PCO_2 can sometimes be achieved rapidly and should usually be attempted first. If the patient is on a ventilator, change the rate and/or tidal volume in the appropriate direction. If the patient is not on a ventilator, consider intubation, or a rebreather mask or paper bag to raise PCO_2 acutely (note: chronically raising PCO_2 is generally not feasible). Next, correct [HCO$_3^-$]. For acidosis, use a bicarbonate infusion; for alkalosis, use NaCl and KCl or other, more aggressive, means (p 303).*

4. "Subtractive pH change" metabolic-respiratory disturbances

When the primary disorders move pH in opposite directions (e.g., metabolic acidosis and respiratory alkalosis), acidemia or alkalemia are relatively mild, and therapy can be undertaken more leisurely. However, treating one of the disorders can unmask the pH-altering effect of the other. It is therefore often desirable to treat both disorders simultaneously. If only one disorder is easily treatable, the clinician may face a dilemma: treat one and suffer a marked pH abnormality or treat neither and have a normal pH. Such dilemmas must be resolved on a case-by-case basis.

---

* **Clinical note.** If the patient has mixed metabolic and respiratory acidoses and you give bicarbonate, remember that the buffering reaction liberates CO_2. If the patient cannot increase ventilation, PCO_2 may rise. Thus, a patient who is not mechanically ventilated must be watched closely.

Topic F

Additional Comments on the Blood Gas Report

This topic has three parts, each of which will increase your facility in interpreting blood gas reports. The first part shows how to check the blood gas report for errors. The second presents five clinically useful generalizations about compensation. The third looks closely at normal ranges for the three variables.

Checking for errors

As described in the main text (p. 239), the blood-gas laboratory measures pH and PCO_2 and then calculates $[HCO_3^-]$. In some laboratories, blood-gas machines calculate $[HCO_3^-]$ automatically; in others, technicians perform this calculation manually. In either method, a miscalculation will give an erroneous $[HCO_3^-]$ value. Thus, when dealing with a critical blood gas, you should check the calculation. Two simple ways to do this check are described here: mathematical and graphical.

Mathematical. Plug the reported PCO_2 and $[HCO_3^-]$ values into the Henderson-Hasselbalch equation, $pH = 6.1 + \log ([HCO_3^-]/0.03\ PCO_2)$, and solve for pH with a calculator. If the calculated and reported pH values match, then $[HCO_3^-]$ was calculated correctly. *Graphical.* Most people find this approach easier. Take any two of the three reported acid-base variables (pH, PCO_2, $[HCO_3^-]$), plot the point on an acid-base map, and read off the third variable. If this "read-off" variable matches the reported one, the laboratory has correctly calculated $[HCO_3^-]$.

It is important to recognize that these approaches assure only that the three acid-base variables are "internally consistent" in terms of the limitations imposed by the Henderson-Hasselbalch equation; they do not rule out other types of errors, such as mismeasurement by the laboratory of pH or PCO_2, deficient blood-drawing technique, or mishandling of the sample.

Can arterial $[HCO_3^-]$ be checked by comparing it with venous Total CO_2? To some extent, yes. Start by recognizing that the two values will always be somewhat different, for three reasons. First, Total CO_2 quantifies not only bicarbonate, but also dissolved CO_2 and a few other minor sources of plasma CO_2 (p. 222). Second, venous PCO_2 is slightly higher than arterial PCO_2. The higher PCO_2 pushes the equilibrium point of the $CO_2 + H_2O \rightleftharpoons HCO_3^- + H^+$ system to the right, slightly raising venous $[HCO_3^-]$. Third, the passage of time between venous and arterial sampling may be enough for endogenous processes to alter $[HCO_3^-]$. In fact, if plasma $[HCO_3^-]$ is changing rapidly, non-contemporaneous samples may yield very different $[HCO_3^-]$ values (e.g., during severe lactic acidosis or treatment of alcoholic ketoacidosis).*

This said, the difference between venous Total CO_2 and arterial $[HCO_3^-]$ is usually small, and a large disparity in approximately contemporaneous samples generally suggests an error in one of the values. On the other hand, if the blood gas proves to be internally consistent, and arterial $[HCO_3^-]$ matches venous Total CO_2 fairly closely (especially if Total CO_2 is slightly higher), then it is usually safe to assume that both the blood gas and Total CO_2 assays are accurate.

Generalizations about compensation

Five statements about compensation follow. Reading and thinking about these will increase your ability to identify anomalous blood gas profiles, even without looking at the acid-base map, confidence bands, or rules of thumb.

1. Respiratory disturbances are usually better compensated than metabolic ones. In simple chronic respiratory disturbances, the final pH is usually within 0.1 pH units of 7.4. More severe acidemia or alkalemia suggests either that inadequate time has passed for compensation to develop fully or that a mixed disturbance is present.

2. Chronic respiratory alkalosis is the only simple disturbance where pH can be normal. In the other disturbances, pH is only returned *toward* normal, and a completely normal pH indicates a mixed disturbance.

3. Compensation never overshoots. In simple disturbances pH is returned towards normal, and in respiratory alkalosis pH can reach normal, but it *never* goes beyond. For example, a simple alkalosis, whether metabolic or respiratory, will never have a low pH. An overshooting pH always indicates a mixed disturbance.

4. The most predictable compensation occurs with metabolic acidosis. Even a modest deviation from the mean of the predicted range for PCO_2 indicates a mixed disturbance. Put differently, the normal band on the map is very narrow.

---

* **Food for thought.** However, if the *same* blood sample (either arterial or venous) is divided, with half sent for Total CO_2 measurement and half sent for blood gas analysis, then Total CO_2 will be very close to $[HCO_3^-] + 0.03 \times PCO_2$.

5. The least predictable compensation occurs with metabolic alkalosis; the normal band is very wide. Because hypoventilation tends to produce hypoxemia, the body "resists" and compensation is highly variable. For this reason, some clinicians do not attempt to quantitatively assess this compensation. Instead, they look for *some* elevation in PCO_2, a pH somewhat (but not too much) above normal, and a maximum PCO_2 below 60 mm Hg (because PCO_2 almost never reaches 60 without a superimposed respiratory acidosis).

Can two rights make a wrong?

In the main text (p. 239), we saw that the three acid-base variables each have a fairly wide range of normal values. Because a low PCO_2 and a high $[HCO_3^-]$ can independently raise pH, we might expect that a low-normal PCO_2 occurring with a high-normal $[HCO_3^-]$ would raise pH markedly. For example, if we plug a PCO_2 of 45 mm Hg and an $[HCO_3^-]$ of 23 mmol/l (both these values are within the normal range) into the Henderson-Hasselbalch equation, we find that pH is 7.33, which is below the normal range. Conversely, a low-normal PCO_2 (35) and a high-normal $[HCO_3^-]$ (28) give an abnormally high pH (7.53). It looks like two normals can make an abnormal.

However, healthy individuals don't have this sort of pH abnormality. Why? A physiologic "linkage" exists between the normal set-points for $[HCO_3^-]$ and PCO_2. Thus, an individual whose set-point PCO_2 is relatively high will also have a relatively high set-point $[HCO_3^-]$, and vice versa. The result is that pH will also remain in the normal range. What accounts for this "linkage" phenomenon? An important factor seems to be PCO_2 itself, which directly affects renal cells involved in bicarbonate handling. For example, raising PCO_2 increases the rate of bicarbonate reabsorption. This same mechanism mediates the renal compensation of respiratory disturbances (p. 135). Other mechanisms may also be involved.

Topic G

Is Compensation Really Compensatory?

The secondary changes in PCO_2 or $[HCO_3^-]$ that occur following the onset of a simple acid-base disturbance have traditionally been understood to have a beneficial, stabilizing effect on pH; hence the term "compensation." However, a body of data has been collected that indicates this view may be only partly correct. These data suggest that compensation may be of transient value. In a nutshell, it appears that secondary, "compensatory" changes may themselves cause subsequent (tertiary) changes in the PCO_2-HCO_3^- system, and these tertiary changes may offset the benefits provided by the secondary changes. Our goal here is to describe this provocative view in detail. We will look at metabolic and respiratory disturbances separately.

Metabolic disturbances

We begin with metabolic acidosis. The data suggest that the secondary ("compensatory") hypocapnia that occurs with metabolic acidosis induces a subsequent decrease in plasma $[HCO_3^-]$, which exacerbates the primary hypobicarbonatemia. This tertiary decrease in $[HCO_3^-]$ may offset the beneficial effect of the hypocapnia. The proposed sequence is as follows: (1) the primary disorder lowers $[HCO_3^-]$; (2) compensation lowers PCO_2; (3) because CO_2 crosses cell membranes freely, intracellular PCO_2 falls; (4) reduced PCO_2 in renal tubular cells acts to lower the kidney's reabsorptive threshold for bicarbonate*; (5) bicarbonate spills into the urine, lowering plasma $[HCO_3^-]$. The final $[HCO_3^-]$ is thus lower than it would have been if compensation had not occurred, and the new $[HCO_3^-]/PCO_2$ ratio, and hence plasma pH, is about the same as it was before the onset of respiratory compensation.

A similar sequence has been proposed for metabolic alkalosis: the secondary rise in PCO_2 leads to a fall in renal intracellular pH, raising the bicarbonate threshold and increasing plasma $[HCO_3^-]$. In sum, the data suggest that respiratory compensation is of substantial value only during the relatively short "window" before the secondary changes in PCO_2 produce tertiary changes in $[HCO_3^-]$.

---

* **Reminder.** High PCO_2 raises the threshold, whereas low PCO_2 lowers it (p. 135).

These data come from experimental animal studies only; human clinical studies have not been done. Nonetheless, the data are striking. If the proposed sequences are correct, then ongoing hyperventilation during sustained metabolic acidosis might be only a tremendous waste of energy. And hypoventilation during sustained metabolic alkalosis might elevate PCO_2 and, more importantly, reduce PO_2 for no good reason.

If these tertiary changes in plasma $[HCO_3^-]$ do occur, could secondary changes in PCO_2 nonetheless be viewed as homeostatic? Yes. To start with, severe metabolic acidosis is usually acute (ketoacidosis, lactic acidosis, and toxic ingestions), and thus falls within the window described. Furthermore, it is possible that sustained compensatory alterations of PCO_2 in both metabolic acidosis and alkalosis continue to stabilize *intracellular* pH, even though they do not stabilize extracellular pH. Intracellular pH stabilization would be important because the effects of pH changes are greatest inside cells (p. 13). Intracellular pH stabilization might occur because CO_2 crosses cell membranes more easily than bicarbonate. If the tertiary change in plasma $[HCO_3^-]$ is not fully reflected inside cells, the intracellular ratio of $[HCO_3^-]/PCO_2$, and hence intracellular pH, would be closer to normal than they would be in the ECF. This possibility, while appealing and plausible, has not been tested.

Respiratory disturbances

A small set of similar data pertains to respiratory acidosis. These data suggest the following sequence: (1) the primary disorder raises PCO_2; (2) renal compensation raises plasma $[HCO_3^-]$; (3) the rise in $[HCO_3^-]$ is transmitted to the CNS, which (4) raises CNS pH; (5) since ventilation is influenced by brain interstitial pH (p. 134), ventilation slows and PCO_2 rises. The underlying hypercapnia worsens, returning the plasma $[HCO_3^-]/PCO_2$ ratio and, hence, pH to their precompensatory levels.

Assuming, again, that this sequence does occur, could compensation for respiratory acidosis still be of value? Possibly. Although PCO_2 is higher than it would have been if compensation had not occurred, plasma pH is the same. Thus, the same pH is maintained, but at a lower rate of ventilation than would otherwise have been possible. Put differently, the secondary rise in $[HCO_3^-]$ allows the body to function at a higher PCO_2 without a further fall in pH. The physiologic burden shifts from the lung (which can ventilate slower) to the kidney (which must regenerate and then reabsorb additional bicarbonate). Because in most cases of chronic respiratory acidosis the lung is damaged and already functioning at a relatively high level of hypercapnic and hypoxic stimulus, this shift of burdens seems desirable.*

To date, no similar data have been collected that pertain to the compensation for respiratory alkalosis.

---

* **Going further.** Nonetheless, the reduced rate of ventilation still lowers alveolar PO_2. It would thus appear that any "shift of burden" that does occur has a cost: the possible exacerbation of hypoxemia.

Topic H

Laboratory Diagnosis of Intoxicant-Induced Metabolic Acidosis

This topic is designed to help clinicians more effectively use the hospital laboratory to diagnose or rule out toxic ingestion as a cause of metabolic acidosis. As explained below, many laboratories cannot assay for methanol or ethylene glycol; therefore, special attention is given here to the osmolar gap. Our discussion builds directly on related material in the pathophysiology (p. 146) and diagnosis (p. 255) sections.

"Panels" and "screens"

Toxicology "panels" (or "screens") are offered by many hospital laboratories. These panels represent an administrative decision by the laboratory to carry out several separate assays without the physician having to order each by name. There is nothing special about the tests themselves: the analytic methods do not change simply because the test is included on a panel. Some laboratories can assay for all common toxins yet have no panel. Other laboratories can assay for only a few toxins yet offer the tests as a package deal. Therefore, it is important to know (1) what tests your laboratory offers and (2) which, if any, are on a panel. You can get this information by calling the laboratory.

For example, Yale-New Haven Hospital's plasma "tox panel" comprises assays for phenobarbital, tricyclics, acetaminophen, salicylate, methanol, ethanol, and isopropanol—but *not* ethylene glycol. Thus, to rule out all the intoxicants that commonly cause metabolic acidosis, you would have to order the panel plus an ethylene glycol assay (or order the desired tests individually).

Tests and their limitations

To understand the diagnostic value of a test you must know its limitations. Knowing these limitations is crucial whether you order the test individually or as part of a panel. What follows are brief discussions of the assays for toxins that are commonly associated with metabolic acidosis.

Alcohols

Two tests are commonly used to assay for alcohols: an enzymatic assay and gas chromatography. In the enzymatic assay, a plasma sample is exposed to alcohol dehydrogenase, which converts alcohols into aldehydes. A colorimetric (i.e., color-changing) indicator shows if aldehydes are present. This assay is designed for ethanol. It may also detect methanol and isopropanol but, because the dehydrogenase has a much lower affinity for alcohols other than ethanol, only very high blood levels of methanol or isopropanol will give a positive result. Given these facts, the following guidelines can be used to interpret results of an enzymatic assay:

1. A positive finding strongly suggests ethanol.

2. A positive finding may also represent (a) a mixture of ethanol plus methanol or isopropanol or (b) very high levels of only methanol or isopropanol.

3. Quantitative results obtained from a positive enzymatic assay are valid only for ethanol intoxication. If a positive result is caused by intoxication with only methanol or isopropanol, quantitations will be falsely low.

4. A negative assay never rules out lethal doses of methanol or isopropanol. This important point is often not recognized.

Although the enzymatic assay is diagnostic only for ethanol, if you order an "alcohol" quantitation, some laboratories may perform the enzymatic assay, and you may falsely conclude that *all* alcohols have been ruled out. To avoid this mistake, always order alcohol assays by name: ethanol, methanol, isopropanol.

The other test for alcohols is gas chromatography ("GC"). This method reliably detects and quantitates methanol, ethanol, and isopropanol (it generates separate chromatographic "peaks" for each). In most laboratories, GC is the only way to rule out methanol and isopropanol.

Ethylene glycol

GC can reliably detect ethylene glycol. However, you must specifically request the ethylene glycol assay, because a different chromatographic technique is required than for the standard GC alcohol assay (which simultaneously tests for ethanol, methanol, and isopropanol). The time required to set up for this technique may cause additional delays, and some laboratories with GC are unable to perform the ethylene glycol assay at all.

Where there is no GC

Most hospital laboratories don't have GC equipment, and some laboratories that have GC can't run the assays at night. If there is no GC, or it is not available when you need it, you have two general options. First, in most areas, you can "send out" blood samples to a commercial laboratory or a larger hospital laboratory for analysis. Second, if no referral laboratory is available, or if there will be a significant delay in getting the results, you will have to rely at least temporarily on the enzymatic assay to rule out or quantify ethanol, and a calculation of the osmolar gap to suggest whether methanol, isopropanol, or ethylene glycol is present.*

Osmolar gap

Technical issues

Clinicians who use the osmolar gap need to be aware of two technical issues that can lead you to conclude falsely that the osmolar gap is normal, when in fact it is elevated.

1. Two types of osmometers are used in hospital laboratories: freezing point depression and vapor pressure. However, only freezing-point-depression osmometers can detect volatile alcohols such as ethanol, methanol, and isopropanol. If a laboratory uses the vapor-pressure method, the osmolar gap may appear normal even if high levels of these alcohols are present. To find out what kind of osmometer is used in your hospital, contact the laboratory. Because vapor-pressure osmometers cannot detect key toxic alcohols, they should be replaced. Note: both types of osmometers can detect ethylene glycol.

2. False normals can also occur in another way. Some modern serum chemistry analyzers (the machines that perform venous electrolyte assays) can automatically calculate osmolarity by inputting data on venous [Na+], [Glucose], and [BUN]. If this capability is used, the laboratory may report *calculated* osmolarity when an osmolarity determination is requested. An unsuspecting physician may think this value represents measured osmolarity and unwittingly calculate the osmolar gap as (calculated osmolarity) − (calculated osmolarity), which, of course, will always equal zero. Some laboratories are aware of this problem and either specify "calculated osmolarity" on the serum chemistry report or, bet-

---

* **Clinical note.** If you need to send out a sample for analysis, your own hospital's laboratory may be able to make the arrangements. If they can't, and you don't know the closest referral laboratory, try calling the 24-hour poison control center in your area for advice on who can do the analysis.

ter yet, have disabled the analyzer's osmolarity output entirely. You can easily determine if a potential problem exists at your hospital by contacting the laboratory.

Thus, before calculating the osmolar gap, you must be sure that "measured" osmolarity is (a) actually measured and (b) measured by a freezing-point-depression osmometer.

Causes of elevated osmolar gaps in patients with anion gap acidosis

It has traditionally been taught that an elevated osmolar gap in a patient with anion gap metabolic acidosis indicates one of three possibilities: methanol, ethylene glycol, or acetone from ketoacidosis (either diabetic or alcoholic). However, it appears that chronic renal failure (CRF) patients who do not receive maintenance dialysis may have osmolar gaps up to around 20 mOsms/l. In addition, it has been suggested (but not proven) that lactic acidosis also might raise the osmolar gap up to about 20 mOsms/l.

The osmolar gap is not usually elevated in acute renal failure, dialysis-treated chronic renal failure, hyperglycemia, or dehydration. In these conditions, the responsible solutes (e.g., BUN, glucose, Na^+) are included in the formula for calculated osmolarity, so measured and calculated osmolarity are both elevated; thus, the gap does not rise. Salicylates do not raise the osmolar gap because they are ionic; only neutral species raise the osmolar gap. Therefore, salicylates must be assayed by specific methods, which are available in virtually all clinical laboratories.

Correcting for ethanol

Patients sometimes ingest ethanol along with methanol or ethylene glycol. Because ethanol can raise the osmolar gap markedly, its presence can complicate the interpretation of an elevated osmolar gap. For example, in an ethanol-intoxicated patient, the osmolar gap will be elevated whether or not other toxins have been ingested. If GC is available, a definitive diagnosis can be established even if ethanol is present. However, if GC is not available, it may be helpful to quantitate ethanol by enzymatic assay and then calculate the osmolar gap using the following modified formula:

$$gap = \text{measured osmolarity} - (2Na^+ + Glucose/18 + BUN/2.8 + Ethanol/4.6)$$

Thus calculated, the osmolar gap reflects abnormal solutes other than ethanol.* Be aware, however, that in patients with alcoholic ketoacidosis, ace-

---

* **Technical information.** 4.6 is used because the molecular weight of ethanol is 46. See footnote on p. 256 for details. If glucose, BUN, and ethanol are measured in mmol/l, the divisors are not needed.

tone and other non-ionic solutes may be present, raising the osmolar gap. Thus, in a patient with suspected alcoholic ketoacidosis, finding an elevated osmolar gap with this modified formula should not automatically lead you to conclude that methanol or ethylene glycol is present. Conversely, the absence of ethanol should not lead you to rule out alcoholic ketoacidosis; perhaps surprisingly, most patients with alcoholic ketoacidosis have low or undetectable ethanol levels.

Progression from osmolar gap to anion gap

Methanol and ethylene glycol are neutral molecules. They raise the osmolar gap but do not cause metabolic acidosis and do not raise the anion gap. However, when methanol and ethylene glycol are metabolized, they give rise to organic acids. These acids are dissociated at body pH and exist as ions. They therefore cause acidosis and raise the anion gap, but do not raise the osmolar gap. Thus, in methanol and ethylene glycol intoxications, normal metabolism leads to a gradual progression from (a) osmolar gap without gap acidosis to (b) gap acidosis without osmolar gap.

Most intoxicated patients present in the middle of this progression, with elevations in both the osmolar and anion gaps. Why? Patients tend not to present at the very beginning of their course, with only an osmolar gap, because symptoms do not become prominent until significant metabolism has occurred (it is the aldehydes and acids that cause most symptoms). Patients also tend not to present at the end of their course, with only a gap acidosis, because symptoms may be prominent for some time while both osmolar and anion gaps are elevated. However, some patients do present at one extreme or the other, with only an osmolar gap or only an anion gap. Thus, although a simultaneous elevation in both the osmolar gap and anion gap is the usual presentation, an elevation in just one of these gaps may be the only clue the physician will get.

After ingestion of methanol or ethylene glycol, a detectable gap acidosis may not appear for hours. For methanol, this "latency period" may be as long as 24 hours or, rarely, even longer. Ethylene glycol is metabolized more rapidly, with the acidosis usually obvious within 12 hours (sometimes in less than 1 hour). However, if ethanol has been ingested along with methanol or ethylene glycol, acidosis may be delayed even longer, because ethanol inhibits the metabolism of methanol and ethylene glycol (p. 294). As the ethanol is itself metabolized, and blood [ethanol] falls, gap acidosis and major symptoms will develop.

It is important to recognize that in patients intoxicated with methanol or ethylene glycol, the metabolism-produced fall in the osmolar gap is not a laboratory artifact but is an accurate reflection of falling plasma [methanol] or [ethylene glycol]. Thus, by the time the osmolar gap approaches baseline, even specific assays such as GC will not detect the toxins. In such patients, you must rely on the history, physical exam, and an anion gap acidosis to make the diagnosis. Note: a very few laboratories can assay for metabolites of methanol (formate) and ethylene glycol (glycolic acid).*

Finally, bear in mind that an elevated, ethanol-adjusted osmolar gap in a patient without metabolic acidosis does not necessarily suggest methanol or ethylene glycol intoxication in the pre-metabolism phase. Most commonly, an elevated osmolar gap without acidosis is caused by isopropanol ingestion. Ingestion of ethyl ether or acetone, or infusion of dextran or mannitol, can also raise the osmolar gap without causing acidosis. Patients with multi-organ failure may also have osmolar gaps up to around 30, due largely to spillage of neutral molecules from cells to plasma.

A "normal" osmolar gap?

Following toxic ingestions, the osmolar gap is often very large. Osmolar gaps above 100 for methanol and above 50 for ethylene glycol have been reported, and values even close to these should immediately suggest the possibility of massive intoxication. However, a normal-range osmolar gap does not rule out relatively small but still potentially lethal ingestions. This is certainly true after metabolism, when little of the original toxin is left. But it is also true before metabolism. For example, a plasma level of 25 mg/dl (a significant ingestion) raises the osmolar gap by just 4 mOsms/l with ethylene glycol and 8 mOsms/l with methanol. These low numbers have special meaning because the pre-intoxication osmolar gap may be below zero (the normal range is sometimes said to be 0 ± 10). Thus, even during the early, pre-metabolism "latency period," when the osmolar gap is most elevated, a "normal" gap does not rule out lethal levels of ethylene glycol or blinding levels of methanol. Consequently, it is possible (but, fortunately, not common) for a serious intoxication to present without discernable elevations in either the osmolar or anion gaps. To summarize:

1.   A normal osmolar gap never rules out toxic ingestion and it should not be thought of as a "screen." Toxins may be present in low but lethal levels, or the toxin may have been metabolized to poisonous, dissociated acids, which do not raise the osmolar gap.

2.   An elevated osmolar gap in a patient with anion gap metabolic

---

* **Going further.** Because methanol is converted to formate, and formate is the anion responsible for raising the anion gap, the numerical rise in the anion gap from an assumed baseline should roughly equal the mmol/l fall in [methanol] from its postabsorption level. This assumed mmol/l decline can be converted to mg/dl by multiplying by 3.2 (because molecular wt. methanol = 32 grams). Adding this assumed mg/dl decline to the current mg/dl [methanol] gives an estimate of postabsorption, premetabolism [methanol]. Although conceptually simple, this calculation has many hidden assumptions (e.g., quantitative methanol-formate conversion, no accumulation of formaldehyde, equal volumes of distribution and no excretion of either methanol or metabolites) and has not been validated clinically. Therefore, it may be prudent to consider the calculation as an intellectual exercise, or at most a very rough guide; it should not be assumed to provide precise quantification.

acidosis does not necessarily indicate a toxic ingestion. A modestly elevated osmolar gap can occur with diabetic or alcoholic ketoacidosis, undialyzed chronic renal failure, and, possibly, lactic acidosis (especially if accompanied by multiorgan failure).

3. An elevated osmolar gap in a patient without metabolic acidosis may indicate ingestion of ethanol, isopropanol, or other non-ionic substances. However, the lack of acidosis does not rule out ingestion of methanol or ethylene glycol.

4. Any suspicion of toxic ingestion should be investigated immediately by specific assay, if available, regardless of osmolar gap findings. However, if extensive metabolism of the parent toxin has occurred, even specific assays may be negative.*

---

* **Clinical note.** Because methanol and ethylene glycol are so toxic, therapy must be started quickly. Thus, arrangements for ethanol therapy and dialysis should be made as soon as methanol or ethylene glycol is *suspected*. Ethanol can be started and then discontinued, and the dialysis session can be cancelled, if definitive assays later come back negative. In addition, multiple ingestions are common, so whenever you suspect one of the toxins discussed here, you must also consider the possibility of co-ingestants. Questioning the patient and family members, and making use of appropriate laboratory assays and screens, can reduce the risk of missing an important co-ingestant.

Topic I

More on Renal Tubular Acidosis

This topic is for readers who wish to deepen their understanding of RTA. It explores aspects of pathophysiology, terminology, and diagnosis not covered in the text. We presume the reader has already digested Chapters 16, 21, and 23, which discuss the pathophysiology and diagnosis of RTA. Our discussion has four main parts, beginning with . . .

What causes [K$^+$] to be abnormal in RTA?

Type 1 RTA

In Type 1 RTA, there may be a link between plasma [K$^+$] and the type of pump defect responsible for the acidosis. In hypokalemic patients, the defect might be in the H$^+$–K$^+$–ATPase. Such a defect could simultaneously account for the acidosis and potassium wasting. In normokalemic patients, the primary defect might be in the H$^+$–ATPase. Such a defect would have no direct effect on [K$^+$]. This proposed link between the type of pump defect and kalemic presentation is appealingly simple, but there is little direct evidence either for or against it.

Other explanations for the kalemic pattern do not assume a link between pump defect and [K$^+$]. Two such mechanisms have been proposed. (1) Metabolic acidosis from all causes, including RTA, reduces proximal Na$^+$ reabsorption (several mechanisms may be involved). This reduction causes urinary Na$^+$ wasting and volume depletion, which leads to a homeostatic rise in plasma [aldosterone]. Aldosterone limits further volume losses by stimulating distal Na$^+$ reabsorption, but it also raises K$^+$ excretion, leading to hypokalemia. (2) Elevated distal Na$^+$ reabsorption (just described) raises the negative charge of luminal fluid. This high charge is not well dissipated by secreted H$^+$, as it is in normal individuals, because H$^+$ secretion is low. The high luminal negative charge augments K$^+$ secretion by electrostatic attraction. It is not clear why some patients have normal [K$^+$].

Type 2 RTA

There is no proximal H$^+$–K$^+$–ATPase, so a proposed defect in this pump cannot account for hypokalemia in Type 2. At least three explanations have been proposed to account for [K$^+$]. Some are similar to those proposed for Type 1. (1) Bicarbonate spillage is accompanied by Na$^+$ spillage to maintain electroneutrality. Both HCO$_3^-$ and Na$^+$ are osmotically active, so spillage increases fluid flow through the distal nephron. High fluid flow keeps the concentration of secreted K$^+$ from building up in the luminal fluid, and this results in a favorable gradient for rapid K$^+$ secretion. (2) Increased distal Na$^+$ delivery, which is secondary to decreased proximal reabsorption, raises distal Na$^+$ reabsorption and, hence, luminal negativity. This increased negativity facilitates K$^+$ (cation) secretion. (3) Because Na$^+$ is lost in urine (not all of the extra distal Na$^+$ is reabsorbed), ECF volume falls slightly. The resulting rise in plasma [aldosterone] further stimulates K$^+$ secretion. Note that the first two mechanisms presume that bicarbonate is being spilled. Thus, once Type 2 enters the steady-state phase, and bicarbonate spillage ceases, we would expect K$^+$ wasting to slow markedly. In fact, in Type 2 patients, plasma [HCO$_3^-$] and [K$^+$] decline together, and then both stabilize at a reduced level. Once [K$^+$] stabilizes, a normal dietary K$^+$ intake can gradually raise plasma [K$^+$] toward normal.

Type 4 RTA

The cause of hyperkalemia in aldosterone-deficiency Type 4 is described in the pathophysiology section (p. 154).

The Type system

With the growth of pathophysiologic knowledge, there has been a gradual move away from the Type (i.e., 1, 2, and 4) system of nomenclature towards one based on an identification of specific cellular and hormonal defects. Nonetheless, the Type system is used clinically and is often referred to in journal articles, so it must be understood by those with an interest in RTA. The following discussion builds directly on the presentation in the pathophysiology section of the text (p. 149). Note: not all clinicians and authors use the same terms in the same ways. The definitional scheme presented below is based on dominant trends in the journal literature.

Type 1 RTA

An exception to the general rule that Type 1 presents with high urine pH is a rare entity called *incomplete distal RTA*. In this disorder, metabolic acidosis and high urinary pH occur only when an acid load, experimental or disease-caused, is imposed.

Type 2 RTA

In addition to the proximal reabsorptive defect that characterizes Type 2, proximal ammonium production, and hence bicarbonate regeneration, may also be slightly reduced.

Type 3 RTA

The term "Type 3" is no longer used. It was previously applied to a particular clinical entity, present in some infants, which is now considered a variant of Type 1. This entity consists of a defect in distal proton secretion plus delayed maturation of the proximal bicarbonate-reabsorptive apparatus. This combination results in a distal RTA with significant bicarbonaturia. In general, the proximal tubule matures as the infant grows, so the entity converts spontaneously to the more typical non-bicarbonate-wasting distal RTA.

Type 4 RTA

Type 4 requires more extensive comment. There are three main varieties of hyperkalemic RTA. As described in the text, the first and most common is hypoaldosteronism, either secondary to reduced renin secretion or due to a primary adrenal defect. When aldosterone is the only adrenal steroid affected, the term "selective aldosterone deficiency" (SAD) is sometimes used. In contrast, patients who also have impaired glucocorticoid secretion (e.g., Addison's disease) do not have SAD. Most patients with Type 4 have SAD. Hyporeninemic hypoaldosteronism, which is the most common RTA entity in adults, is a subgroup of SAD.

The second variety of hyperkalemic RTA is aldosterone resistance, also known as "pseudohypoaldosteronism." Hypoaldosteronism and aldosterone resistance are sometimes lumped together under the aegis of "reduced aldosterone activity." Insofar as the specialty literature continues to use the Type system of nomenclature, hypoaldosteronism and aldosterone resistance are almost universally classified as Type 4.

The third variety of hyperkalemic RTA was not discussed in the text. It is usually called hyperkalemic distal RTA (HDRTA). This entity is relatively uncommon but is mentioned frequently in the journal literature. We discuss it now.

Hyperkalemic distal RTA

Recall that "distal RTA" is generally used as a synonym for Type 1, which presents with high urine pH (> 5.5) and hypo- or normokalemia. The name hyperkalemic distal RTA therefore suggests an entity with high urine pH, like Type 1, but with hyperkalemia, like the aldosterone-deficiency states. Thus HDRTA falls between the usual presentations of Type 1 and Type 4.

Because of this intermediate status, HDRTA is not typed consistently. Some writers consider it a hyperkalemic variant of Type 1, whereas others consider it a high-urine-pH variant of Type 4. In this text, we have implicitly categorized HDRTA under the umbrella of Type 4, because it seems simplest, for both mnemonic and diagnostic reasons, to group all the hyperkalemic RTAs together. In addition, most patients with HDRTA have modest elevations in creatinine and BUN, just like patients with "normal" Type 4. Regardless of how one classifies HDRTA, it is important to recognize that the combination of high plasma [K$^+$] and high urine pH is unique among the RTAs. To avoid possible confusion, the usual (i.e., non-hyperkalemic) forms of distal RTA are sometimes referred to as *classic* distal RTA. The two major causes of HDRTA are obstructive uropathy (i.e., renal dysfunction caused by urinary obstruction) and sickle cell anemia.*

At least four mechanisms have been proposed to cause HDRTA. Each may be responsible in a particular subset of patients. The first mechanism involves a "voltage-dependent defect." In the distal nephron, the reabsorption of Na$^+$ leaves the luminal fluid with a slight negative charge, which attracts positive charges and hence facilitates proton secretion by the H$^+$–ATPase. A defect in sodium reabsorption impairs the formation of this luminal negative charge (this is the "voltage defect"), slowing secretion of the cations H$^+$ and K$^+$, thus causing acidosis and hyperkalemia. Unlike the H$^+$–ATPase, which is "electrogenic" (i.e., it generates an electrical charge by transporting a lone proton), transport by the H$^+$–K$^+$–ATP is electrically neutral, so its operation is not affected by Na$^+$ reabsorption. Note: some patients with voltage-dependent defects also have SAD. For clarity, SAD patients who do not have voltage defects are sometimes described as having "pure" SAD.

For some years it was thought that the voltage-dependent defect was the main cause of HDRTA. However, recent studies raise the possibility that, in many patients, HDRTA might simply represent a defect in the distal H$^+$–ATPase (just as may occur in classic Type 1) *plus* an independent defect in K$^+$ excretion caused either by low aldosterone levels (e.g., SAD) or by damage to the distal K$^+$-secreting mechanisms that is secondary to generalized (e.g., tubulointerstitial) renal injury.

The two other proposed mechanisms for HDRTA, both variations on the voltage-dependent theme, are intended to account for specific clinical patterns present in particular subsets of patients. One is a reversible form of

---

* **Clinical note.** Although most Type 4 patients have creatinines around 2–3 mg/dl, some (especially those with HDRTA from obstructive uropathy) may have creatinines of 5 mg/dl or higher. These high creatinine values can overlap with those seen in CRF. In attempting to differentiate high-creatinine Type 4 from CRF, the following can help. First, CRF patients usually do not develop hyperkalemia until their disease is end stage and [creatinine] is very high (unless they are eating a high-potassium diet or subject to other acute potassium loads). In contrast, Type 4 always causes hyperkalemia, and [creatinine] rarely reaches levels typical of end-stage CRF. Second, although the acidosis of advanced CRF may be hyperchloremic, it is more commonly anion gap. In contrast, Type 4 never raises the anion gap. Third, urine pH in CRF is usually below 5.5. In contrast, in patients with HDRTA, which generally accounts for the highest creatinine levels in Type 4, urine pH is above 5.5. Therefore, hyperkalemia with a non-gap acidosis suggests Type 4; the additional finding of high urine pH indicates HDRTA; and normokalemia, elevated anion gap, and very high [creatinine] all indicate CRF. Note: although Type 4 is the only RTA consistently associated with elevated [creatinine], Type 1 RTA may lead to nephrocalcinosis, which can cause a secondary rise in [creatinine].

RTA that can occur with volume depletion. Volume depletion reduces Na^+ delivery to the distal tubule, apparently by stimulating proximal Na^+ reabsorption. The reduced availability of distal Na^+ lowers the rate of distal Na^+ reabsorption, thereby causing a functional voltage-dependent defect. This RTA can usually be corrected by giving NaCl solutions, which repair the volume depletion, or loop diuretics, which decrease loop Na^+ reabsorption, leaving more Na^+ in the lumen for distal delivery.

The other mechanism applies to a subset of HDRTA patients who experience volume expansion caused by renal salt (i.e., Na^+ and Cl^-) retention. In these patients, hypertension sometimes occurs and can be a diagnostic tip off. This pattern may be due to increased reabsorption of Cl^- from the distal luminal fluid ("chloride shunt"). The efflux of the anionic chloride from the lumen is said to decrease luminal negativity, impairing H^+ and K^+ secretion, and to promote excess Na^+ reabsorption (by facilitating electroneutral transport of Na^+ and Cl^- out of the lumen), thus expanding ECF volume.

Diagnosis

The major varieties of RTA can be differentiated fairly easily. Many approaches exist. The following approach is relatively simple yet provides good discrimination.

1. Rule out other causes

Attempt to exclude the other common causes of hyperchloremic metabolic acidosis (i.e., diarrhea and non-gap renal failure) as well as, if possible, any potentially relevant uncommon causes (see Appendix Topic K). Also, assess the possibility that a urinary tract infection with a urea-splitting organism is present (the conversion of urinary urea to NH_4^+ consumes protons and can raise urinary pH even when renal proton secretion is normal).

2. Check plasma [K+]

An RTA with low or normal [K^+] represents either Type 1 or Type 2 (unless hypokalemia is caused by factors unrelated to the RTA); to determine which, skip to step 3, below. A high [K^+] indicates Type 4 (unless hyperkalemia is caused by factors unrelated to the RTA); to further differentiate Type 4, check urine pH and continue as follows:

A. If pH is low

If urine pH is below 5.5 in a Type 4 patient, reduced aldosterone activity is probably the cause. This diagnosis is supported by finding a slightly elevated plasma [creatinine]. To differentiate hypoaldosteronism from aldosterone resistance, plasma [aldosterone] can be measured. Low [aldosterone] suggests hypoaldosteronism; high [aldosterone] suggests resistance. However, because hyperkalemia stimulates aldosterone secretion, you must interpret the aldosterone level carefully. For example, a Type 4 patient with a normal aldosterone secretory response will have a high plasma [aldosterone], whereas a Type 4 patient with a subnormal response will likely have a normal-appearing [aldosterone]. If both cortisol and aldosterone are low, the underlying cause is likely generalized adrenal insufficiency (Addison's disease).

B. If pH is high

If urine pH is above 5.5 in a Type 4 patient, the disorder is probably hyperkalemic distal RTA. Creatinine elevated to a degree consistent with that found in hypoaldosteronism (about 2 mg/dl) is the typical presentation. Volume depletion (actual or effective), assessed either clinically or by low urinary [Na^+] or [Cl^-], suggests that the RTA is reversible and caused by volume depletion. Hypertension, especially in the setting of a normal plasma creatinine level, suggests the salt-retention form.

3. For low or normal [K^+]

Continue here for RTA patients who have either low or normal [K^+]. Check urine pH. If pH is low, the diagnosis is probably proximal RTA in its steady-state phase. If pH is high, the diagnosis is either classic distal RTA or proximal RTA in its early, non-steady-state phase. It should be easy to differentiate these last two entities because proximal RTA is usually (a) due to acetazolamide (Diamox; typically administered for glaucoma) or multiple myeloma or (b) is part of the Fanconi syndrome (typically in children). A patient who is not receiving acetazolamide, does not have multiple myeloma, and lacks the classic Fanconi plasma and urine profiles (p. 154) is unlikely to have proximal RTA.

Another way to differentiate Types 1 and 2 RTA is to observe the response to bicarbonate therapy. In proximal RTA, bicarbonate therapy will quickly raise plasma [HCO_3^-] above the abnormally low reabsorptive threshold. As a result, urinary [HCO_3^-] and pH will increase sharply (urine pH > 7.5). Plasma [HCO_3^-] will rise only gradually and will fall quickly once bicarbonate is discontinued. In contrast, in distal RTA (which has a relatively normal reabsorptive threshold), bicarbonate therapy results in a progressive rise in plasma [HCO_3^-] up to normal levels, and bicarbonaturia will not occur until normal levels are exceeded. Furthermore, in distal RTA, once [HCO_3^-] normalizes it will fall slowly, over a period of days, as physiologic endogenous acid production gradually consumes plasma bicarbonate.

How to measure urine pH

Like blood, urine contains dissolved CO_2; and, as with blood, a fall in PCO_2 causes a rise in pH. It is therefore important when measuring urine pH to minimize the loss of dissolved CO_2. Loss of CO_2 can be minimized in one of two ways: (1) Place a few drops of mineral oil into the voiding receptacle before the patient urinates. The oil, which is less dense than water, floats to the surface, where it slows the egress of CO_2. (2) Draw the urine into a syringe, tap out and express any bubbles, replace the threaded plastic cap, and put the syringe into a cup of ice. With either method, take the sample to the laboratory for immediate analysis and be sure pH is measured by electronic meter, because a high degree of discrimination (especially near a pH of 5.5) is necessary and cannot be achieved by dip stick. The preferred time for measuring urine pH is morning, before breakfast, when urine pH is normally at its lowest.

Diarrhea vs. Distal (Type 1) RTA

As described in the text (p. 258), it is usually fairly simple to rule out the common non-RTA causes of hyperchloremic acidosis. However, in certain cases of severe diarrhea, a difficulty can arise. The difficulty, and the solution, are as follows:

Diarrhea and distal RTA both present with hyperchloremic acidosis and hypokalemia. This similarity does not usually complicate diagnosis because, to determine which condition is present, you need only check for a history of diarrhea. And if the history is ambiguous, a urine pH often provides the answer: low pH (i.e., the normal renal response to metabolic acidosis) suggests diarrhea, whereas high pH suggests Type 1. However, if diarrhea causes severe volume depletion, a reversible voltage-dependent defect may appear, raising urine pH.

Thus, in a patient with hypokalemic, hyperchloremic metabolic acidosis, who presents with an ambiguous history and a high urine pH, it can be difficult to differentiate diarrhea from Type 1. The solution is to evaluate urinary ammonium excretion, which in diarrhea remains high (the normal homeostatic response to metabolic acidosis) even if pH is elevated, but is low in Type 1. The urinary ammonium assay is not available in all hospitals and, where available, is a special-order test. However, urine $[NH_4^+]$ can be estimated by calculating the *urinary anion gap*. This variable, which is analogous to the plasma anion gap, is discussed in detail in the next topic.

Topic J

Urinary Anion Gap

The goal of this topic is to explain the concept and clinical application of the urinary anion gap. The major urinary ions are Na^+, K^+, NH_4^+, and Cl^-. Urea is the major uncharged solute. Unlike in plasma, ionic concentrations and total osmolarity in urine vary greatly, depending on various factors, including the rate of NH_4^+ excretion and the levels of dietary Na^+, K^+, and water. Here are two typical urinary ionograms with different levels of NH_4^+:

Low ammonium   High ammonium

Ca^{2+}, Mg^{2+}	Phosphate
NH_4^+	Organic anions
	SO_4^{2-}
K^+	
	Cl^-
Na^+	

Ca^{2+}, Mg^{2+}	Phosphate
NH_4^+	Organic anions
	SO_4^{2-}
K^+	
	Cl^-
Na^+	

Notice that the additional NH_4^+ in the high-NH_4^+ ionogram has replaced Na^+ and K^+. As a result, in the low-NH_4^+ ionogram, the column height of $[Na^+] + [K^+]$ exceeds that of $[Cl^-]$, whereas in the high-NH_4^+ ionogram the column height of $[Cl^-]$ exceeds that of $[Na^+] + [K^+]$. These "height" differences can be quantified via a *urinary anion gap*, calculated as $[Na^+] + [K^+] - [Cl^-]$. Notice that when more NH_4^+ is present, the anion gap becomes smaller (because the sum of $[Na^+] + [K^+]$ decreases whereas $[Cl^-]$ does not). Therefore, as $[NH_4^+]$ rises, the gap decreases, then becomes zero and, eventually, negative. Pause for a moment to make sure you grasp these points both visually and mathematically.

We can now formulate a general rule: when urinary $[NH_4^+]$ is low, the urinary anion gap, defined as $[Na^+] + [K^+] - [Cl^-]$, is positive (e.g., +30 meq/l), and when urinary $[NH_4^+]$ is high, the gap is negative (e.g., −50 meq/l). Because various minor ions in the urine are not included in the anion gap formula, the gap provides at best only a very rough estimate of urinary $[NH_4^+]$. Note: urine $[Na^+]$, $[K^+]$, and $[Cl^-]$ are obtained by ordering a urinary electrolyte assay ("urine lytes").

How is the gap used clinically? During metabolic acidosis, the healthy kidney homeostatically excretes large quantities of NH_4^+, and therefore produces urine with a markedly negative anion gap. However, renal ammonium excretion is impaired in chronic renal failure and in Types 1 and 4 RTA, thus leading to a positive urinary anion gap (note: NH_4^+ excretion is relatively normal in Type 2). It is generally unnecessary to calculate the urinary anion gap in renal failure (because plasma creatinine is always markedly elevated, and thus suggests the diagnosis) or in Type 4 (because hyperkalemia suggests the diagnosis). However, for Type 1, calculating the gap can sometimes help. As we saw in Appendix Topic I, if diarrhea is accompanied by significant volume depletion, it may present with a high urine pH and therefore be confused with Type 1 RTA. However, in Type 1 RTA, NH_4^+ excretion is impaired, whereas in diarrhea it is not.

This Type 1 vs. diarrhea differentiation provides the primary clinical use for the urinary anion gap. However, even in this setting, the urinary anion gap is often not needed: simply finding out if the patient has diarrhea will usually suffice. The gap is most useful when you are concerned that both diarrhea and Type 1 RTA may be present, or when a reliable history, which might otherwise suggest or rule out diarrhea, cannot be obtained. In most other settings, calculating the gap may help salvage a dull morning but it won't help you make the diagnosis.

A caveat. Chloride is the only major anion in normal urine and, therefore, is the only anion included in the gap formula. If other anions are present in high concentrations, the gap formula becomes inadequate and NH_4^+ will be underestimated by an amount roughly equal to the concentration of the abnormal anions. Clinically, this underestimation may occur in two situations: (1) When urine pH is high (above 6.5), urinary $[HCO_3^-]$ is substantial, and (2) during ketoacidosis, urinary organic anion concentration is elevated. In theory, the gap formula could be modified to account for these anions (i.e., $[Na^+] + [K^+] - [Cl^-] - [HCO_3^-] - [\text{organic anion}]$). In practice, however, this modification is unworkable because urinary $[HCO_3^-]$ and [organic anion] are not normally measured. Thus, the urine anion gap does not provide reliable information, and should not be used, when urine pH is high (> 6.5) or when the patient has ketoacidosis.

Finally, it should be noted that studies which have attempted to validate the urinary anion gap have not produced consistent results. In fact, one study found that within the $[NH_4^+]$ range of about 0–90 mmol/l the urinary anion gap was *positively* correlated with urinary $[NH_4^+]$, just the opposite of what "should" have occurred. Thus, while it is probably reasonable to differentiate between markedly negative (high $[NH_4^+]$) and markedly positive (low $[NH_4^+]$) urinary gaps, it can be a mistake to attempt fine discriminations or to consider the gap a definitive diagnostic modality. Remember: quantitative urinary ammonium assays, while not routine, are available.*

---

* **Food for thought.** Since unmeasured anions (in plasma) are assessed via an anion gap, it might be conceptually simpler to assess unmeasured cations such as NH_4^+ (in urine) via a "cation gap." By transposing the (Cl^-) and ($Na^+ + K^+$) terms of the urinary anion gap formula, one can obtain a positive value when $[NH_4^+]$ is high. That is, Urinary cation gap = $Cl^- - (Na^+ + K^+)$.

Topic K

Rare Causes of
Acid-Base Disorders

The main text discusses all common, and some less common, causes of acid-base disturbances. Here, we briefly describe some of the uncommon and rare causes not previously considered, although even this list is not exhaustive. Only metabolic disturbances are discussed because rare respiratory causes can generally be inferred from the text discussions (e.g., rare causes of respiratory center suppression will cause respiratory acidosis). The topic ends with a brief overview of the diagnosis of volume-resistant metabolic alkalosis.

Metabolic acidosis

Hyperchloremic metabolic acidosis

Oral CaCl$_2$ can cause acidosis by reacting with secreted bicarbonate, forming insoluble calcium carbonate in the intestinal lumen via the reaction CaCl$_2$ + 2HCO$_3^-$ → CaCO$_3$ + 2Cl$^-$ + H$_2$O + CO$_2$. To keep gut-lumen pH from falling, more bicarbonate is secreted, thereby raising gastrointestinal acid production (GAP). In intestinal ileus or obstruction, bicarbonate-rich fluids can be secreted into the gut lumen and sequestered there, raising GAP; fistulas of the pancreas and biliary tract may also increase GAP by a similar mechanism. Following surgical removal of the bladder, the surgeon may establish a new urinary path by implanting the ureters into either the sigmoid colon (uterosigmoidostomy) or, and now more commonly, the ileum or jejunum. Colonic implantation almost always causes acidosis; small bowel implantation causes acidosis in about 10% of cases. The mechanism appears to be an exchange of urinary Cl$^-$ for HCO$_3^-$ across the apical membrane of the gut epithelium. The absorption and hepatic metabolism of urinary NH$_4^+$ (p. 85) may play a secondary role. "Dilutional acidosis" can occur when large volumes of bicarbonate-free saline are infused, thereby lowering extracellular fluid [HCO$_3^-$]; the fall in [HCO$_3^-$] is mild, at most 2–3 mmol/l. Mechanistically, dilutional acidosis is the exact opposite of contraction alkalosis (p. 166). Hyperkalemia, by a mechanism described elsewhere (p. 154), has at times produced acidosis.

Anion gap metabolic acidosis

Paraldehyde was once commonly used as a sedative-hypnotic. Poisoning can cause high levels of poorly-characterized organic acids, which may give a positive nitroprusside reaction, falsely suggesting ketoacidosis. Patients often have a distinctive, pungent odor on their breath. Paraldehyde poisoning is now rare. Overdoses of isoniazid and, in large amounts, iron supplements also can cause gap acidosis. D-lactic acidosis can occur when patients with preexisting gastrointestinal pathology, especially short-bowel syndrome (e.g., jejunoileal bypass), develop colonic bacterial overgrowth. The acidosis may be intermittent, accompanied by neurologic symptoms, and precipitated by ingestion of carbohydrate, yogurt, or lactobacillus supplements, which leads to the absorption from the gut of large amounts of bacteria-produced D-lactic acid (the endogenous human form is L-lactic acid). A special D-lactate assay or gas-liquid chromatography must be used for detection and quantitation of the lactate. D-lactic acidosis should be suspected when patients with preexisting gut pathology develop an unidentified gap acidosis.

Gap acidoses can also be caused by various inborn enzyme disorders, which are often referred to, collectively, as congenital organic acidoses. These include the following: Glucose-6-phosphate deficiency, which, by inhibiting gluconeogenesis and glycogenolysis, can result in severe hypoglycemia on fasting. The hypoglycemia may, in turn, cause an exaggerated starvation ketoacidosis, which is typically preceded by lactic acidosis. Fructose-1,6-bisphosphate deficiency, by inhibiting gluconeogenesis, has a similar result. Other rare defects in enzymes such as phosphoenolpyruvate carboxykinase and pyruvate carboxylase also cause exaggerated fasting hypoglycemia and starvation ketoacidosis. Disorders of fat-metabolizing enzymes can cause accumulation of various organic acids.

Metabolic alkalosis

Volume-responsive metablolic alkalosis

Two rare causes of volume-responsive metabolic alkalosis involve unusual forms of diarrhea (recall that diarrhea usually causes metabolic *acidosis*). In infants, a disorder known as congenital chloride diarrhea, characterized by large volumes of unformed stool rich in chloride, can cause metabolic alkalosis. In adults, villous adenoma of the large bowel results in diarrhea and can cause metabolic alkalosis; this tumor is usually large and easily detected by rectal exam or sigmoidoscopy. These two disorders should be suspected when metabolic alkalosis is accompanied by severe diarrhea.

Volume-resistant metabolic alkalosis

Primary hyperaldosteronism and Cushing's syndrome are discussed in the text (p. 168). Bartter's syndrome (p. 169) is a genetic salt-wasting disorder, usually diagnosed in childhood or adolescence, which is characterized by metabolic alkalosis, severe hypokalemia, and elevated plasma [renin] and [aldosterone]. Renal artery stenosis and certain other causes of hypertension are associated with secondary hyperaldosteronism and can cause very mild metabolic alkalosis. Several rare congenital syndromes increase secretion of deoxycorticosterone, an aldosterone agonist. High levels of ACTH from a pituitary adenoma or an ectopic ACTH-secreting tumor may overstimulate the adrenals, leading to hyperaldosteronism (or excess of other steroids with aldosterone activity). Ingestion of large amounts of natural licorice, which contains glycyrrhizic acid as a flavoring agent, can cause metabolic alkalosis; this is usually not a problem in the United States because most licorice is flavored artificially. Magnesium depletion can cause the kidney to waste potassium, and may be associated with mild metabolic alkalosis. Other rare causes also exist.

The diagnosis of volume-resistant metabolic alkalosis

A detailed diagnostic algorithm for volume-resistant metabolic alkalosis is beyond the scope of this book. However, a few basics can be noted. Most causes of volume-resistant alkalosis present with elevated blood pressure secondary to volume expansion from excess aldosterone (or aldosterone-agonists). In contrast, Bartter's syndrome causes urinary salt wasting and therefore does not expand volume or present with hypertension. Thus, a patient with metabolic alkalosis, normal or elevated urinary [Cl$^-$], and normal or low blood pressure, is likely either to be surreptitiously abusing diuretics or to have Bartter's syndrome. If a urinary diuretic screen is negative, Bartter's should be suspected.

Among the hypertension-associated causes (i.e., almost all causes except Bartter's), broad categories can be distinguished based on plasma levels of renin and aldosterone: primary defects of high renin secretion present with high levels of both renin and aldosterone; primary defects of high aldosterone secretion present with low [renin] and high [aldosterone]; and primary increases in aldosterone agonists such as deoxycorticosterone present with low levels of both aldosterone and renin. However, accurate testing of plasma levels of renin, aldosterone, cortisol, and related substances is complex and, if not done using specified procedures, can easily lead to erroneous results.

Topic L

Local Anesthesia for Arteriopuncture

Arteriopuncture requires that a needle penetrate the skin, subcutaneous tissues, and arterial wall. The level of pain varies, depending on the patient's pain threshold, the depth of the artery, the skill of the operator, and the number of "sticks" required to obtain the blood sample. For some patients, the arteriopuncture for blood gas is the most painful part of the hospital experience.

To reduce pain and anxiety, some physicians advocate the routine use of local anesthesia, especially when it is anticipated that more than one clean "stick" may be needed. In general, patients are very thankful for this anesthesia; they appreciate the pain relief itself as well as the concern for their comfort that pain relief represents. Two methods of local anesthesia have been widely used: needle instillation of local anesthetic and topical application of skin-penetrating anesthetic. Both methods have been shown to provide significant pain reduction. A brief discussion of each method follows.

Needle instillation of local anesthetic

In this approach, a small syringe with a very fine needle is used to instill a small amount of local anesthetic into the skin and/or subcutaneous tissues at the arteriopuncture site. A 1 ml tuberculin syringe with a needle between 27 and 30 guage is ideal for this purpose. The usual anesthetic is lidocaine in a concentration of 1%, without epinepherine, but other anesthetic agents can be used. Although different physicians use different techniques, one typical set of instructions follows:

> Clean skin with alcohol swab and let dry. Using a tuberculin syringe filled with 1 ml of a local anesthetic solution, raise a superficial skin wheal by injecting a few tenths ml of anesthetic intradermally, just below the surface of the skin. This superficial anesthesia may be sufficient in some patients. When additional anesthesia is desired, after raising the skin wheal, penetrate *slightly* deeper with the needle, beneath the level of the skin, and inject the remaining contents of the syringe into the superficial subcutaneous tissues near the artery, taking care not to inject the artery itself.

After penetrating the skin with the needle, but before instilling the anesthetic, it is advisable to withdraw the plunger of the syringe slightly to check for blood, to ensure that the needle tip is not in a small blood vessel or the artery itself. After injection, at least two minutes are waited for the anesthetic to take effect before arteriopuncture.

Advantages: The anesthetic effect of needle instillation is reliable and strong, and the procedure adds only a few minutes to the time required for unanethesized arteriopuncture. *Disadvantages:* Some patients (including most children) are afraid of even small needles. The instillation of some anesthetics (including lidocaine) causes mild pain, both from the needle puncture and because of the chemical properties of the anesthetic. During the pre-procedure explanation, therefore, patients should be told that a transient burning sensation may follow the instillation of anesthetic.* It is sometimes stated that the instillation of anesthetic, by changing the superficial appearance of the puncture site, makes accurate arteriopuncture more difficult; however, many physicians feel that this is not a significant problem.

Topical application of skin-penetrating anesthetic

Special skin-penetrating topical anesthetic creams have recently been developed. Their use is rapidly becoming standard practice for pediatric venepuncture and arteriopuncture, and they are being increasingly used in adult patients as well. A few grams of the cream are applied to skin at the puncture site and covered with an occlusive dressing (e.g., Tegaderm). After a waiting period to allow for skin penetration, the occlusive dressing is removed and the site is cleaned for arteriopuncture.

Waiting time varies with the anesthetic used. The only skin-penetrating agent currently available in the U.S. is a specially formulated mixture of lidocaine and prilocaine (EMLA). This agent usually requires 90–120 minutes waiting time for optimal effect at the arterial site, although less time may be of some benefit. In Europe, but not in the U.S., a skin penetrating tetracaine gel has been marketed, which may be effective in 30–40 minutes.

Advantages: Topical anesthetics are painless and involve no needle. These agents do not usually change the appearance of the puncture site, except for transient blanching of the skin. *Disadvantages:* The time needed for good skin penetration makes topical anesthesia inapplicable in some acutely ill patients.

---

*Going further. The chemical pain produced by local anesthetics appears to be partly related to the low pH of the solutions, which are required for long shelf life. Raising the pH of the anesthetic by adding a small amount of sodium bicarbonate solution can reduce both pain and shelf life. Readers interested in details on the preparation and storage of buffered anesthetic solutions will find relevant articles in the bibliography.

Annotated Bibliography

This bibliography has two parts. The first, "General Reading," is designed for readers of the main text. It describes works that I believe readers will find especially useful and interesting if they choose to explore acid-base further. I have even included (at the end) a few personal favorites that don't pertain directly to acid-base. Some of the listed texts are revised periodically, so look for the latest editions. Note: PB = paperback, HC = hardcover.

The second part of this bibliography, "Appendix Reading," is designed for those who have read an appendix topic and wish to explore further. There are 12 short lists, one for each of the topics. These lists, which comprise both journal articles and book chapters, can be thought of as self-directed reading programs for additional study.

General Reading

First are books of special relevance to the clinician with a strong interest in acid-base:

> *Acid-Base Disorders* by Heinz Valtin and F. John Gennari helps readers hone clinical skills by providing basic diagnostic and management problems, with detailed solutions; see especially chapters four through eight (PB, Little, Brown, Boston, 1987, 195 pp). *Repairing Body Fluids* by Jerome P. Kassirer, Donald E. Hricik, and Jordan J. Cohen is a concise, readable text that focuses on practical and conceptual issues in the treatment of acid-base and electrolyte disturbances (HC, WB Saunders, Philadelphia, 1989, 174 pp). *Clinical Physiology of Acid-Base and Electrolyte Disorders* by Burton David Rose is a clear, detailed text and reference on acid-base and electrolytes; a fine resource for the thoughtful clinician (PB, McGraw-Hill, New York, 4th ed., 1994, 914 pp).

Next are "academically" oriented works. These books emphasize cellular mechanisms and specialized topics, but also contain a wealth of clinically useful information:

Acid-Base by Jerome Kassirer and Jordan Cohen is an invaluable classic for the serious student of acid-base; it also contains a short section of challenging clinical problems involving mixed or progressive disturbances (HC, Little Brown, Boston, 1982, 510 pp). *The Regulation of Acid-Base Balance,* edited by Donald W. Seldin and Gerhard Giebisch, is a gold mine of information difficult to obtain elsewhere (HC, Raven, New York, 1989, 603 pp). *Fluid, Electrolyte, and Acid-Base Disorders,* edited by Allen I. Arieff and Ralph A. DeFronzo (HC, Churchill Livingstone, New York, 2nd ed., 1995, 946 pp) and *Fluids and Electrolytes,* edited by Juha P. Kokko and Richard L. Tannen (HC, WB Saunders, Philadelphia, 3rd ed., 1996, 899 pp) both contain several interesting chapters on acid-base. *Acid-Base Balance* by A. Gorman Hills provides, among other things, an interesting history of acid-base theory (PB, Williams & Wilkins, Baltimore, 1973, out of print).

Among multi-volume sets, *Diseases of the Kidney,* edited by Robert W. Schrier and Carl W. Gottschalk, contains detailed review articles on basic science and clinical aspects of renal acid-base (HC, Little Brown, Boston, 5th ed., 1993, 3 vols). *The Kidney,* edited by Donald W. Seldin and Gerhard Giebisch, reviews a variety of interesting topics not found in other texts (HC, Raven Press, New York, 2nd ed., 1992, 3 vols). *Textbook of Respiratory Medicine,* edited by John F. Murray and Jay A. Nadel, has detailed discussions of the lung and respiratory diseases (HC, WB Saunders, Philadelphia, 2nd ed., 1994, 2 vols).

The following will be of interest to scientific iconoclasts, innovators, and free thinkers. They pose thought-provoking challenges to the conventional acid-base paradigm:

"Metabolic aspects of the regulation of systemic pH" by Daniel E. Atkinson and Edmund Bourke created a fury when it appeared in the American Journal of Physiology. The authors argue that the *liver* (and not the noble kidney) is the organ responsible for regulating plasma $[HCO_3^-]$. In a published reply, an eminent authority hinted that—to prevent students from being corrupted by false doctrine—Atkinson and Bourke should be poisoned. The article, along with two of the many critical responses, can be found on the following pages of Am J Physiol: 1987;21(6):F947-F956. 1987;22(1):F199-F202. 1987;22(6):F1308-F1310.

In contrast to this violent reaction, hardly an eyebrow was raised when Peter A. Stewart published *How To Understand Acid-Base* (HC, Elsevier, New York, 1981, 186 pp). In this innocently titled "primer," Stewart makes the astonishing assertion that extracellular $[HCO_3^-]$ is not an independent variable in determining pH, and he proposes a new way of conceptualizing acid-base regulation. He also argues that, when used to analyze titrations, pH (as opposed to [H$^+$]) curves are misleading. This rigorous book makes rewarding reading, even for those who remain unconvinced by the more provocative points.

Finally, for those who want a break from the usual approach to science, I wish to recommend four personal favorites:

"The Creative Mind," the first essay in mathematician Jacob Bronowski's *Science and Human Values,* is a remarkable exploration of the common essence of art and science (PB, Harper Collins, New York, 1972). The *Structure of Scientific Revolutions* by Thomas Kuhn, hailed in Science as a "landmark in intellectual history," gives a fascinating view of how scientific theories develop (PB, University of Chicago Press, Chicago, 1970). "The philosophical basis of peer review and the suppression of innovation" by David Horrobin gives an intriguing, and sometimes disturbing, perspective on how journal articles are selected for publication (JAMA 1990;263:1438–1441). And last, Arthur Koestler's *The Case of the Midwife Toad,* which recounts a strange and amazing chapter from the history of evolutionary biology, is arguably the best true-life scientific mystery thriller ever written. This short book is out of print but is available through public and academic libraries.

Appendix Reading

For brevity, journal citations include only the first author. When a book is listed by title only, details can be found above in the "General Reading" bibliography.

Topic A

Madias NE. "Acid-base chemistry and buffering." Chapter 1 in *Acid-Base* □ Boron WF. "Chemistry of buffer equilibria in blood plasma." Chapter 1 in *The Regulation of Acid-Base Balance* □ Gunn RB. "Buffer equilibria in red blood cells." Chapter 3 in *The Regulation of Acid-Base Balance* □ Roughton FJW. "Transport of oxygen and carbon dioxide." *Handbook of Physiology,* 1964 ed. Chapter 31, section 3, volume 1, see pp 799–807 □ Klocke RA. "Carbon dioxide transport." *Handbook of Physiology,* 1987 ed. Chapter 10, section 3, volume 4, pp 173–197 □ *How To Understand Acid-Base.*

Topic B

Halpern ML. "Biochemistry and physiology of ammonium excretion." Chapter 76 in *The Kidney* □ Knepper MA. Ammonium transport in the kidney. Physiological Reviews 1989;69:179–249.

Topic C*

Gennari FJ. "Determinants of plasma bicarbonate concentration and hydrogen ion balance." Chapter 4 in *Acid-Base*. See pp 57–59 and 83–88 □ Charney AN. "Internal exchanges of hydrogen ions: gastrointestinal tract." Chapter 5 in *The Regulation of Acid-Base Balance* □ Halperin ML. Metabolism and acid-base physiology. Artif Org 1982;6:357–362 □ Lennon EJ. The effects of diet and stool composition on the net external acid balance of normal subjects. J Clin Invest 1966;45:1601–1607 □ Gonick HC. Reexamination of the acid-ash content of several diets. Am J Clin Nutr 1968;21:898–903 □ Oh MS. A new method for estimating G-I absorption of alkali. Kidney Int 1989;36:915–917 □ Camien MN. A critical reappraisal of "acid-base" balance. Am J Clin Nutr 1969;22:786–793.

Topic D**

Winter SD. The fall of the serum anion gap. Arch Intern Med 1990; 150:311–313 □ Sadjadi SA. A new range for the anion gap. Ann Intern Med 1995;123:807 □ Gabow PA. Disorders associated with an altered anion gap. Kidney Int 1985;27:472–483 □ Madias NE. Increased anion gap in metabolic alkalosis. N. Engl J Med 1979;300:1421–1423 □ Paulson WD. Anion gap-bicarbonate relation in diabetic ketoacidosis. Am J Med 1986;81: 995–1000 □ Orster JR. Use of the anion gap in clinical medicine. South Med J 1988; 81:229–237 □ DiNubile MJ. The increment in the anion gap: overextension of a concept? Lancet 1988 Oct 22;951–953 □ *Clinical Physiology of Acid-Base and Electrolyte Disorders*, 4th ed. See pp 548–551 □ Wrenn K. The delta gap: an approach to mixed acid-base disorders. Ann Emerg Med 1990;19:1310–1313 □ Badrick T. The anion gap: a reappraisal. Am J Clin Pathol 1992;98:249–252 □ Iberti TJ. Low sensitivity of the anion gap as a screen to detect hyperlactatemia in critically ill patients. Crit Care Med 1990;18:275–277. See follow-up correspondence in: Crit Care Med 1991; 19:129–131 □ Salem MM. Gaps in the anion gap. Arch Intern Med 1992;152: 1625–1629 □ Varon J. Reflections on the anion gap in hyperglycemia. West J Med 1992;157:670–672.

---

* Most authors cited here use the term "endogenous acid production" to indicate strong acid production from all sources (i.e., MAP + GAP). However, some use other definitional schemes, which are either explicitly stated or apparent from the context. Also, some authors do not include the metabolism of dietary organic anions as part of MAP. Instead, they consider both GAP and absorbed organic anions as part of an integrated gut effect on acid-base. Since the alkalinizing impact of dietary organic anions exceeds the acidifying effect of gut net bicarbonate secretion, these authors speak of the gut as a net alkalinizing organ.

** Some authors arrange R and F not as a ratio, but as the subtractive formula R − F. For example, when R/F = 1.0, R − F = 0.

Topic E

"Mixed acid-base disturbances: clinical examples." Chapter 8 in *Acid-Base Disorders* □ Harrington JT. "Mixed acid-base disorders." Chapter 12 in *Acid-Base* □ "Acid-base." Chapter 12 in *Repairing Body Fluids*. See pp 163–167 □ Hamm L. "Mixed acid-base disorders." Chapter 7 in *Fluids and Electrolytes*.

Topic F

Gennari FJ. "Normal acid-base values." Chapter 6 in *Acid-Base* □ Frassetto L. Age and systemic acid-base equilibrium: analysis of published data. J Gerontol: Biol Sci 1996;51A(1):B91-B99.

Topic G

Madias NE. The maladaptive renal response to secondary hypocapnia during chronic HCl acidosis in the dog. J Clin Invest 1977;60:1393–1401 □ Madias NE. Maladaptive renal response to secondary hypercapnia in chronic metabolic alkalosis. Am J Physiol 1980;238(Renal):F283-F289.

Topic H

Sklar AH. The osmolal gap in renal failure. Ann Intern Med 1983;98:481–482 □ Braden GL. Increased osmolal gap in alcoholic acidosis. Arch Intern Med 1993;153:2377–2380 □ Ammar KA. Ethylene glycol poisoning with a normal anion gap caused by concurrent ethanol ingestion: importance of the osmolal gap. Am J Kidney Dis 1996;27:130–133. □ Reuler JB. Anion and osmolar gaps in a patient with alcoholism. West J Med 1993;158:191–194 □ Goldfrank LR. Methanol, ethylene glycol, and isopropanol. Chapter 47 In: Goldfrank LR. *Toxicologic Emergencies*. 4th ed. Appleton & Lange, 1990;481–497 □ Glasser DS. Utility of the serum osmol gap in the diagnosis of methanol or ethylene glycol ingestion. Ann Emerg Med 1996;27:343–346 □ Wargotz ES. Asymptomatic blood methanol in emergency room patients.* Am J Clin Pathol 1987;87:773–775 □ Inaba H. Serum osmolality gap in postoperative patients in intensive care. Lancet 1987;June 13: 1331–1335. □ Palatnik W. Methanol half-life during ethanol administration: implications for management of methanol poisoning. Ann Emerg Med 1995;26:202–207.

Topic I

Kurtzman NA. Renal tubular acidosis: a constellation of syndromes. Hosp Prac (off ed) 1987;22(11):173–188 □ Sabatini S. Pathophysiology of the renal tubular acidoses. Sem Nephrol 1991;11:202–211 □ Arruda JAL. Distal renal tubular acidosis: molecular and clinical aspects. Hosp Prac (off ed)

* The low methanol levels discussed in this article are below the detection threshold of many, but not all, clinical GC instruments.

1994;29(1):75–78, 82–88 □ Schlueter W. On the mechanism of distal acidification in hyperkalemic renal tubular acidosis: evaluation with amiloride and bumetanide. J Am Soc Nephrol 1992;3:953–964 □ Lash JP. Laboratory evaluation of renal tubular acidosis. Clin Lab Med 1993;13:117–129.

Topic J

Richardson RMA. The urine pH: a potentially misleading diagnostic test in patients with hyperchloremic metabolic acidosis. Am J Kidney Dis 1987;10:140–143 □ Goldstein MB. The urine anion gap: a clinically useful index of ammonium excretion. Am J Med Sci 1986;292:198–202 □ Battle DC. The use of the urinary anion gap in the diagnosis of hyperchloremic metabolic acidosis. N Engl J Med 1988;318:594–599. See follow-up correspondence in: N Engl J Med 1988;319:585–587 □ Kim GH. Evaluation of urine acidification by urine anion gap and urine osmolal gap in chronic metabolic acidosis. Am J Kidney Dis 1996;27:42–47 □ Inase N. Is the urine anion gap a reliable index of urine ammonium excretion in most situations? Nephron 1990;54:180–181 □ Dyck RF. A modification of the urine osmolal gap: an improved method for estimating urine ammonium. Am J Nephrol 1990;10:359–362 [see data on urinary anion gap].

Topic K

See chapters on metabolic acidosis and alkalosis in detailed reference texts listed in General Reading bibliography. *The Regulation of Acid-Base Balance* has excellent coverage.

Topic L

Gajraj NM. Eutectic mixture of local anesthetics (EMLA) cream. Anesth Analg 1994; 78:574–583 □ Russell GN. Local anesthesia for radial artery cannulation: a comparison of a lidocaine-prilocaine emulsion and lidocaine infiltration. Journal of Cardiothoracic Anesthesia 1988; 2:309–312 □ Gourrier E. Use of EMLA cream in a department of neonatology. Pain 1996; 68:431–434 □ Russell SCS. A risk-benefit assessment of topical percutaneous local anaesthetics in children. Drug Safety 1997; 16:279–287 □ McKay W. Sodium bicarbonate attenuates pain on skin infiltration with lidocaine, with or without epinephrine. Anesth Analg 1987; 66:572–574 □ Erramouspe J. Buffering local anesthetic solutions with sodium bicarbonate: literature review and commentary. Hospital Pharmacy 1996; 31:1265–1282.

Acknowledgments

This book grew out of a fascination with acid-base that began, ten years ago, when I was a first year student at the Yale School of Medicine. During that year, I was fortunate to have participated in a seminar on renal physiology taught by Drs. Fred Wright and Asghar Rastegar, and then, in a different setting, to have met Dr. Peter Aronson. These three teachers introduced me to acid-base and, later, contributed to this book in many ways.

Dr. Aronson played an essential role during the early stages. He read the first draft of the book and then, as I wrote the second, critiqued each new chapter for form and content. His expertise, pedagogical talents, and persistent good sense helped shape the text and greatly improved its overall quality. Dr. Rastegar shared with me, during a half-dozen interviews, some of his immense pathophysiologic and clinical knowledge. I tape-recorded these discussions for later reference and subsequently incorporated many of his insights into the text. Dr. Rastegar also reviewed many chapters, helping me correct errors and clarify confusing points. Dr. Wright, my first teacher of acid-base, reviewed a complete draft of the text and provided many specific suggestions for improvement. Dr. Wright also advised me on a literature review I conducted on endogenous acid production, the results of which are reflected in several chapters and appendix topics.

Many others provided essential help. The following were kind enough to read complete drafts or substantial portions of the text and provide detailed feedback: Drs. L. Lee Hamm, Richard Donabedian, Mark Siegel, Robert F. Reilly, Peter Stein, Linda Costanzo, Nancy Angoff, and Armen Khechatryan. These reviews, and the oral discussions that followed, significantly improved the overall quality and accuracy of the text.

Others generously read anywhere from one chapter to several sections of the manuscript, or orally discussed aspects of the text with me: Drs. John Brackett, Brian Burke, Alan Charney, Phillip Cheng, Joseph Coleman, Gregg Coodley, Bill Dwyer, C. Gregory Elliot, Kevin Fallon, Lewis and Julie Kay-Foreman, Susan Friedmann, J. Bernard L. Gee, David Glassman, David W. Good, Zouhair Harab, John T. Harrington, Donald E. Hricik, Janet Hilbert, Barry M. Kacinski, Tom Krahn, Neil A. Kurtzman, Charles A. McKay, Constantine A. Manthous, Richard Mathay, Ira Meisels, Eli Merritt, Andriana Natale, Lewis Nelson, Man S. Oh, Petrie M. Rainey, Siegfried Rotmensch, Alan Segal, and Ed Weaver. Some of these individuals provided extensive and detailed feedback, which greatly improved the quality of the text.

The following friends provided expert editorial and/or technical feedback on parts of the text: Haim Chertok, John Hayden, Roxann King-Feuerman, and Robin Shifrin. I am especially grateful to Laurie Magid, Jack Hammer, Dr. Edward Phillips, and Daniel Abelow for providing essential editorial and strategic help. I thank John R. Riina for his indispensable advice. I appreciate the encouragement and support shown me by Donna Sommers, RN, and Terry Santino.

I am grateful to the administration of the Yale School of Medicine, particularly Dr. Robert H. Gifford, for giving me substantial freedom, including several periods of academic leave, to begin my research and writing when I was still a medical student.

I wish to thank scientific illustrator Susan Hochgraf, who worked closely with me, over a period of three years, on the illustrations, layout, and cover. Susan was my partner in actualizing the visual aspects of this book. I also wish to thank Tricia Kim, Naomi Osnos, Ellen Higham, and Nan Adams for their feedback and suggestions on drafts of the illustrations, page design, and cover.

Finally, I wish to thank my family. My parents, Dr. Irving Abelow and Phoebe Abelow, helped fund this project. Their generosity allowed me to work on the manuscript much more consistently than would otherwise have been possible. I also wish to thank my brother, Adam Abelow, who, along with my father, played a key role in teaching me to write clearly and logically. Without this foundation, *Understanding Acid-Base* would have been impossible.

I am indebted to all those listed here. Without their efforts, expertise, and generosity, *Understanding Acid-Base* would be a pale shadow of its current self. I regret if I have inadvertently failed to acknowledge anyone for their contribution. I welcome comments, corrections, and suggestions for future editions. These can be sent by email to: Benjamin.Abelow@Yale.Edu

Index

Note: "n" indicates footnotes. "A" indicates appendix page number.